'Several years ago I was diagnosed with multiple sclerosis … A chance discussion put me on the track of your newsletter, which linked MS-type symptoms with the Pill I'd been taking. Had I listened to my GP and neurologist, I would probably be in a wheelchair. Thank you, *What Doctors Don't Tell You*, for saving my life.' D. J., Norfolk

'Recently, my mother-in-law was diagnosed with breast cancer. I cannot tell you how encouraging your newsletter was to the whole family … She is faring well and confident she is making the right decisions thanks to your timely advice.' J. B., Jersey

'Instead of suffering from asthma, unwillingly forced into the last-ditch resort of taking steroids in order to have any sort of liveable life, I am virtually free of it and, to boot, have lost a surplus two stone. This is all attributable to your informative publications.' M. B. C. P.-B., Cornwall

'After a wonderful uncomplicated start in life, my baby contracted whooping cough. Thank you, WDDTY, for putting together so much information. It was you and your publication which put me on the path of being informed. My son made a full recovery. I will be for ever indebted.' Janet, Berkshire

'My husband was given three months to live two years ago due to prostate cancer. By reading your newsletter and the information you provide, I contacted the right people and he started an alternative therapy. It succeeded and he was later told that he was clear of cancer. Thank you for being you.' M. R., Dyfed

'Two months ago I could barely walk more than 50 yards or stand in the queue at the Post Office. Chronic lower back pain was the problem … now thanks to WDDTY I ramble and cycle miles and miles without pain.' R. P., Norfolk

'I was told I had glaucoma and was going blind. I developed a diet and supplement programme based on your information, and two months later I had my eyes examined again, and there was no sign of glaucoma any more.' G. R., Edinburgh

Praise for *What Doctors Don't Tell You*

'This groundbreaking book ... has potential to save lives. Stunning stuff!' Kathryn Marsden, author of *The Food Combining Diet*

'A hugely impressive book, and the finest critique of modern medical practice I have yet read. Lynne McTaggart takes a scalpel straight to the heart of medicine's most cherished dogmas. Essential reading ...' Peter Cox, health campaigner and bestselling author

'A mine of subversive information ... irresistibly argued. Lynne McTaggart is a very big thorn in the side of the medical propaganda machine.' Dr Keith Mumby, allergy specialist and author of *The Allergy Handbook*

'Introduces some welcome sanity by its critical appraisal of the value of many diagnostic and treatment procedures, especially the unbelievable escalation in the use of symptom-suppressive drugs. Excellent, stimulating ... and a thoroughly good read.' Dr John Mansfield, former President of the British Society for Allergy and Environmental Medicine

'Extremely provocative and meticulously researched ... should be part of the medical cabinet in every household in this country. I have long admired Lynne McTaggart's pioneering spirit, vision and courage, and this book exemplifies it.' Kitty Campion, practitioner and author

'A courageous book! I congratulate Lynne McTaggart on her passion, research and indefatigable efforts to bring information to the public that can help people to take control of their own lives.' Leslie Kenton, broadcaster and bestselling author

'This book dispels so many harmful medical myths and gives people back the freedom of informed choice. Essential reading for those facing medical intervention.' Patrick Holford, director of the Institute for Optimum Nutrition

WHAT DOCTORS DON'T TELL YOU

The truth about the dangers of modern medicine

LYNNE McTAGGART

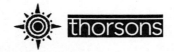

Every illness and every patient is unique. This book is intended as a source of information only. Readers are urged to work in partnership with a qualified, experienced practitioner before undertaking (or refraining from) any treatments listed in these pages.

Thorsons
An Imprint of HarperCollins*Publishers*
77–85 Fulham Palace Road,
Hammersmith, London W6 8JB

The website address is: www.thorsonselement.com

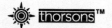

and *Thorsons* are trademarks of
HarperCollins*Publishers* Ltd

First published by Thorsons 1996
This revised and updated edition 2005

1 3 5 7 9 10 8 6 4 2

© Lynne McTaggart

Lynne McTaggart asserts the moral right to
be identified as the author of this work

A catalogue record of this book is
available from the British Library

ISBN 978 0 00 717627 4

For Bryan

Contents

Part V: Surgery

Part VI: Taking Control

Acknowledgements

In 1988, my husband Bryan, also a journalist, mentioned one day that he thought we should launch a newsletter called *What Doctors Don't Tell You*. We both shared a conviction that modern medicine was unproven and sometimes dangerous, and a passion to share this information with the public. I am sorry to admit this, considering how closely I am now identified with this title, but at the time I told him, quite emphatically, that the idea wouldn't fly. Also, I am sorrier to admit, I thought that title wasn't any good. So Bryan, who knew who he was dealing with, asked if I knew another good editor who might want the job. I snatched the baited hook and all these years later, here I am.

Although many books result from the silent collaboration of many parties, this one is smudged with the fingerprints of most of the people who have been involved with *What Doctors Don't Tell You*, the newsletter. Much of the information contained in this book has been published, in another form, in our newsletter over the years, and this is an attempt to pull it together into a central statement about medicine.

Although not all of our collaborators shared our intense interest in medical matters, all shared our commitment to working as a team. In a sense, this book is the product of every person who contributed in some way to the complicated business of starting a publication – and publishing company – from scratch.

I am grateful, first, to all the support teams we've had since those early days, who have willingly involved themselves with every aspect of our company, when that largely entailed packing envelopes from the top floor of our house. I am particularly grateful to our present indefatigable team: Mark Brandwood, Michelle DeVilliers, Kristy Downton, Andrew Miller, Kathy Mingo, Wajeeha Nolan, Pat Thomas and Nicolette Vuvan. Thanks and acknowledgement are due to the many contributors of our newsletter, particularly Fiona Bawdon, Clive Couldwell, Tony Edwards, Deanne Pearson, and Pat Thomas, whose insights and investigative skills have helped to inform mine. I'm also grateful to our designer John Clement for his visual skills over the years; and to our production editor Sharyn Wong, who performs small miracles with copy and research every month.

For this latest edition, I owe a special debt to Henrietta Cole, who helped to collate research and, with Wajeeha Nolan, performed a vital cross-checking of the approximately 1000 medical references which support the ideas of this book.

I am also indebted to a number of doctors and practitioners for their help with research and ideas, most particularly Patrick Kingsley, Ellen Grant, Harris Coulter, John Mansfield, Harald Gaier, Tony Newbury, Jack Levenson, Melvyn Werbach, Annemarie Colbin, Michel Odent and Leo Galland. Our family has been privileged to be cared for by a number of special healers in both alternative and orthodox medicine, whose knowledge helped to inform my views. I am also grateful for the panel members of *What Doctors Don't Tell You*, particularly the many doctors among them who had the faith in us to put their name to a controversial project before they'd seen one word of it.

All of the case histories mentioned in this book come from real letters we've received from our readers. With the exception of several cases which have been well publicized, the names of all such patients have been changed or shortened to protect their identities. For all their confidence in allowing me access to their private stories and pain, I am especially grateful.

I am also indebted to all our other wonderful subscribers here and in America for supporting us through the years and for wanting to read what we had to say.

The entire staff of HarperCollins have my deep gratitude for their enthusiasm and courage in backing this project, most particularly Wanda Whiteley and Simon Gerratt. Barbara Vesey made vital contributions in her dedicated work in copyediting the manuscript. Carter-Ruck took a special interest in this book and spent many arduous hours offering wise legal counsel.

I also owe a special debt to my agent Russ Galen, who is always there batting for me when I need him, and my foreign agent, Daniel Benor.

A special mention must be made of my daughters Caitlin and Anya, who continue to teach me more about life and health than a roomful of paediatricians ever could.

Three others stand out as particularly vital to the undertaking of this project. As a young journalist, I was privileged to edit the work of Dr Robert Mendelsohn, whose staggeringly prescient views about medicine have largely informed mine. Dr Stephen Davies, a nutritional pioneer, not only contributed to my own good health but provided me with a new way of looking at health and disease.

This book and my work owes its largest debt to my husband Bryan Hubbard, whose thoughts and words are so entwined with mine that this is virtually a work of co-authorship. For his love, for his knowing what I was made to be doing before I did, for the daily joy he gives me in living and working side by side, I am forever grateful.

About the Author

Lynne McTaggart is an award-winning journalist and author of the best-selling book *The Field*. As co-founder and editorial director of *What Doctors Don't Tell You* (www.wddty.co.uk), she publishes the most successful health newsletters in Britain. She is also editor of *Living the Field*, a course that helps to bring the science of *The Field* into everyday life. Her company holds highly popular conferences and workshops on health and spirituality.

She has become a well-respected national spokesperson on the practices of conventional and alternative medicine and a favourite with the media and as a public speaker in both Britain and America.

Ms McTaggart is also author of *The Baby Brokers: The Marketing of White Babies in America* (The Dial Press) and *Kathleen Kennedy: Her Life and Times* (The Dial Press/Weidenfeld & Nicolson in the UK). *The Field* and *What Doctors Don't Tell You* each have been translated into languages around the world.

She and her husband, WDDTY co-founder Bryan Hubbard, live and work in London with their two daughters.

Introduction

This book was born from a grand passion I once had: a passion to get better.

In the early eighties, after an extraordinary patch of bad choices, I underwent a prolonged bout of stress. In every profoundly important area of my life, green lights I'd always taken for granted suddenly began turning red. If I had taken one of those little tests you find in women's magazines that add up your stress quotient – with death, marriage, divorce and moving the most stressful situations – my sums would have leapt off the chart.

In rapid succession I'd struggled under an impossible book deadline, married Mr Wrong, divorced Mr Wrong, bought the wrong flat, accepted the wrong job, suffered the death of a close friend, incurred several large debts, and spent a prolonged period of intense isolation in a foreign country. I couldn't, in those days, even get a good haircut.

Shortly after emerging from the eye of this personal squall, I began to experience strange symptoms, at first your workaday 'female problems' – everything from ferocious premenstrual tension and irregular periods to cystitis and almost constant vaginal infections.

As time wore on, my symptoms multiplied: eczema, hives and allergies to a load of food and chemicals; diarrhoea and an irritable bowel; insomnia and night sweats; and severe depression. I had felt powerless for so long that my body seemed to be reacting in parallel, caving in under any sort of microbial onslaught.

For nearly all of the three years that I was ill, I made the rounds of medical circles – first the standard ones, then the periphery, with nutritionists and homoeopaths, and finally the very outer rim, from breathing specialists to Bioenergeticists. By the autumn of 1986 I was hacking my way though the dense thicket of New Age therapies. I tried breathing from the abdomen. I had the negative emotions Rolfed out of me. Somebody tried to diagnose me by subjecting my hair sample to radio waves. I ploughed through autogenic training, colonic irrigation and even a form of psychotherapy – a mixture of Wilhelm Reich and what felt like being tickled on the face. I learned something about my relationship with my mother. But I did not, at any point, get better.

By the summer of 1987 a sense of hopelessness descended over me. The worst part of being chronically unwell without a diagnosis legitimatizing it is that a lot of people don't believe you, or view your symptoms as imaginary – as a puerile sort of attention-getter. And in this land of stoics, if your illness isn't hard-core, like cancer or leprosy, you're supposed to learn to live with it, to dysfunction quietly, without complaint.

At some point it began to dawn on me that there was no miracle remedy out there that was going to turn my health around. If I was going to get better, I was going to have to take charge of the entire process myself – from diagnosis to, possibly, even the cure. Somehow I would have to figure out what was going wrong with my body and find whatever tools were necessary to cure myself. It began to make sense that I should take control of my health, since no one else would care about its outcome so passionately.

I began reading up on allergies and female problems, and one day came upon a newly discovered illness whose symptoms matched almost every one of mine. When a specialist I consulted wasn't familiar with it, I searched out a renowned GP specializing in allergies and nutritional medicine, whose battery of tests and diagnostic sensitivity confirmed my own suspicions, and rooted out other contributory problems besides.

What I seemed to have inside me was, essentially, thrush of the body, or polystemic chronic candidiasis. Candida albicans is a yeast that lives in the upper bowel of most of us without doing good or harm, kept in line by our immune systems and the friendly bacteria that coexist with it. But, according to current theories (and that's all they are at the moment), when the immune system is weakened and the good-guy bacteria fall in numbers, these yeast can start multiplying out of control, sending out toxins that eventually interfere with a range of bodily functions.

Whether or not candida was the main cause of my illness, the root of the problem appeared to be an immune system that wasn't functioning at full throttle. Prolonged severe stress tends to have a depressant effect on the immune system. That, and a bunch of long dormant allergies, including an allergy to wheat, which probably came to the fore as a result of stress, meant that I was poisoning my body every day with substances it could no longer tolerate. I'd also become sloppy about my diet, and was low in a large number of nutrients.

My treatment consisted of taking large doses of a well-tolerated drug for a time, plus a batch of specially tailored doses of supplements and a restrictive healing diet of fresh, unrefined food. A month after I'd started, my dry cleaner asked me if I'd had a face lift.

However good these initial results, I soon realized that getting better wasn't going to be an overnight affair. For a year healing became, in effect, my career. Fortunately I had teamed up with an extraordinary doctor, and we worked together as a partnership in recovering my health, and with it, my sense of control. That year was heady and instructive, with plenty of opportunities to meditate on the science and art of healing, as well as the nature of the doctor-patient relationship. It seemed to me that patients were more likely to get better, so long as they were in charge of the decision-making about their care. True healing could only begin if there existed a dialogue between doctor and patient, a democracy of shared responsibility. I also experienced first-hand that people can get well without drugs and surgery, just by altering what they eat and how they live. Healing isn't simply a matter of finding the right drug or right operation, but a complex process of accepting responsibility for your own life.

This personal experience stirred up dormant memories that had affected me deeply early in my career. As a young journalist in New York, I had headed the editorial department of the Chicago Tribune – New York News Syndicate. There I'd met the late Dr Robert Mendelsohn and helped to launch his column 'The People's Doctor' in the mid-seventies. As former medical director of a national programme for underprivileged children, and chairman of a state licensing committee for doctors,

Mendelsohn had been entrenched in the very heart of the American medical establishment. Nevertheless, here was this kindly, mild-mannered man, your prototypical Jewish grandfather, blowing the whistle on all his peers by denouncing medicine as excessive and unproven. Every week his column would savage yet another medical sacred cow. Most famously, it was Bob who likened medicine to the new religion. 'Medicine', he wrote, 'is not based on science – it's based on faith.'

Bob sent tremors through the very foundation of my belief system. I had been a product of the post-war American baby boom, the Kennedy New Frontier, brought up to regard American science and technology as the saviours of mankind. As a teenager I had believed in the principles of Lyndon Johnson's American dream. Most of the big problems of mankind – racism, poverty, illness – could be eliminated by social engineering and science, there in the best country in the world.

In my own journalism, when I began examining some of the social 'goods' that medical science engages in – such as 'breakthroughs' like the Pill – I came to realize that at times they amounted to a great deal of dangerous meddling. But it wasn't until I began to investigate my own health problems that the prescience of Mendelsohn's views really came home.

Once I got better (which took, all told, a year), I became drawn in my freelance work to medicine. I began studying the professional literature in medical libraries and learned how to read medical studies. I followed around exhausted junior doctors working a standard 84-hour shift in a special baby unit, to get a taste for the extreme conditions which young doctors had to endure (and the kind of questionable care their patients would receive under these conditions).

In time I began to feel I'd walked through the looking glass. Nothing in my university training prepared me for the peculiar, often tortured logic of medical studies. Treatments had been adopted with little or no scientific basis in fact. Studies which cast doubt on a drug's effectiveness were nevertheless applauded as evidence of success. Many of the gravest, sloppy mistakes in study design had been overlooked. Studies clearly showed that certain drugs cause cancer, yet here were top scientists dancing all around the numbers to avoid acknowledging the obvious. Medicine's own scientific literature offered overwhelming evidence that some of it not only didn't work, but was highly dangerous. This was not a 'science'. This was a belief system so fixed, so inherent, that any truth to the contrary was dismissed as virtual blasphemy.

Fired by the missionary zeal of the newly converted, at some point I became extremely boring on the subject. Probably out of desperation, my then new partner (now my husband), Bryan, suggested that I start a newsletter about the true risks of medical practices – so I didn't have to tell him anymore, but could tell the world.

At the time, we didn't expect that this newsletter, which we planned to call *What Doctors Don't Tell You*, would be much more than a hobby. I was pregnant by that time, and we thought it might be a way for me to stay home with our child and make a modest living.

From the outset, after our launch at the 1989 *Here's Health* show, people showed keen interest in subscribing. By then I had assembled an advisory panel of 25 top doctors, chosen because they themselves had blown the whistle on unproven medical practice or pioneered less invasive medical procedures. Although we rarely advertised during the first year, the newsletter seemed propelled forward by its own steam and the zealous faith of our initial subscribers; by the end of that first year we had somehow managed to accumulate 1,000 readers, and now we have many thousands of loyal subscribers in Britain, the United States, and all over the world.

Outrage is now the passion that powers the newsletter – as well as this book. I am livid every time I open my post. Each morning I wade through piles of letters containing heart-rending stories of personal catastrophe – children who have been killed, or husbands and wives mutilated or incapacitated through medicine. Whenever we study their cases we usually discover that the dangers of the treatments given to them were well known. Their doctors just hadn't bothered communicating this vital information to them.

The problem is, by the time they write to us, it is too late.

I have written this book because I don't want you to be another statistic in my morning post. I do not promise you a comfortable read. Many of the facts in this book are likely to unsettle you. You may learn that much of what your doctor tells you isn't true. But that is my intention. I want to help you to become a more informed medical consumer by determining when you actually need your doctor and when his advice is best ignored. I want to save you from unnecessary treatments and dangerous cures, from 'preventive just-in-case medicine' that will leave you damaged even before you've actually become ill. Besides being alerted to the hazards of many accepted practices, you'll also find many proven, safe alternatives for diagnosing, preventing or treating many illnesses. I want to help you to learn not to be a 'good' patient. Good patients, the kind who blindly follow orders instead of demanding answers, sometimes die.

The following pages will open up to you the trade secrets of what has been largely a closed shop. You'll have a chance to listen to the private conversation that medicine conducts with itself. And, once you discover just how much hokum resides in your doctor's medicine cupboard, just how much medicine relies on blind faith, received wisdom and selective facts, not reason, science or common sense, you can grab the power away from this false shaman and begin to take back control of your health.

PART I

MEDICINE'S FALSE SCIENCE

1

The Un-science
of Modern Medicine

It's comforting in life to have certainties. One of the cosiest of certainties we've grown up with is that modern medicine works miracles and doctors cure diseases. In the stories we tell ourselves, Dr Kildare, Marcus Welby, Dr Finlay, clad in symbolically pure white, engage in the business, all day, every day, of saving lives. And even though more people die in our modern-day equivalents like *ER* and *Casualty*, those doctors in the emergency room still have gadgets capable of raising the dead.

Our greatest certainty about medicine is that it is a lofty and reputable science, arrived at by scientists in laboratories by exhaustive testing and review. We proudly point to the fact that science has progressed and triumphed over chaos and darkness, over the time when doctors didn't even know that they had to wash their hands.

Since the Second World War, and the discovery of the two great miracle drugs of this century – penicillin and cortisone – medicine has indeed worked miracles. People who would have died from hormone-related deficiencies such as Addison's disease, and life-threatening infections such as pneumonia or meningitis, can now recover easily and return to normal lives. Most of the great medical discoveries – painless surgery, antiseptic hospital environments, x-rays – only discovered in the last century, have given us in the West the best emergency medicine in the world. If you have an unforeseen heart attack, an operable brain tumour, a near fatal car accident, an emergency in childbirth, then Western medicine, with its array of space-age gadgetry, is without parallel for sorting you out. If a

3

building ever falls on me, I'd like all the very latest in Western gee-whizz technology to put me back together. Indeed, if it hadn't been for 20th-century drugs, my mother would have died in her early twenties and I never would have been born.

It was also these discoveries during the Second World War, ending abruptly with the ultimate scientific discovery, the atomic bomb, which left us with a great expectancy about science. The aftermath of victory was also the dawning of the scientific age of medicine. Science had helped us to conquer our human enemies. Now it would do battle with our microscopic ones. We were beginning to conquer space; it wouldn't be very long, as *Life* magazine promised my generation in America, before we conquered disease.

Doctors and medical authorities contribute to this view of infallible medical science. Whenever discussing its own track record, especially against that of alternative treatments, medicine stakes out the moral high ground, flying the territorial flag of established scientific fact. In mounting an attack on alternative medicine, a *British Medical Journal* editorial self-congratulatingly trumpeted medicine's 'record of objective evaluation of claims.'[1]

By the same token, orthodox medicine denounces alternative medicine as not following suit. The Royal College of Physicians and the Royal College of Pathologists once denounced alternative treatments for allergies as unscientific, warning that 'until the methods have been evaluated by reputable, randomized, double-blind, placebo-controlled trials they cannot be accepted into routine clinical practice.'[2]

Our faith in medical science is so ingrained that it has become woven into the warp and woof of our daily routine. In any average day in Britain, a family may place its entire future in the hands of medical advance. For a pregnant mother, the result of prenatal tests may determine whether she carries her pregnancy to term. Her child may be given his vaccine and her husband his blood-pressure lowering drugs on the premise that this medicine will prevent them from getting future disease. Medical tests determine whether we can have children, continue working, have operations, are eligible for insurance, require caesareans, or, as with an HIV test that comes back positive, are shunned as pariahs. It is doctors with their miracle treatments, we believe, who will deliver us

4

from evil, which, these days, is not temptation so much as the frightening randomness of disease.

But much as we cling to the notion of science as a force of redemption, our faith is misplaced. The truth of it is that medical science actually isn't working too well. The United States and Britain are losing the 'War on Cancer'.[3] Despite state-of-the-art mammogram screening equipment and surgical techniques, breast cancer mortality rates stubbornly refuse to fall. Despite millions of people following low-fat diets, heart disease is still the biggest killer in the West. With all the fancy chemicals and computerized testing equipment we have to hand, asthma, arthritis, diabetes, cancer – virtually all the chronic degenerative diseases known to mankind – are thriving, and medicine hasn't affected their incidence one tiny bit.

One glance at the statistics shows that, except in the case of getting run over or needing an emergency caesarean, orthodox Western medicine not only won't cure you but may leave you worse off than you were before. In fact, these days, scientific medicine itself is responsible for a good percentage of disease. If you're in hospital, there's a one in six chance that you landed there because of some modern medical treatment gone wrong.[4] Once you get there, your chances are one in six of dying in hospital or suffering some injury while you're there. Since half this risk is caused by a doctor's or hospital's error, you've got an 8 per cent chance of being killed or injured by the staff.[5] At last count, about 1.17 million Britons end up in hospital each year because of doctor error or a bad reaction to a drug. In the United States, if we extrapolate the results of a 1984 study, over one million Americans are being injured in hospital every year, and 180,000 die as a result.[6] Recently, the *Journal of the American Medical Association*, the official organ of the primary organization representing physicians in America, recently admitted that doctor-induced disease is the third leading cause of death in America, responsible for a quarter of a million deaths per year.[7] Dr Allen Roses, the only worldwide vice-president of genetics at GlaxoSmithKline (GSK), shocked the world by recently admitting that 90 per cent of his company's – or any other drug company's products – don't work on the majority of patients.[8] In Britain, the latest statistics are that 10,000 Britons die every year from a reaction to a drug, and one in every 16 patients is put in hospital because of an adverse reaction to everyday drugs – even aspirin. To put the magnitude of the problem in perspective, the entire population of a city the size of Birmingham is put in a hospital bed every year by medical error. If you live in the US, where about 40,000 people are shot dead every year, you are nevertheless three times more likely to be killed by a doctor than by a gun.[9]

This appalling track record has nothing to do with incompetence or lack of dedication. Most doctors are extremely well-intended, and probably a majority are highly competent in what they've been taught.

The problem isn't the carpenter, but his tools. The fact is that medicine is *not* a science, or even an art. Many of your doctor's arsenal of treatments don't work – indeed, have never been proven to work, let alone to be safe. It is a false science, built upon conjuring tricks, supposition and blind preconception, whose so-called scientific method is a vast amount of stumbling in the dark.

Many of the treatments we take for granted – for breast cancer or heart surgery, even treatments for chronic conditions such as arthritis or asthma – have been adopted and widely used *without one single valid study demonstrating that they are effective or safe.* The so-called 'gold standard' respected by medical scientists as the only scientific proof of the true worth of a drug or treatment is the randomized, double-blind, placebo-controlled trial – that is, a study in which patients are randomly assigned to receive either a drug or a sugar pill, with neither researchers nor participants aware of who is getting what. Nevertheless, despite the fact that thousands of studies are conducted every year, very few of the treatments considered to be at the very cornerstone of modern medicine have been put to this most basic of tests – or, indeed, to any test at all.

For all the science-speak in medicine about risk-factors and painstakingly controlled data, the stringent government regulation, the meticulous peer review in professional literature – for all the attempts to cloak medicine in the weighty mantle of science – *a good deal of what we regard as standard medical practice today amounts to little more than 21st-century voodoo.*

In their own literature, medical authorities openly acknowledge this fact. *New Scientist* once announced on the cover of one issue that 80 per cent of medical procedures used today have never been properly tested.[10]

6

Medicine as it is practised today is largely a conspiracy of faith. Probably because of the miracle of drugs such as antibiotics, doctors have come to believe that their little black bag ought to be filled, in effect, with magic. The late medical critic Dr Robert Mendelsohn was one of the first to liken modern medicine to a church, with doctors its high priests following the teachings with blind faith: 'Modern Medicine is neither an art nor a science. It's a religion,' he wrote in his book, *Confessions of a Medical Heretic* (Contemporary Books), 'just ask *why?* enough times and sooner or later you'll reach the Chasm of Faith. Your doctor will retreat into the fact that you have no way of knowing or understanding all the wonders he has at his command. *Just trust me.*'[11]

Doctors believe so fervently in the power of their tools that they are willing to suspend all reasonable scepticism about current and new medical treatments – so long as these treatments fit in with orthodox medical practice. Most doctors and researchers operate on the assumption of *a priori* benefit, whether or not a given remedy has actually been proven: *we know what we're doing is right.* Enthusiasm for statins, the current favourite for high cholesterol, is so great, for instance, that doctors are willing to ignore the grossest of scientific lapses in safety testing in order to promote what is looked upon *prima facie* as a good thing. *We know what we're doing is right.*

Even if studies have been done demonstrating that a treatment is ineffective or even downright dangerous, so powerful is this faith that these results often get ignored. Virtually every good study of foetal monitoring – devices employing ultrasound testing supposedly to measure the condition of the foetus during labour and birth – all show that this procedure produces a worse outcome for mother and child.[12] This information appears well known to many senior obstetricians – the former head of the Oxford Perinatal Unit repeatedly has written widely about this fact – yet foetal monitors continue to be employed in every delivery room in the land. *We know what we're doing is right.*

This is probably why doctors make such rotten logicians. Many in medicine get tied into logical knots, attempting to justify apparent contradictions with the most arcane Alice-in-Wonderland reasoning. Robert Mendelsohn used to say that his favourite line spouted by doctors was: 'Breastfeeding is best, but bottlefeeding is just as good.'

'High serum cholesterol levels are an important risk factor for coronary disease,' once wrote noted heart researcher Dr Meir J. Stampfer of the Harvard School of Public Health, repeating the prevailing view. In the next breath, however, he added, parenthetically: *'but most patients with [heart attacks] have normal cholesterol levels'* (my italics).[13]

The faith in the infallibility of their tools allows doctors to adopt as the 'gold standard' what are usually little more than experimental treatments, and employ these on millions before their effects are fully understood or the procedure has stood the test of time. The favourite line of doctors, when steam-rolling ahead without proof, is that if they had always waited until they had proper evidence, goodness knows how many advances in medicine would have been held up (and how many millions of people would have died). That argument does not, of course, take into account the vast number of people who *have* died taking unproven treatments later found to be dangerous. The new Cox 2 arthritis drug Vioxx, one of the biggest money spinners of all drugs, was withdrawn by its manufacturers Merck after it was discovered that it doubled the risk of heart attacks. Still others, such as amalgam in dental silver fillings and the radical mastectomy, are treatments devised a century ago and never properly tested or reviewed to determine whether they are as safe or effective as has always been presumed.

Medicine as it is now practised relies entirely on numbers. When judging the worth of any treatment, researchers must weigh the risks of the drugs or treatments (and all treatments in orthodox medicine carry some risks) against their likely benefits and against the risk of the illness being treated. A drug known to be effective but with serious side-effects might be worth taking if you have a life-threatening illness, but not if your medical problem is a hangnail.

Medical science is, in the main, a triumph of statistics over common sense. When bumping up against unpalatable truths in the study, medical scientists, who again always assume a medical treatment to be beneficial, are inclined to put the best face on the whole exercise, or cut and paste, refine and edit, to fit the premise or explain away an undesirable result.

Some years ago, a large study from the Netherlands Cancer Institute showed that all women taking the Pill, no matter what their age, had an increased risk of breast cancer. Most worryingly, 97 per cent of women under aged 36 who contracted breast cancer had taken the Pill, for any

8

length of time.[14] For more than 30 years, doctors have been touting the Pill as the safest drug ever developed. The Dutch study, now the fifth and possibly most damning to show a link between the Pill and cancer, was a colossal embarrassment to an entire industry devoted to contraception at all costs.

However, once they trumpeted the negative findings in the beginning of their article, the Dutch researchers began back-pedalling, by qualifying the overall implications of their findings. They emphasized that the increased risk mainly occurred among certain subgroups. Because the numbers supposedly showed no increased risk of breast cancer after long-term use among women in their latter thirties, their study was, in effect, *good* news: 'Our findings accord with the mass of evidence that [oral contraceptive use] by women in the middle of their fertile years [25–39 years] has *no adverse effect* on breast cancer risk' (my italics).

Doctors can often minimize the risks of drugs by magnifying the risk of not using them. Most studies have been able to justify that the Pill is safe by turning pregnancy into a dangerous disease. This risk-benefit equation only works if you believe it is better to risk breast cancer, cervical cancer, a stroke or thrombosis – all known risks associated with the Pill – than to have an unwanted baby or to use a condom instead.

A spokeswoman from the British Family Planning Association, which has probably handed out its fair share of Pills to teenagers, dismissed any breast cancer risk out of hand, arguing that this theoretical risk had to be weighed against the 'evidence that the Pill protects against endometrial and ovarian cancer'.[15] This is a typical example of medical reasoning. This drug is beneficial because it may 'protect' you against one kind of fatal cancer (a highly questionable conclusion, in any event), even though it may give you another potentially fatal cancer.

And because they live and breathe medicine by numbers, and believe in the infallibility of their tools, doctors are willing to hand out dangerous medication on the confident assumption that new tests will pick up any side-effects that they cause, and yet other drugs will be able to treat these new problems. Hence the reason why family planning enthusiasts will usually patiently explain that, even though the Pill may cause cervical cancer, cervical smears should pick up early changes, at which stage things are mainly treatable. Like many in medicine, they make the fatal error of requiring medicine to be infallible. This reasoning works *if* a test that can be wrong more than half the time picks up the cancer early, and *if* medicine can always cure cancer, which thus far it has singularly failed to do.

This kind of tortuous logic was once used to minimize evidence showing a link between vasectomy and the development of prostate cancer. The two studies, which examined over 74,000 men who had had vasectomies, showed that vasectomy increases the prostate cancer risk by 56 to 66 per cent.[16] Those patients who'd had their operation done 20 years ago faced a whopping increase in risk of between 85 and 89 per cent. In other words, having a vasectomy 20 years ago nearly doubles your risk of getting cancer.

Pretty damning evidence, one would have thought. Nevertheless, after it was published, some professional magazines encouraged doctors to tell their patients that the risk of prostate cancer following a vasectomy was minimal. The article attempted to claim that, compared to other methods of birth control (*the condom? natural family planning?*), vasectomy is 'still one of the safest'. A Family Planning Association spokesperson concurred: 'These studies *do not tell us* that vasectomy causes prostate cancer' (again, my italics).

A similar situation has occurred with HRT. Although two major studies were stopped when it was found that women on HRT are more likely to have heart attacks, cancer and stroke, the British medical establishment refused to recant or admit that this might not be the treatment of choice for women going through the menopause.

Doctors and medical researchers have been known to hype up the risks of a disease compared with the risks of the drug used to treat it. Dangerous drugs look good if you turn an ordinarily benign problem into a killer disease. In 1992, the UK Department of Health (DoH) announced the hasty withdrawal of two of the three brands of the combined measles, mumps and rubella (MMR) vaccines. The official line circulated to the press about why these drugs were withdrawn, after having been jabbed into millions of 15-month-olds, were allegedly the results of a study showing that the two withdrawn brands had a 'negligible' (1 in 11,000) risk of causing a 'transient' and 'mild' (all DoH words, these) case of meningitis. The third brand, made from a different strain of the mumps virus, supposedly did not pose this risk.

In 1989, when I first interviewed Dr Norman Begg of the UK's Public Health Laboratory Service, which recommended the vaccine in Britain, he assured me that mumps on its own was a very mild illness in children. Mumps, he said, 'very rarely' leads to long-term permanent complications such as orchitis (where the disease hits the testicles of adult males, very occasionally causing sterility). The mumps component had only been added, he said, to give 'extra value' to the jab.[17]

By 1992, however, when the two versions of the MMR were withdrawn, the British government painted a very different picture, announcing that mumps leads to meningitis in 1 in 400 cases. Hence, even though the old vaccine was dangerous (and it must have been pretty dangerous to get hauled off the market virtually overnight), *it was not as dangerous as catching mumps.*

But of course, two-thirds of medical practices don't have any proof at all. There is no such regulatory agency like the Food and Drug Administration or the Committee on Safety in Medicines to monitor surgery, screening or diagnostic tests – nothing but peer review through national medical associations. Run by doctors for doctors, these organizations tend to rule by consensus, and by a peculiarly circular logic: if a practice is universally employed, it must be safe, even when many studies point otherwise.

In the case of surgery, most treatments get the nod without any kind of clinical trial (partly because it is very difficult to have either a randomized or double-blind trial or to reverse an operation with an unfavourable result). Consequently, some new techniques get adopted with very little in the way of proof to show they are doing any good or at least not doing drastic harm.

Medicine as it is currently practised is a private conversation by doctors, for doctors. There's no doubt that medicine maintains a double standard. Doctors often privately voice their doubts, disappointments and fears about particular treatments in their own literature, yet fail to disclose this in any discussion with patients or the press. For instance, some years ago an especially alarming piece of information came to light about vaccines. The US Centers for Disease Control and Prevention in Atlanta, Georgia, discovered that children receiving the triple jabs for diphtheria/tetanus/whooping cough or for measles/mumps/rubella were three times more likely to suffer seizures. Nevertheless, this information was only announced to nine scientists and was never otherwise publicized.

Another prime example of this double standard surrounded the issue of treatment for breast cancer. An editorial in *The Lancet* published a scathing attack on the failure of mammography as a technology to halt the rising breast cancer death rates, and organized a conference to talk over new solutions[18] – at the same time that various government bodies were calling for *increasing* the frequency of mammograms.

The greatest reason that medical research is tainted is that the majority of it is funded by the very companies who stand to gain by certain results. These drug companies not only pay the salaries of researchers, but they can often decide where – indeed, whether – they get published. It's wise to keep in mind that this industry, in a sense, has a vested interest in ill health: if drug companies found cures, rather than lifelong 'maintenance' therapies, they'd soon be out of business.

The constant exposure of medicine to the pharmaceutical industry, and the reliance of future medical research on these companies, has bred a climate in which much of mainstream medicine refuses to consider any other treatment options besides drugs and surgery, even when copious scientific evidence exists to support those options. Many conventional doctors are especially vituperative in their dismissal of important work by innovators, while uncritically embracing many surgical or drug-based solutions that are little more than modern-day snake oil. This has bred a climate into which healers are polarized into 'alternative' and 'orthodox' camps, rather than into one common group approving of anything that has a solid basis in science or clinical practice. Dr Peter Duesberg, a leading University of California professor in molecular biology, was one of many publicly vilified for suggesting, with a well-reasoned argument backed up by a 75-page published paper, that HIV is not the cause of AIDS.

To give you some idea how medicine handles heretics, witness how it still reacts to scientific evidence supporting alternative medicine. A study conducted scientifically, with all the usual gold-standard double-blind, placebo-controlled checks and balances that medicine prides itself on, showed that homoeopathy for asthma actually works. Scientists now had some proof: *homoeopathy works*. In fact it was the third study carried out by the same man since 1985 to show exactly the same result.

12

Nevertheless, in his published report the leader of the trial distanced himself from his results, pointing out in his conclusion that tests such as these just might end up producing false-positive, or wrong, results.[19] Despite the scientific design of the trial, an editorial in *The Lancet* flatly refused to accept the results: 'What could be more absurd than the notion that a substance is therapeutically active in dilutions so great that the patient is unlikely to receive a single molecule of it? … Yes, the dilution principle of homeopathy is absurd; so the reason for any therapeutic effect presumably lies elsewhere.'[20] In other words, the scientific method works only when it applies to things we have faith in, but not, it seems, with anything we don't understand or agree with.

The problem with this dogmatic adherence to preconception and dismissal of dissension or doubt, as far as you and I are concerned, is that it covers up the fact that much of standard medical practice may not work very well. It makes dangerous drugs look safe and effective. It makes it seem like people who don't need drugs should take them. It justifies a lot of useless surgery that may very well kill you, and certainly isn't going to make you better. It explains away many promising treatments that don't require dangerous drugs or surgery. Despite the very best of intentions, it sometimes causes untold pain and suffering, rather than contributing to your health. In fact, you are in grave danger from the moment you walk into your doctor's surgery, particularly at the point when he tells you he'd like to take a few tests.

PART II

DIAGNOSIS

2

Diagnostic Excess

Your modern-day doctor has at his disposal an array of high-tech gadgetry that allows him to monitor and measure virtually every nook and cranny of your body. He and his fellow doctors are now completely reliant upon these tests to diagnose disease. As patients, we trust tests so implicitly to provide us with a definitive view of our state of health, even to predict when we're going to get ill at some distant point in the future, that most of our children begin having tests as soon as they've been conceived.

At last count, there were more than 1,400 of these, ranging from the simple blood-pressure cuff to the most sophisticated computerized nuclear magnetic imaging devices. Back in the relatively dark ages of 1987, some 19 billion tests were performed on Americans that year alone, which works out to be 80 tests for each man, woman and child.[1]

Despite the kind of gadgetry that would put NASA to shame, the problem is that the technology doesn't really work very well. Most tests are grossly unreliable, giving wrong readings a good deal of the time. A false-positive test sets in motion the juggernaut of aggressive treatments at your doctor's disposal, with all their attendant risks. But the tests themselves can be as risky as some of the most dangerous drugs and surgery, risks that are magnified because so many of these tests are patently unnecessary. In many cases (more so in the United States), doctors protect themselves against potential lawsuits by ordering every test they can. In fact, in the US, many orders for tests are motivated by a doctor's own self-interest, since so many physicians either own or have substantial shareholdings in the facilities to which they refer their own patients.

Another problem is that, these days, technology has replaced the fine art of diagnostics – of examining a patient's clinical history and having a good look at his eyes and the state of his tongue. The problem often comes down to trainee doctors, who often order tests under the mistaken notion that their consultant superiors desire such 'just-in-case' medicine. But in many cases senior doctors do flog their juniors if they fail to request particular tests, engendering the view that more is better and that massive test-taking is what constitutes good doctoring.[2]

Tests also make the fundamental error of assuming not only that all people are alike, but that people (and their measurements) always stay the same.

The other problem is that, unless your doctor has a particular feeling for taking apart computers in his spare time, he can get a bit muddled by this gee-whizz technology. One study found that virtually all doctors and nurses don't know how to work a pulse oximeter, a monitoring system which is vital for monitoring patients recovering from anaesthesia and recording potential life-threatening situations.[3] Consequently, they make serious errors in evaluating readings. The medics reported not being 'particularly worried' when patients had levels indicating that they were seriously deprived of oxygen and needed immediate attention if they were to live.[4]

BLOOD-PRESSURE READINGS

Your problems can start even when your doctor brandishes his blood-pressure cuff to record your blood pressure. Professor William White, chief of Hypertension and Vascular Diseases at the University of Connecticut, refers to this gizmo, known in medicalese as the 'sphygmomanometer', as 'medicine's crudest investigation'. Blood pressure, he says, can vary tremendously – as much as 30 mm Hg over the course of any day.[5] In fact, the time it's most likely to rise is in your doctor's surgery, when you're waiting to have the test – a phenomenon known as 'white-coat hypertension'. A recent study comparing blood-pressure readings taken at home, at work and at the doctor's surgery found that the most inaccurate were those performed in the doctor's surgery.[6] Such an artificially high test reading at the doctor's surgery can launch a patient onto a lifetime of blood-pressure medication.[7] The latest studies into blood pressure and hypertension have concluded that true high blood pressure is more related to average levels over 24 hours and also the degree of fluctuation between day and night than any particular or casually-made blood-pressure readings.[8]

These days, your doctor is more likely to give you a home-monitoring device or even to strap you up with a portable electronic device, which will measure your blood pressure at pre-set intervals over 24 hours. This is now thought to be the more accurate way of assessing your average blood pressure, although there is still a great deal of evidence that this system, called 'ambulatory monitoring', likewise doesn't provide accurate enough information for doctors to decide whether a patient needs treatment for high blood pressure.[9]

Even the World Health Organization recommends that ambulatory monitoring is best conducted with multiple readings over six months. But because no one has yet bothered to do proper large-scale scientific studies, no one can agree over how long you should go on doing the ambulatory monitoring before making a diagnosis, or what actually constitutes high blood pressure over this period, or even how much blood pressure should be lowered by to make it 'normal'.[10]

The values used today are still hypothetical, gleaned from studies of populations with normal blood pressure.[11] With home-monitoring systems, accuracy also remains a large problem. Only about a fifth of self-recording devices evaluated in recent studies have met acceptable criteria.[12]

In the US, the Food and Drug Administration mandates that any hypertension medication must be shown to lower blood pressure over 24 hours through ambulatory monitoring. Nevertheless, neither doctors nor drug companies really understand which reading – morning average, evening average, ambulatory reading, difference between day and night, degree of variation – shows that things are finally under control. Furthermore, many patients have different degrees of variability, depending on the nature of the stress they confront on the job.[13] Older patients also have more exaggerated differences in day and night readings – the significance of which is anyone's guess.[14]

A task force of participants at the 1999 Consensus Conference on ABP monitoring, sponsored by the International Society of Hypertension, recommended against using ambulatory monitoring for routine screening purposes.[15] The latest recommendations are that patients use ambulatory monitoring for initial diagnoses of hypertension, and self-monitoring for long-term follow-up.[16]

Even the variation between the arms influences a blood-pressure reading. One doctor from City General Hospital in Staffordshire, England discovered a variation of more than 8 mm Hg in systolic blood pressure between the two arms of nearly a quarter of his patients. In one case, the difference was 20 mm Hg.[17]

Things are just as confusing for pregnant women and children. Doctors and health-care workers can't even agree over how to record the second beat of blood pressure (called the diastole), which measures when blood fills up the heart,[18] or whether certain sounds accurately reflect diastolic pressure. This was even the subject of a heated debate at a world congress of hypertension in pregnancy in Italy, calling for an 'international consensus' on how to record blood pressure in pregnant women. In fact, some researchers have claimed that doctors have been using the wrong type of blood-pressure test on pregnant women: obstetricians and midwives prefer the blood-pressure gauge called Korotkoff phase 4, but research shows that phase 5 testing is far more reliable – the reverse of the prevailing view. In one test, virtually nobody agreed on the reading from a K4 test, while everyone was in agreement on the K5 test.[19] As for children, the latest recommendations are that they, too, have ambulatory monitoring.[20]

This potential for different interpretations in readings can cause problems for you if your blood pressure is being monitored by several people who may have had different training in how to read the cuffs.

CHOLESTEROL TESTS

Today, a cholesterol test is the most-often sought diagnostic test of all. In a general check-up a doctor will routinely offer you one to determine whether if you are at risk of heart disease. The test measures the amount of cholesterol and triglycerides in the serum (the non-cellular part) of your blood.

A total cholesterol test, which is rarely used these days, will examine all the blood fats, including the overall cholesterol level, the LDL (low-density lipoproteins, or 'bad' cholesterol), HDL (high-density lipoproteins, or 'good' cholesterol), VLDL (very low-density lipoproteins), chylomicrons (fats that are present right after a meal but ordinarily disappear within two hours) and triglycerides (compounds in the body that shift fatty acids through your blood). However, the typical cholesterol test only examines the LDL cholesterol.

The test requires a relatively straightforward blood test. You are asked to fast for 9–12 hours before the test is taken. A tourniquet is applied to your arm, so that the lower veins will pool with blood, and the blood is drawn from a vein either on the inside of the elbow or the back of the hand.

All fat tests (lipids, as they are known in medicalspeak) are measured in terms of milligrams per deciliter of blood (mg/dL). Medicine rates as acceptable a total cholesterol count of less than 200 mg/dL. The current medical wisdom is that the higher the cholesterol count, the greater the risk of heart disease or atherosclerosis (clogged arteries), and that if your levels are over 240 mg/dL you nearly double your risk of heart disease, compared with someone in the normal range.

The (largely unsubstantiated view) is that high LDL cholesterol levels may be the best predictor of risk of heart disease; if you have no other risk factors, your LDL count should come in at below 160 mg/dL. People with diabetes, heart or vascular disease, other risk factors or a family history of heart disease should try to keep their cholesterol levels even lower, say doctors.

Medicine loves statistics, and nowhere is this more evident than with this test, where a high LDL is thought to be countered by a high HDL, and vice versa. HDL cholesterol levels of 60 mg/dL are thought to counteract other risk factors; HDL levels below 40 mg/dL themselves become a risk factor.

Even if you have low LDL and high HDL cholesterol, high triglyceride levels may put you at risk. For instance, a normal triglyceride level should be less than 150 mg/dL. A vast array of conditions can result in an inaccurate test – liver disease, an underactive or overactive thyroid, kidney problems, liver disease, malabsorption of your food (say from a leaky intestinal tract), pernicious anaemia, infection and diabetes that isn't under control.

Pregnant women and those who have had their ovaries removed also will register high on the test. An array of prescription drugs – beta-blockers, thiazide diuretics, steroids, phenytoin, sulphonamides, the Pill, even vitamin D – can also throw off your test.

The other problem is the inherent inaccuracy of the lab test itself. According to one study, some 70 per cent of samples analysed have evidence of bias in the computation of results[21]; other research shows the products themselves used to measure blood cholesterol have major drawbacks.[22] In one Canadian study of total cholesterol tests, nearly one-quarter were misclassified (as, say high risk), nearly a fifth registered a false-positive (a high cholesterol level when it wasn't) and among those in the 'high risk' category, half had a false-positive reading.[23]

A few people in medicine are waking up to the fact that LDL levels alone are not an accurate predictor of heart disease. A large British Health Survey for England found that forecasting heart disease was far more accurate when factoring in the HDL levels, too.[24]

ECG Readings

Besides blood-pressure and cholesterol measurements, your doctor's next favourite activity is listening to the state of your heartbeat. However, these days, the all-purpose stethoscope (never proved to have any advantages over the naked ear) has been replaced by a number of space-age gadgets, all designed to record the most minute changes in your heart's ability to do its job.[25] The stalwart of any cardiac specialist is the electrocardiogram (ECG), even though studies demonstrate enormous potential for error in recording or interpreting correct results. One study showed that computers, often used to interpret ECG readings, were only right two-thirds of the time, and missed 15 per cent of cases of enlargement of the right ventricle. Nevertheless, human beings didn't fare much better; even trained heart specialists misinterpreted one out of every four readings.[26] This is largely because, as with blood-pressure, readings can be affected as much as 20 per cent by recent activity, time of day, and even factors such as fear of the cardiologist's findings! The late Dr Robert Mendelsohn wrote of a study in which electrocardiography detected only a quarter of proven cases of heart attack, and another study in which the tests found

22

gross abnormalities in more than half of perfectly healthy people.[27] As Stephen Fulder, author of *How to Be a Healthy Patient* (Hodder & Stoughton), notes, an incorrect ECG has led to 'vague diagnoses of organic brain disease in healthy but unruly children, turning them into medical cases'.[28]

More state-of-the-art these days than the ECG is *echo-cardiography* – a diagnostic test on the heart, often using a mixture of contrast agents and soundwaves. The procedure had been gaining acceptance for its safety and accuracy. However, as with much 'perfectly safe' new technology, doctors have only recently realized that it is more dangerous than had been thought, possibly leading to life-and-death complications.

The first major study into the procedure discovered that it can be life-threatening in one in 210 cases, requiring special treatment or a stay in hospital; two people of the 3,000 studied suffered a heart attack after the procedure had been completed.[29]

The procedure often employs the use of microbubbles of a contrast agent like octafluoropropane, which are useful in visualizing the tiniest blood vessels of the heart. In laboratory research, rats have developed cardiac arrhythmias after being exposed to echocardiography because the contrast agent interacted with ultrasound, causing the alterations in heart rhythms. Although animal models often don't apply to humans, this effect on a living being demonstrates that pulsed ultrasound can interact with bubbling contrast agents.[30] There's also evidence that the microbubbles cause destruction of capillaries, leaking red blood cells into skeletal muscle.[31] Furthermore, the act of using pulse-sound waves with contrast agents in the brain has been shown to cause tissue damage to vascular walls, causing haemorrhage and tissue death.[32]

ANGIOGRAPHY

If your doctor suspects that something is awry, he may trot you off for angiography, an x-ray test supposed to examine the state of your arteries via a contrast dye. The doctor will place a catheter into a blood vessel in your arm or leg, guide it towards the heart, and inject what is usually an iodinated dye like isosorbide dinitrate, which then travels into the main pump of the heart. Once all this is in place, the doctor will then snap pictures of your heart from different angles, all the while replenishing the supply of dye.

There's plenty of evidence that this test also has a poor batting average, wrongfully setting in motion one of a number of potentially lethal heart operations. In one test in Boston, half of the 171 patients recommended to have a coronary angioplasty (the operation where furred-up veins are opened by tiny inflated balloons) on the basis of their angiograph were found not to need the operation. In the end, only 4 per cent of the patients advised to have the angiograph really needed one.[33]

Angiographs are also especially open to misinterpretation. In another study in which the pathology reports of deceased patients were compared with prior angiographs, two-thirds were found to be wrong.[34] A number of critics blame the test itself, which only examines the main coronary arteries, will not show any vessel smaller than a 0.5 mm in diameter and will only highlight, at best, a quarter of all the blood flowing to the heart.

Many patients with an abnormal angiogram are referred for surgery, when, at best, the procedure can locate the site of a block and its severity, but not overall heart function. Angiography, for instance, cannot distinguish between patients with stable and unstable angina.

There's also a problem with accuracy. In one instance, after the deaths of three patients unsuccessfully treated by angioplasty, pathology reports found that the angiography on which the procedure was recommended had given misleading information about the patients' conditions.[35]

Finally, this nasty little test is not without its own dangers. The procedure itself causes death in two of every 1,000 patients or, at very least, can trigger a heart attack, stroke or severe blood loss.

Serious side-effects occur, regardless of the type of dye used,[36] and reactions to the dye often appear up to a week later. In one study, nearly half the patients involved complained of delayed reactions – including itchiness, rash and nausea – from one hour to seven days later.[37] More than 5 per cent of patients suffer reactions to the dye of moderate intensity, particularly those who have had the test before,[38] and one in ten will have a reaction of some sort. Although most are mild, at least 1 in every 2,500 is quite severe.[39]

If you have to have such a test, the less dangerous option may be magnetic-resonance-imaging angiography, which doesn't require either x-rays or dyes, but a magnetic field and pulses of radiowave energy to produce pictures of soft body tissues.[40] And as it provides pictures in three dimensions and on multiple planes, it shows better differentiation of tissues.

X-RAYS

X-rays are the most common procedure you're likely to be exposed to at least once in your lifetime. Today they represent approximately 10 per cent of any Western nation's health expenditure. Ionizing radiation is actually comprised of very high-frequency waves, which pass through living tissue. Depending on how dense the tissues are, the body retains some of this radiation. These absorbed rays are what gets recorded on the film as white or grey; those that pass completely through hit a plate of photographic film and show up as dark grey or black. Besides mammograms, bone x-rays and dental x-rays, the newest kind of x-rays include CAT scans, in which a moving beam of x-rays creates a three-dimensional picture, usually of the brain, and fluoroscopy, which sends the x-ray shadow picture onto a television screen. Occasionally contrast dyes like iopamidol or mediums like barium are used to provide a clearer picture.

Although the newest equipment uses lower and more precisely targeted doses, there is still no such thing as a safe x-ray (that goes for dental x-rays, too). In all of medicine there is virtually no disagreement that ionizing radiation is damaging – and those risks are multiplying as our understanding of the medium grows. 'Medical irradiation is by far the largest man-made contribution to the radiation burden of the population of developed countries,' R. Wootton, professor and director of Medical Physics at Hammersmith Hospital in London, wrote in a textbook on the subject. In the UK, he says, x-rays ordered by doctors account for over 90 per cent of the total radiation exposure of our population.[41]

X-rays harm people in three ways. First, they can damage individual cells (although the harm caused by the lower doses is usually quickly repaired). Rarely (but depending on exposure), this damage can convert the cell to a cancer cell. Although we don't know exactly how this works, it has been proposed that, since a cell is 75 per cent water, most of the radiation will be absorbed by the water, forming free radicals, which are known to be carcinogenic.[42]

25

Second, if a woman is pregnant, it can injure the developing foetus, causing death or malformations.

Finally, x-rays can damage the sperm or ovaries of children or adults, causing abnormalities in future generations. We also know that x-ray exposure is cumulative; the danger of something going wrong may increase every time you get another one.

We're still coming to grips with exactly how dangerous x-rays are, however. Unnecessary radiation from x-rays may be responsible for 700 cancer deaths in the UK every year, and perhaps 5,700 cancer deaths per year in the US, according to a recent Oxford University study.[43] But these figures may still be conservative. A UK National Academy of Science committee reviewed the usual assumptions that x-rays were responsible for 1 per cent of all leukaemias and 1 to 2 per cent of all other cancers, and concluded that the real risk could be as much as four times higher[44] – a conclusion also reached that same year by the International Commission on Radiological Protection.[45] Recently, multiple x-rays have even been linked with multiple myeloma – a form of bone cancer now sharply on the rise. Those who'd had the most exposure had a four times increased risk, the National Cancer Institute found.[46]

As far back as the 1950s, medicine discovered a link between leukaemia and prenatal x-rays. X-raying pregnant woman used to be routine, on the ludicrous notion that x-rays could tell a doctor whether her pelvis was 'wide enough' for the foetus to fit through during birth. We now know that if children are exposed to x-rays in utero their risk of all cancers is increased by 40 per cent, of leukaemias by 70 per cent, and of tumours of the nervous system by 50 per cent.[47] There also may not be a safe 'dose threshold'; single babies who'd received five to six times less radiation than twins who'd been x-rayed more frequently had the same incidence of cancer.[48] To put these numbers in perspective, for every million babies exposed in the womb to even a single rad of x-rays – the equivalent of a single picture of the stomach and intestines – between 600 and 6,000 could develop leukaemia.[49] John Gofman, Professor of Molecular and Cell Biology at the University of California, believes that women who undergo yearly mammograms receive cumulative doses not unlike the Japanese atomic bomb survivors.[50]

Gofman estimates that women's breasts receive 0.4 rad of medical x-rays a year for each year of life. If you compare that dosage with the levels suffered by Japanese atomic bomb survivors, he says, 114,000 women, from 62 to 75 per cent of those diagnosed every year with breast cancer, could blame x-rays as the cause. Besides cancer and genetic deformities, x-rays of the brain can lead to abnormal hormonal function, possibly causing under-active thyroid and infertility, or resulting in subtle changes in your adrenal glands.[51] The US Food and Drug Administration has also lately received a number of reports of patients suffering skin burns after radiation, so severe in some instances that the skin has died. The problem is complicated by the fact that these injuries don't show up for weeks after exposure. Your typical dose of fluoroscopy can result in skin injury after less than an hour.[52]

Even the offspring of those exposed to x-rays suffer. Exposure to x-rays increases a woman's risk of giving birth to a Down's syndrome baby.[53]

Although x-ray risk is cumulative over a lifetime of exposure, even single shots are not innocuous. According to the United States' Health Research Group, a consumer group which reports on risks in medicine, topping the list are x-rays of the upper intestine, which give an equivalent dose to the entire body of 400–800 millirads; the next highest (apart from the risk associated with x-raying the other organs) is the spine (100–500 millirads); stomach, breast and pelvis (100–200 each); skull or shoulder (25–75); chest (20–60); with whole mouth dental x-rays taking up the rear at 10–30 millirads.[54]

In case you are feeling complacent about that low dosage from dental x-rays, a single bite-wing dental x-ray is equivalent to smoking half a ciga-rette every day for a year. The US Academy of Sciences figures that one barium meal shot of the intestines carries the same risk as smoking up to a pack of cigarettes a day for a year. This means that, with x-rays of the lower back, which some 700,000 people undergo in Britain alone every year, 19 people could die each year as a direct result.[55]

Even if everyone in medicine knows that x-rays are dangerous — possi-bly dazzled by another of their 'miracles', the ability to 'see' through living tissue, Superman style — doctors blithely downplay the dangers and make few efforts to minimize exposure when ordering up a set, even on your teeth. Most GPs and orthopaedists have a kneejerk approach to ordering x-rays.

A joint working party established between the UK's Royal College of Radiologists and National Radiological Protection Board (NRPB) reviewed the existing evidence in 1990 and estimated that up to one fifth of the x-ray exams done in the UK were unnecessary or downright useless.[56] In one examination of patients given x-rays of the lower back, more than half were absolutely unnecessary[57] In the US, the Food and Drug Administration reckons that a third of all radiation is unnecessary.[58]

The most common unnecessary x-rays are those of the chest, limbs and joints. This translates into some seven million unnecessary x-ray exams in a single year. The UK's more modest wastefulness has worrying implications for the rest of the West, since the UK performs only about half the number of x-rays per person as other countries such as France or the US,[59] where seven out of every 10 people get subjected to at least one x-ray every year.[60] In Canada the figures are even worse: virtually everyone gets an annual x-ray of some sort.[61] (It's also no cause for complacency in the UK, since British doctors order twice the number of certain types of x-rays – barium meal and enema – as their American counterparts.[62]) The NRPB has recently announced that overall radiation in the UK could be halved without reducing diagnostic effectiveness.

For instance, doctors routinely x-ray for back pain, when it has never been found to do any good at all.[63] Skull x-rays have a poor batting average in detecting bleeding in the brain,[64] and even the good old chest x-ray, used to detect tuberculosis, is considered a waste of time by the World Health Organization.[65] The prestigious medical journal *The Lancet* admitted that most chest x-rays routinely performed on patients awaiting surgery other than on their heart or lungs were of so little benefit that over a million pounds' worth of x-rays would have to be done to end up saving a single life.[66]

The decision of whether you need an x-ray or not also depends on the whim of the individual doctor. An audit of nearly a million day and in-hospital patients has shown that referrals for x-ray varied by 13-fold in general and up to 25-fold for chest x-rays, depending on which consultant was in charge.[67]

Because the reproductive organs are susceptible to radiation damage, they should always be protected from exposure during x-ray by a lead shield. Nevertheless, in a Consumers' Association (*Which?*) report, in 40 per cent of cases the men surveyed had not had their testes shielded, and women were unprotected two-thirds of the time.[68] (In a third of cases, no attempt was made to find out if the women were pregnant.) In another study of children, three-quarters of the time the lead shields used to protect the reproductive organs hadn't been used or placed properly.[69]

Obviously there are times when x-rays are invaluable – particularly when limbs are first broken (though many doctors insist on constant new shots to check the progress of healing). However, even if your doctor is responsible about 'dose constraints' – the new buzzword among radiologists for the least amount of radiation necessary for individual snapshots – you still could be getting more radiation than necessary, largely from ageing equipment. The NRPB has reported that patients in some hospitals receive doses 20 to 30 times higher than necessary for obtaining diagnosis from machines that were, in some cases, 15 years old.[70] Just a few years ago Liz Francis, NRPB information officer, said 'physicists were saying that old x-ray equipment was giving out doses bigger than Chernobyl'.[71]

Even dental x-rays can subject you to unnecessary risks, since they are often performed by untrained staff who can't use the equipment properly and who may either need to repeat the exercise or will set the dosage unnecessarily high. Two dentists in the West Midlands escaped suspension by their professional body for using untrained school-leavers to take their x-rays when it became clear that dentists throughout Britain were doing exactly the same thing.

As with most tests, there is a strong likelihood of human error in interpreting the results. One study of Harvard radiologists found they disagreed on the interpretation of chest x-rays half of the time. There were significant errors in 41 per cent of their reports.[72]

Myelograms and X-ray Dyes

The other danger with x-rays are the contrast agents often used to highlight soft tissue of the body. These dyes have been associated with anaphylactic shock, cardiac instability, and poisoning of the kidneys, particularly among diabetics. In one study, of 319 patients with abnormal kidney function after being given 'high osmolality contrast agents', nearly one in 10 required kidney dialysis.[73]

Contrast agents like iopamidol, used for urographs and angiographs, have also been linked with pulmonary oedema (fluid in the lungs).[74] Barium, used for barium enemas, has been known to remain in the bowel and harden. In a patient with with a weakened bowel from diverticulitis, ulcerative colitis or Crohn's disease, the impacted material could cause the colon to split open.

Many hundreds of thousands of cases of chronic, debilitating back pain have been caused by spinal x-rays, called myelograms. This diagnostic tool involves the use of a contrast medium or dye injected into the canal space and trickled into and around all the discs and nerve roots in the back, which is then x-rayed. Mounting evidence shows that a number of myelogram patients will develop a condition called arachnoiditis, causing permanent, unrelenting pain and rendering many virtually unable to move.

Arachnoiditis is a little-understood condition in which the middle membrane protecting the spinal cord becomes scarred. Nerves atrophy and become enmeshed in dense scar tissue, which presses constantly on the spine. US orthopaedic surgeon Dr Charles Burton of the Institute for Low Back Care in Minneapolis, Minnesota, one of the few doctors to make a study of lumbar sacral adhesive arachnoiditis (LSAA), estimates that it accounts for 11 per cent of patients with 'failed back surgery syndrome'– where surgery has left them worse off than before.

Although LSAA results from a number of different causes, in Dr Burton's view it is mainly caused by the introduction of foreign substances into the human sub-arachnoid space. The foreign body most often identified in victims, he says, is iophendylate (known as Myodil in the UK; Pantopaque in the US), the oil-based dye used for myelograms. In LSAA, he says, iophendylate is often found in a cyst within the scar tissue mass.

An estimated one million people worldwide suffer from arachnoiditis caused by this dye, and even this figure could be conservative. Until the 1980s, nearly half a million myelograms were being performed in the US every year.

This is exactly what happened to Brian from Massachusetts. In 1980, after a staphylococcus blood infection causing paralysis, fever and pain, Brian had to undergo back surgery. Before his operation, a myelogram was performed on him, which left residual dye in Brian's coccyx.

In 1993, after spraining his back, he developed severe muscle spasticity, which caused pain in his legs and lower back. Each night now, the pain forces him out of bed every one or two hours. An MRI scan and x-ray finally revealed that Brian had arachnoiditis and that the myelogram he'd had left residual dye in his coccyx. 'Eighteen months, and several doctors later, with muscle relaxants, physical therapy, epidermal injections, chiropractic and even seizure drugs like Dilantin, nothing seems to work,' he says.

Pantopaque was introduced in the US in 1944 after the medical profession was convinced that it was safe. This was despite animal studies showing that Pantopaque caused arachnoiditis (the Swedes banned the product from use in humans in 1948).[75] Even though the product was discontinued by Glaxo with the onset of water-based dyes and imaging techniques, iophendylate continued to be used around the world until supplies ran out, and many back specialists continued to maintain that the dye was safe.

At the time, the US Food and Drug Administration and the British government also made no moves to ban oil-based myelograms. 'Despite the fact that iophendylate was identified as being causally related to the production of arachnoiditis from the time of its introduction, its use in the US has never been restricted by industry, government or the medical profession,' says Dr Charles Burton.[76]

It took patients with myelogram-induced LSAA bringing legal suits against the manufacturers before anyone else took notice. In the UK, the Arachnoiditis Society has some 1,000 members, and a class action suit was taken against Glaxo. After detailed negotiations, Glaxo reached a settlement with the 426 plaintiffs of £7 million, without admission of liability.

The water-based dyes now being used instead are not without risk. One woman being investigated for sciatic pain (back-caused leg pain) with iopamidol (Niopam 200), a water-soluble contrast medium, was immediately rendered paraplegic,[77] as was another middle-aged woman given a myelogram with itohexol (Omnipaque), another water-soluble dye.[78] Dr Burton says that some new mediums have caused such pain that the x-rays have had to be performed under general anaesthesia. 'The medical profession has not yet succeeded in finding a benign, effective myelographic medium,' he says.[79]

BONE SCANS

Besides looking for broken bones, x-rays are now being used to screen for osteoporosis. That might be a good idea – if we had a test that could be relied upon to deliver an accurate result. The problem is, as many medical experts agree, that even the latest techniques in bone scanning should be interpreted with caution, since changes in bone mass may not signify anything.[80]

The instruments are imprecise, multiple measurements may be wrong, even the assumptions upon which we scan bone are open to question – for example, the very notion that bones have a density that can be measured or that we can treat it and effectively reverse bone loss.

The latest souped-up bone scan is the 'dual energy x-ray absorptiometry' or DEXA – a fancy sort of x-ray. Again, you are injected with a radioactive liquid beforehand, then asked to lie flat on a table while you are scanned for between a half-hour to an hour or even more if a full three-dimensional shot is required. Measurements are usually taken from the spine, hip, spine, heel and forearm.

But an accurate reading in this technique can easily be knocked off. 'A walk around the room causes the measurement to change by up to 6 per cent (at the hip), which corresponds to six years of bone lost at the usual rate,' says Susan M. Ott, associate professor in the Division of Metabolism, University of Washington in Seattle.[81] Poor machine quality-control and a high percentage of operator error also throw off results.

The favoured technique, measuring many different areas of the body at the same time – one shot of the top of the leg produces five separate measurements, for instance – also increases the risk of a false-positive reading.

'Apparently dramatic changes can be taken as indicating improvement or dramatic bone loss but may simply be due to the precision of the measurement and poor repositioning technique,' wrote David M. Reid, a rheumatologist at City Hospital in Aberdeen, Scotland, and his colleagues.[82]

Studies show that DEXA tests are not necessarily very accurate. In one study, the scans failed to detect osteonecrosis in one-sixth of confirmed cases.[83] Extremes in weight (under- or overweight), age (over 60) and arthritis can throw off the result of a test. In fact, the entire exercise of measuring bone mass may be useless, because bone mass doesn't necessarily have anything to do with bone strength. For instance, fluoride causes bone mass to increase dramatically, but decreases its strength. This is why elderly populations in highly fluoridated communities show an increase in osteoporosis. Similarly, some drugs may increase bone mass by 5 per cent, but because bone structure has been damaged, it isn't strengthened with the drug. New research shows that only half the people considered to be at most danger from a fracture because of their reduced bone density will actually suffer one.[84]

It's important to understand that bone in healthy individuals is a dynamic entity, constantly undergoing interior remodelling. Two sets of cells are responsible: osteoclasts – the construction workers – which rip down the worn-out bone; and osteoblasts – the architects – which utilize calcium, magnesium, boron and other minerals to build up healthy new tissue. This process is called 'resorption'. All that the usual drugs for osteoporosis such as oestrogen, calcitonin or etidronate (called 'antiresorbing drugs') do is to slow this process of turnover and renewal, preventing the hardhat osteoclasts from doing their job. Eventually, there is no further bone formation.

Some researchers argue that the presence or absence of low bone density is a meaningless indicator of risk of fractures or osteoporosis.[85] In one nine-year study of 1,000 middle-aged women, the group considered at *high* risk of osteoporosis actually had fewer fractures than the group not considered at risk. Bone-density screening has also never been shown to be effective in preventing fractures, according to a large review of published work on bone-density screening.[86]

Bone scans may have a one-time use to help in diagnosing women suspected clinically of osteoporosis, but appear to be too variable to be relied upon as a general screening test for women without symptoms.

CAT SCANS

As with most other industries, the advent of the computer has taken the medical x-ray business to a new level. In the 1970s, computed axial tomography, now usually known as CAT, or CT, scans, revolutionized diagnosis, particularly of bones, blood vessels and soft tissue of the body, offering pictures with up to 20 times the detail of ordinary x-rays. It has now made it possible to scan for diseases of the abdomen, lung, heart, liver and pancreas, and even for early osteoporosis.

Adapted from an image-processing system developed for the Apollo moon landings, CAT scans take a 360-degree series of cross-sectional x-ray images from multiple angles – up to 30 shots – by passing a pencil-thin beam through a particular portion of the body, sometimes with the use of a contrast agent. An X-ray tube on a moveable ring revolves around your body, taking individual 'slices' of images.

This information is then passed through a computer, which reconstructs the slices into a three-dimensional image on a video screen, allowing the operator to see this portion of the body from any angle. It is also stored so that the doctor can take photographs of the video screen or call up the information in the future. Your problem is that now that your doctor has computerized diagnostic toys at his disposal, he's more likely to want to play with them. Although doctors have attempted to claim that CT scanning reduces the need for other tests such as brain scans, arteriography or exploratory surgery, this may be a false saving.

While no doubt CAT scanning represented the height of 20th-century technology, it also poses far more risks than most other tests, blasting you with far higher doses of radiation. In 1991, the NRPB concluded that CAT scans accounted for only 2 per cent of the total UK x-ray examinations but 20 per cent of the overall collective dose, and so were the largest single source of exposure from x-rays.[87] This risk is magnified if you don't stay stock still during the half-minute or so of the test and it has to be repeated. In Japan nearly one-eighth of the population was getting CT-scanned as far back as 1979. Radiation from a single body shot is now considered comparable to that of the low-dose atomic bomb survivors from Hiroshima.[88]

CAT scans are particularly dangerous when used on children. Despite their reduced size, they may receive adult-sized doses of x-rays, up to five times of what is necessary, leaving them prone to cancer. In the US, where 600,000 children under 15 receive CAT scans every year, an estimated 500 die as a result.[89] Furthermore, although all the early studies showed that CAT scans reduced diagnosis time, helped doctors to understand their diagnosis, reassured doctors about their diagnosis or treatment plans and avoided the need for other tests, very few demonstrated that this knowledge in any way reduced illness, shortened hospital stay or prevented death.[90]

There are also questions of accuracy. Despite the dangers of high–dose radiation in children, particularly of their sexual organs, it is often used to diagnose cerebral (brain) hernia after lumbar puncture for meningitis. Nevertheless, one study found that one-third of children with hernias were misdiagnosed as normal.[91] As with other contrast mediums, the dyes used can permanently damage the kidneys.[92]

Despite any real demonstration of value, other than as a diagnostic toy, use of CT scanning has moved briskly apace. Patients who have a seizure are scanned, even before a clinical history is taken, to rule out alcohol withdrawal.[93] So beloved is this gadgetry that it has even been used to research the cause of the common cold, the researchers concluding that their study patients had – wait for it – swelling of the mucous membranes.[94] Besides megadoses of radiation, CT scans (indeed all x-rays) have long been known to cause cataracts and other lens opacities, such as nuclear sclerosis,[95] and could affect thyroid function.[96]

MRI SCANS

The dangers of CAT scans and the use of computers led to the development of nuclear magnetic resonance, which developed into magnetic resonance imaging (MRI). This screening procedure was hailed as a promising alternative to x-rays for providing detailed pictures of soft body tissue, particularly the brain and spinal cord.

In MRI, you are placed inside a massive cylindrical magnet weighing up to 500 tons – large enough to envelope the entire body. While you are inside the magnet a quick pulse is applied, creating a magnetic field some 50,000 times stronger than that of the earth.[97] The effect of this is to excite the nuclei of atoms within body cells. These hyped-up nuclei produce radiofrequency echoes, which get translated into images on a computer.

The MRI scan works by focusing on the water molecules, which largely make up the tissues of your body. The scan excites the hydrogen and oxygen molecules and, as they begin moving in a certain pace and direction, the scanner is able to detect and measure them and then reconstruct a picture of your body from them, displaying it in real time on a television monitor. Although it was originally believed that the good 'pictures' afforded by MRI would eliminate the need for injectible dyes, this hasn't proved so. Contrast agents are needed to detect brain tumours, for example. Unlike the contrast materials used for CAT scans, which contain iodine, those used for MRI are magnetically-active substances.

Currently, the only MRI contrast materials approved by the American Food and Drug Administration are chelates, containing a rare earth element called gadolinium. When injected into a patient's veins, this works similarly to iodine contrast agents, but is supposed to be far safer, with severe reactions occurring in about 1 in 350,000 patients.

MRI is mainly used to view the nervous system, for suspected strokes, brain tumours, multiple sclerosis, brain infections such as meningitis, epilepsy, developmental disorders of the brain such as hydrocephalus, and problems of the spinal cord or vertebrae. Its advantages over CAT scans are that it shows better tissue contrast, enables you to get images in multiple planes, has no radiation, employs a safer contrast medium, and enables you to view veins and the top and front joining of the skull. The big drawback is that you must undergo a much longer scanning time, and results can be flawed if you move at any time during the procedure. However, these days the latest MRI scanners can work faster and take in more detail in one go.[98] MRI is reputed to be fairly accurate for detecting multiple sclerosis; one study of MS patients showed a 95–99 per cent accuracy in detecting the disease.[99]

But, again, large question marks remain about its accuracy. According to a medical textbook on CT and MRI, many initial reports that MRI gave more detailed images than CT were 'overly optimistic'. All the initial fanfare, which came from individual cases of patients, could not be confirmed by subsequent larger studies using full scientific methods. The earlier studies turned out not to be well controlled.[100]

Lately, MRI has shown to be less than accurate in detecting early prostate cancer[101] or coronary artery disease.[102] It is now thought that MRI is better than CT for the brain and spine, because of its ability to take shots of the top of the head and front of the skull and to detect subtle tissue changes, but CT is better for studying any sort of trauma – such as blows to a body part – or the bones or calcium.

The problem is that no one yet knows the likely long-term effects of subjecting the body to a magnetic field powerful enough to send magnetic objects flying across the room. So far, the National Radiological Protection Board has sounded a warning about the heating effects of the magnetic field and its ability to influence magnetic matter inside the body or to damage tissues.

Microbiologist Wendell Winter and colleagues at the University of Texas Health Center at San Antonio stated that exposure to these types of electromagnetic fields may not be totally harmless. They subjected a number of living things to a range of electromagnetic fields and found that they stimulated the growth rate of cancer cells.[103]

Research on chick embryos has demonstrated that they are at risk with the increased temperatures; female mice chronically exposed showed changes in their white blood cell count. Other animal studies show that MRI can cause birth defects in the eyes[104] and damage to the ears.[105] In the States, several patients with pacemakers died when the magnetic forces altered them.[106]

Another potential danger concerns any metallic substances on your body. Complications can occur if you have any metal prostheses or implants, surgical clips or artificial heart valves, you are wearing any metal object, like a watch, have any metal on your clothing, wear a shade of eye shadow that contains metallic substances or even have your ATM card in your wallet.

One of the big problems with MRI scannings is claustrophobia. Up to one-third of patients given MRI scans have felt so claustrophobic that the tests had to be abandoned.[107] 'After an MRI scan for my neck, I had appalling claustrophobia (during it), with memory loss,' writes Jill from Aberdeen. 'I kept crying, shaking, couldn't write, stammered, had nightmares for two weeks afterwards. It was 55 minutes of hell – worse than the two previous CAT scans. It must affect the brain cells with all that magnetism.'

Perhaps the most unsuspected problem caused by radiofrequency fields of MRI is localized heating, a risk that is magnified among babies or patients who are anaesthesized.[108] For instance, in one poll of 10 US American departments of radiology, the overwhelming majority of serious injuries relating to MRI imaging were burns.[109] This heating can also cause future fertility problems in men, since sperm are rendered sterile if heated up to body temperature. One study found that average scrotal skin temperature was significantly raised by an average of 2°C, with the highest change 4°C.[110] Four separate studies support Jill's contention that the technique causes memory loss.[111]

The National Radiological Protection Board concludes that a magnetic field of 2.5 tesla (T) is safe for all patients. Between 2.5 and 4 T, evidence of harm is doubtful, but from 4 T upwards, likely to occur.

If you are pregnant, have a pacemaker or have a metal prosthesis such as an artificial hip, retained shrapnel or cochlear, carbon-fibre implants, you should avoid MRI. Implants in particular can either move or become foci for the heating effect of MRI, causing discomfort and local tissue damage. Besides the dangers of metal inside your body, every metallic object in the scanning room becomes a potentially lethal missile once the MRI device is turned on. The most serious reported injury with MRI occurred when an oxygen tank near the magnet started flying and struck a patient's face.[112]

Doctors are also increasingly worried about the contrast agents used for all the 'nuclear' imaging techniques.

Of all the reports made to the UK Adverse Reaction Reporting Scheme in the six years between 1977–83, nearly half concerned methylene diphosphonate for bone imaging and one-third concerned colloids for liver scans. The majority of complaints concerned hypersensitivity to the dyes. The most conservative estimate is one in 1,000 people react – a figure far higher than originally believed.[113]

If your doctor wants you to undergo the procedure you should make sure he first takes your full medical history, since the protocol for using MRI differs depending on what you are investigating. According to multiple sclerosis specialist Dr Patrick Kingsley, when diagnostic toys like MRI weren't available, any reasonably experienced neurologist could make a confident diagnosis of MS based on a patient's symptoms and history. The only reason perhaps to proceed with an MRI scan is if the neurologist wishes to rule out a brain tumour which might be amenable to surgery.

LAB TESTS

Besides x-rays, laboratory tests of all persuasions are subject to the grossest sort of error. The Centers for Disease Control and Prevention in Atlanta, Georgia, studied a representative sampling of laboratories all over the US and found that about a quarter of all tests had incorrect results.[114]

An editorial in *The Lancet* once concluded that many routine laboratory diagnostic tests are a waste of time and money.[115] This includes blood counts and biochemical screening when you're admitted to hospital. One study, it said, showed that the illnesses of only six out of 630 patients were diagnosed from routine blood and urine tests. In another study of over 1,000 patients in an adult psychiatric unit, routine blood and urine tests contributed to less than 1 per cent of diagnoses; nearly three-quarters of diagnoses were made on the basis of the patient's medical history or a physical examination.[116]

Doctors can't even agree on blood sugar levels in people with diabetes.

A Scottish study found marked differences in the results between the two tests – one which measures carbohydrates in the blood, the other, just glucose – used to assess control of blood sugar levels and whether good blood sugar control has been achieved.[117]

THE HIV TEST

The most shameful instance of an unreliable lab test used for diagnostic purposes is the AIDS test. The enzyme-linked immunosorbent assay (ELISA) test is most frequently used to test your HIV status, and is usually considered proof-positive that you are infected with HIV. A test called Western Blot is often used as a confirmation. For the ELISA test, a sample of the patient's blood is added to a mixture of proteins. It is assumed that if HIV antibodies are present in the blood, they will react to the HIV proteins in the test.

The proof that HIV causes AIDS hinges entirely on the idea that detection of an antibody response to the virus is proof of its actual presence. Doctors assume that if your body has made antibodies specific to HIV, it must mean that a protein of the virus – and so the virus itself – is present. In other words, the so-called AIDS tests cannot test for the presence of HIV, just the presence of antibodies to it – the usual sign that the body has fought off infection and won.

With the Western Blot, these HIV proteins are isolated in bands; when mixed with a blood sample, each protein band will show up if it has bound to an antibody.

Besides being unable actually to detect HIV, these tests are notoriously unreliable; in Russia, in 1990, out of 20,000 positive ELISA tests, only 112 could be confirmed using the Western Blot, according to Australian biophysicist Eleni Papadopulos-Eleopulos, who has studied both tests in depth.[118] The French government considers these tests so unreliable that it withdrew nine of the 30 HIV tests that were once available.

The other problem is that neither test is specific to HIV; both react to many other proteins caused by other diseases. For example, the protein p24, generally accepted to be proof of the existence of HIV, is found in all retroviruses that live in the body and do no harm. This means that p24 is not unique to HIV, as Dr Robert Gallo, co-discoverer of the HIV virus, has stated repeatedly. Hepatitis B and C, malaria, papillomavirus warts, glandular fever, tuberculosis, syphilis and leprosy are just a few of the conditions that are capable of producing biological false-positives in ELISA tests.[119]

In one study, antibodies to p24 were detected in 13 per cent of patients with generalized papilloma virus warts, 24 per cent of patients with skin cancer and 41 per cent of patients with multiple sclerosis.[120] In one study, half the patients with a positive p24 test later tested negatively.[121]

Western Blot, supposed to be the more accurate of the two, has proven no better than ELISA. Dr Max Essex of Harvard University's School of Public Health, a highly respected AIDS expert, found that the Western Blot gave a positive result to some 85 per cent of African patients later found to be HIV-negative. Eventually, he and his researchers discovered that proteins from the leprosy germ – which infects millions of Africans – can show up as a false-positive on both ELISA and Western Blot, as can malaria.[122] In one study of Venezuelan malaria patients, the rate of false-positives with Western Blot was 25–41 per cent.[123]

This poor track record is disturbing when you consider that the main AIDS 'risk' groups – gay men, drug-users and haemophiliacs – are exposed to many foreign substances such as semen, drugs, blood transfusions and blood components, hepatitis, Epstein Barr virus and many other factors or diseases known to cause false-positives in HIV tests. Other populations exposed to a greater than normal amount of disease – such as Africans and drug-users – also make many more antibodies than the rest of us and therefore are likely to end up with a false reading.

Blood transfusions can also produce a false-positive HIV test result. In one study, the amount of HIV antibody detected in ELISA tests was greatest immediately after blood transfusion, and thereafter decreased.[124] One volunteer was given six injections of donated HIV-negative blood at four-day intervals. After the first injection his HIV test was negative, but the HIV-positive antibody response increased with each subsequent transfusion.[125]

Of course, the greatest problem with an HIV test is that a positive test labels you HIV positive for life. Being HIV positive can bar you from insurance, employment, marriage or even entry into another country. The HIV test can also launch many healthy patients on the inexorable road to 'just-in-case' AIDS treatment with drugs whose considerable, even life-threatening side-effects bear uncanny resemblance to the list of symptoms doctors describe in HIV infection or full-blown AIDS.

'OSCOPY' TESTS

Most other tests you're likely to encounter are more invasive, requiring that your doctor inject or penetrate your body with something. These can include 'oscopy' tests, where an optic tube or 'scope' is passed through a bodily orifice in order to inspect the inside of the appropriate body cavity – the stomach (endoscopy), abdomen and pelvis (laparoscopy), lungs (bronchoscopy), colon (colonoscopy), cervix (colposcopy), rectum and lower colon (flexible sigmoidoscopy, or even the knee joint (arthroscopy).

Although doctors consider the common endoscopy routine, there are enormous risks, including perforation of the wall of the oesophagus, stomach or duodenum (the small intestine), infections and adverse reactions to anaesthetic – even death. Up to one in 36 patients ends up with a perforation, and nearly one in 100 patients will suffer one so serious that it proves fatal.[126] Overall, it's estimated that endoscopy is killing one in 2,000 patients. This poor batting average only came to light because a special audit of UK hospitals was carried out to look into the long-term effects of the technique.[127] The study discovered that patients were dying up to 30 days after having the test, usually from heart or respiratory complications. Complications are occurring because the test requires the patient to be sedated, which means the patient can still respond but cannot feel any pain. Nevertheless, sedated patients must be carefully monitored; inadequate monitoring is the cause of 20 per cent of all deaths related to anaesthesia.

Another recurrent problem with 'oscopy' tests, such as endoscopes and bronchoscopes, are outbreaks of infection occurring in American hospitals caused by inadequately sterilized flexible fibre-optic endoscopes and bronchoscopes. According to the US Food and Drug Administration, up to one-quarter of all endoscopes, even those that are sterilized, contain 100,000 or more different types of bacteria, a fertile ground for cross-contamination. Although there are no known cases of HIV infection due to endoscopy, there is evidence of the transmission of hepatitis B and C, and Creutzfeldt-Jakob disease.[128]

The devices are cleaned and disinfected either manually, which is time-consuming for a busy hospital, or, increasingly, by automated machines. After investigating an outbreak of *Pseudomonas aeruginosa*, causing infection of the gall bladder, which occurred in one American hospital, the American Centers for Disease Control and Prevention found the culprit to be a thick film of *P. aeruginosa* which had formed in the detergent-holding tank, water hose and air vents of the automated disinfecting machine. Attempts to disinfect the machine according to the manufacturer's instructions using commercial preparations of glutaraldehyde were unsuccessful.

After the second outbreak, the American Food and Drug Administration (FDA) requested that one of the manufacturers send out a safety alert to all hospitals with its products, recommending that a stringent rinsing programme be adopted for the cleaning of the machines. The FDA has also suspended the further sale of any of the machines until the contamination problem is resolved. In the meantime, even disinfectant has caused side-effects such as bloody diarrhoea among patients and hospital staff alike.[129]

As for laparoscopy, three out of every 1,000 of these procedures cause complications, and even death. Between 1995 and 1997, more than 500 patients suffered nearly 600 injuries, and 65 died.[130] A goodly number have to do with doctors being unable to use the equipment properly. In a survey of gynaecologists, one in every 25 had injured a major vessel during laparoscopy at some point in their career.[131]

One of the main culprits is the common use of the trocar (a sharp implement which withdraws fluids by puncturing the abdominal wall), which frequently injures major blood vessels and major organs, sometimes causing death due to vascular injuries.[132]

Arthroscopy, another 'oscopy' used to examine the knee, can cause deep vein thrombosis. Nearly a fifth of patients undergoing the procedure develop the condition.[133]

BIOPSIES

When the mere image of a body part won't yield up the problem, doctors resort to nicking off a piece of you and studying it under the microscope. These types of tests include those in which one or more of the body's tissues or fluids are withdrawn for examination, such as biopsies, bone marrow aspiration or spinal tap (also called lumbar puncture). There are four types of biopsies, ranging from removal of a few cells to excising a good-sized chunk with a scalpel or through the use of an endoscope with a tiny set of forceps, for those body parts conventional methods can't reach. Even such a seemingly simple test as a tissue sample is not without risk. About a fifth of lumbar punctures lead to injury. Although it had always been assumed that injuries occurred when a junior doctor carried out the procedure, new evidence now finds that mistakes occur across the board, even with very experienced practitioners.[134]

Spinal taps have also been used to diagnose children with bacterial meningitis, the disease's most dangerous form. But research now shows that, with spinal taps, children are 30 times more likely to develop herniation, a catastrophic complication of bacterial meningitis, with a high risk of death or damage.[135]

As for biopsy, when a sample tissue is being removed to help diagnose suspected cancer, certain types have a terrible batting average. For instance, biopsy of the prostate, one of the most common, is wrong in one of four cases, even when multiple tissue sites are taken.[136] Breast, liver, kidney, lung, pancreas and lymph node (sentinel node) biopsy results all have high rates of false-positives and -negatives. Like mammograms, biopsies aren't discriminatory and cannot distinguish between benign and malignant tumour cells.[137]

As with all medical tests, biopsies also aren't without dangers. The biggest potential risk is when the doctor misses, and punctures the organ itself or ones that sit nearby. For instance, one in three cases of a lung biopsy cause collapse of the lung,[138] and one in 1,000 liver biopsies damage the gallbladder, causing a fatal peritonitis from bile leaking into the abdomen.[139]

Furthermore, doctors are now beginning to realize that, unless the tumour is entirely removed at the same time, such tampering may cause the cancer to 'seed' elsewhere. This is now such an acknowledged risk that doctors performing prostate biopsy routinely offer radiotherapy at the same time. Cancer-seeding occurs in one-third of cases in breast biopsy[140] and a sixth of cases in liver biopsy.[141]

'Such a biopsy on a secondary tumour, which was diagnosed after a "local" needle biopsy, I consider responsible for the death of my beloved wife Geena at the age of 50,' writes Conor from Ireland. 'Geena was then radiant, playing sports and active in the garden. She was also into alternative therapies and fighting her cancer magnificently.' He goes on:

> *However, she was pressurized into that surgical biopsy by arrogant dismissals of our expressed fears, and assurances that such a test carried no risk; the doctors stressed the need to locate the primary tumour immediately so that 'urgent treatment' could start.*
>
> *Tragically, medical dogmatism prevailed over our instincts and better judgement, and the biopsy took place. That biopsy caused the tumour (in her neck) to spread rapidly.*
>
> *It was agonizing to witness. Just two months later, radium had to be prescribed to reduce its growth. From day two of the 'treatment', Geena experienced abdominal pain. After its conclusion in September, her decline was precipitous.*
>
> *A few weeks later, an emergency hysterectomy had to be performed to treat what was finally diagnosed as cancer of the ovaries.*
>
> *Surgery could not extract all the cancer; what remained spread like wildfire. 'Last-ditch' chemotherapy was powerless to prevent it. Geena died on 23rd November.*
>
> *Twelve years ago, my father died within two weeks of a 'routine' biopsy test on his lung.*

With this great potential for error and danger, it is vital that you forego any test – even the most seemingly gentle – unless it is truly vital. Also insist on a thorough verbal and physical exam before you get a test. Oftentimes, taking a good clinical history will give your doctor enough information to pre-empt a routine test. Finally, think twice about annual check-up tests when you are feeling perfectly healthy.

If you are told to have a cholesterol test, insist on a test that will measure *all* your blood lipids and have them compared. The US National Cholesterol Education Panel now recommends that all cholesterol tests should include four components: total cholesterol, HDL, LDL, and triglycerides. Insist on two tests, given at different times at between one and eight weeks apart, preferably by another lab.[142] This small inconvenience could save you from a life of drug-taking.

Because of the inherent dangers, CAT scans should be used only in exceptional circumstances, when there is no safer diagnostic tool available. If you do need a CAT scan, insist that one is enough. During all x-rays (even benign ones of the hand or finger), ignore the likely ridicule of nurses and insist that your reproductive organs and thyroid gland are shielded, which can reduce scatter radiation by 20 per cent.[143]

Whenever possible, avoid contrast agents in imaging tests and look to the safest alternatives. New techniques like endoscopic ultrasound (where sound waves are used with an endoscope) probably offer the safest alternative.

Resist biopsies whenever possible and look into new and safer imaging techniques, such as thermography for breast cancer, ultrasound, MRI or PET scans.

TESTING THE TEST

Before you agree to the simplest test, including one for your blood-pressure, ask your doctor some of the following questions:

- **Do I really need this test?** Is there another, safer way of determining the same thing (such as a thorough interview and physical exam by an experienced medic)?

- **What will you advise me to do if the tests are normal/abnormal?** If your doctor cannot do anything about any abnormal findings, why take the test?

- **What is this test's track record of accuracy?** What are the risks of the test? Of the subsequent treatment? Again, you may have to do your homework, contacting the medical journals, the internet, our offices and even the manufacturers of the test (see pages 246–8 for more suggestions about how to do your own research).

- **What are the qualifications of the operators (and how many hours are they likely to have been on duty when you take the test)?** If the operators are house officers at the end of a 72-hour stint, you would be wise to insist on more experienced – and rested – parties to handle the equipment.

- **When was the equipment last checked for safety/accuracy?** This is a particularly pertinent question in a health-care system increasingly strapped for cash.

- **What dosage (of radiation or ultrasound, say) will I receive? Are there any protective devices (shields, in the case of radiation) that I can wear?** A protective apron worn when you receive dental x-rays can prevent the rest of your body getting 'zapped' at the same time.

- **Is it possible to use earlier test results so that I am not exposed to further risk?** Insist that your dentist keep your x-rays permanently on file. And if you move, insist that they be transferred to your new dentist. If your former dentist balks at this, get your Community Health Council to intervene, on the basis of your concern about 'dosage constraints'.

- **What is the real risk of my developing the condition you're investigating?** If the doctor suggests a mammogram to investigate a breast lump and you're 15 and have never been exposed to hormones, the risk of your developing breast cancer at your age may be far less than the risk of the test.

All this test-taking presumes that you have symptoms, which is why you went to your doctor in the first place. These days, you're more than likely to get screened for diseases even before there's anything wrong with you – and never more so than from the first moment you are 'diagnosed' as being pregnant.

3

Prenatal Testing: Dead Certainty

The moment you first miss a period, medical science informs you that you will not be able to give birth unless you are subjected to a large round of prenatal tests, all supposedly designed to 'put your mind at rest'. In reality, these tests have the opposite effect. According to medical science, for instance, my daughter, Caitlin, could have had Down's syndrome. If I had listened to the experts I might have aborted her or lost her through a high-tech, test-induced miscarriage. The very thought sends a chill down my spine.

When I got pregnant, I firmly resisted all recommendations to have ultrasound monitoring and amniocentesis despite being a reasonably elderly primagravitas (37) at conception, because of my fears about their known and unknown risks.

Nevertheless, when I was 16 weeks' pregnant my doctor, who respected my wish to avoid amniocentesis, suggested that I take a routine prenatal alpha-fetoprotein (AFP) test. The test measures the level of AFP produced by the foetus and present in the mother's bloodstream.

It was designed to detect babies with rare neural tube defects such as spina bifida, as evidenced by a 'high' reading. Although the test wasn't designed for it, low readings are now thought to be associated with an increased risk of Down's syndrome.

'Just to put your mind at rest,' my doctor cajoled.

Since it only involved taking a blood sample from my upper arm rather than invading the womb as all other prenatal tests do, I let myself be talked into it. After all, I was having a fantastic pregnancy. I was convinced my baby was perfectly healthy. Now I'd know for sure. What was there to lose?

A week or so later, my doctor's secretary rang and asked me to phone him. 'What for? Did the test come back?' I asked apprehensively.

'That's what he wants to discuss with you.'

For an agonizing half-hour I stayed on the phone waiting for him to get on the line. When he did, it was to report the words I'd never even thought to consider: 'The results of the AFP test are borderline low.'

I burst out in hysterical sobbing, and only after five minutes had calmed down sufficiently to ask what I already knew that meant.

'There's a slight possibility of Down's syndrome.'

I don't remember much of the rest of the conversation. My doctor tried a few gentle reassurances − we could find out for sure through a combination of amniocentesis and ultrasound; this combination of tests had a high degree of accuracy; the other borderline situations he'd investigated had turned out all right.

Finally I managed to say that I would call him back. I had a secretary drag my husband out of a meeting to tell him the news, and after he rushed home we considered our options. We could run through the battery of tests with ultrasound and amniocentesis, and risk miscarrying a perfectly healthy baby or damaging it through the test − both known risks of the procedure. We then discussed the ramifications of a test result confirming that I was carrying a handicapped child.

We would be faced with the decision of aborting a five-month-old foetus − not some lima-bean-sized tadpole, but a perfectly formed, nearly viable human being. It meant going through labour and giving birth to a dead baby or, if he wasn't expelled in that manner, having the body removed, piece by piece.

I looked down at my bump. For me, that simply was not a possibility I could contemplate, no matter how deformed this child might be, which made the entire AFP exercise an utter waste of time. If you are not prepared to abort a handicapped foetus, there is no point in going through with the tests.

I was appalled by medicine at that moment for creating a situation that could only be resolved through the high-tech measures I had so wished to avoid. If I had never had the AFP test, I thought, I would never have had to consider subjecting my baby to a battery of possibly damaging tests just to bury the doubts raised by the first test result.

In the end, to our minds, there was only one reasonable path: to ignore the test and to listen to our hearts, which told us that the baby was fine.

This is what we chose to do. I called my doctor to tell him, and my husband and I never spoke about the test again. Sure enough, it turned out that we had been traumatized for nothing. The test was wrong. At the end of my term, out came our perfectly normal, healthy baby.

Despite the murmurs from your obstetrician about the very best in medical technology, most prenatal testing is little more than ritualistic nonsense.

ULTRASOUND SCANS

The mainstay of modern obstetric diagnosis is the ultrasound scan (or sonography) and is the most likely test you'll be given, following hard at the heels of your urine test confirming pregnancy in the first place. Most women these days can show off pictures of their babies in the womb when they are not much past the tadpole stage. First developed during the Second World War to track down enemy submarines, ultrasound scanning began to be used in the 1970s for diagnostic testing and eventually for pregnancy.

Similar to radar, real-time scanners employ very-high-frequency pulsed sound waves (3.5–7 mHz, or 3.5–7 million cycles per second) that are sent to the foetus via a transducer placed on the abdomen. Echoes of the sound waves create moving images on the monitor screen.

In the radiology industries ultrasound is known as the biggest growth area, with equipment manufacturers enjoying a 20 per cent growth in sales over the next few years and some 60 to 90 million investigative tests of all sorts performed every year.[1] Although originally planned to be used for aiding high-risk pregnancies, the exam is now presently looked upon, as New York's Columbia University Professor Harold E. Fox once put it, as the equivalent of a 'physical exam of the foetus in utero',[2] with a good reading the tacit assurance of a healthy baby. Virtually all pregnant women are now scanned and given photos or videos to take home as a pleasantly packaged souvenir of their first baby picture.

It's meant to determine whether your baby is healthy and when you are likely to give birth. Scans supposedly can assess gestational age, size and growth, rule out multiple or tubal pregnancies or ovarian cysts, locate the position of the baby in the womb, and show whether the baby is growing properly or whether it has died.

A scan before 20 weeks also looks for abnormalities such as hydro-cephalus, anencephaly, spina bifida, cleft lip or palate and congenital heart problems. Ultrasound is increasingly being used to pick up so-called 'soft markers' – subtle defects which may or may not be serious. It can identify club foot, low-set ears and even problems with facial development.

It is now the first port of call for checking for chromosomal abnormal-ities such as Down's syndrome. At the bare minimum, women are scanned at 12, 18–20 and 34 weeks of pregnancy. Many are scanned 10 or 12 times before giving birth, starting as early as seven weeks into the pregnancy. In late pregnancy it is used to rule out *placenta praevia*, when a low-lying placenta blocks the birth passage.

Although doctors rely on scanning as an early warning signal of prob-lems that can largely be remedied, babies who are scanned tend to have poorer outcomes, possibly because scans simply invite more invasive procedures that don't appear to aid survival. In one study, more of the scanned babies died, were delivered sooner and spent more time in hospi-tal and on ventilators than babies who were not scanned. Of those with abdominal wall defects, the scanned group were operated on sooner, but had the same outcomes as unscanned babies whose operations were delayed. Furthermore, more of the scanned babies died (23 per cent vs only 4 per cent of the unscanned babies).[3] A German study found that caesarean section and preterm delivery was five times more frequent, and admission into intensive care three times higher, for babies diagnosed by ultrasound before birth.[4]

In the UK and the US, pregnant women are generally told by their doctors that ultrasound is as safe as a television set. The official line of the Royal College of Obstetricians and Gynaecologists is that the wave inten-sity currently used in scans is 'probably' safe. Obstetricians take the airy position that there are 50 million people walking around today who were scanned in the womb, and with no laboratory evidence to indicate that it is a hazard, they must be all right.[5] And it is true that the very short pulses of sound that produce echoes and ultimately the pictures you see on the screen when they hit soft tissue – 1,000 pulses to a second, each lasting one-millionth of a second – have never been definitely shown to cause heating or bubbles in the tissues of human babies.[6]

Nevertheless, this position ignores a growing body of medical evidence to the contrary, so much so that all of the pertinent US regulatory bodies urge obstetricians not to use ultrasound routinely.

The enthusiastic and uncritical embracing of this new technology reminds many of what happened in the US with diethylstilbestrol (DES), the wonder drug of the fifties that was supposed to cure miscarriage. The side-effects of the drug are only now showing up in adult offspring some 30 years later, in the form of reproductive problems and cancer.

The fact is, any woman who has had a foetal ultrasound scan is participating in one of the biggest laboratory experiments in medical history. Both in the US and the UK, the regulatory bodies approved the use of ultrasound without any long-term studies being done, leading the public to assume that the procedures are safe.

'No well controlled study has yet proved that routine scanning of prenatal patients will improve the outcome of pregnancy.' That was the official statement put forward by the American College of Obstetrics and Gynecology (ACOG) in 1984.[7] At a 1988 meeting in London jointly held by the Royal Society of Medicine and the ACOG, several top obstetricians, as well as the executive director of the ACOG, disclosed that of eight major studies attempting to evaluate the effectiveness of ultrasound, 'none has shown [that] routine use improves either maternal or infant outcome over that achieved when diagnostic ultrasound was used only when medically indicated.'[8]

As studies into the effects of ultrasound began to be done in the late eighties and nineties, they confirmed these early suspicions. Two researchers in Switzerland did an analysis of all the scientific (that is, randomized, controlled) studies of ultrasound scanning to evaluate its effect on the outcome of pregnancy. Their conclusion: ultrasound doesn't make one bit of difference to the ultimate health of the baby. This means it doesn't improve the live birth rate or help to produce fewer problem babies.[9] One reason it makes no difference in terms of live births is that the babies who are usually aborted after a scan shows up a severe malformation are usually those who would have died during pregnancy or shortly after birth, anyway.

The only good reason to use ultrasound, the researchers concluded, is to screen for gross congenital malformations – not to ensure your baby is 'all right', the usual vague rationale offered to most pregnant woman with no suspicious symptoms.

Another study of 15,000 American women also found 'no significant differences in the rate of adverse perinatal outcome (foetal or neonatal death or substantial neonatal morbidity)' between those scanned and those in the control group. The number of premature babies were identical in the two groups, as were the outcomes of multiple births, late-term pregnancies and small-for-dates babies.[10] As Dr Richard Berkowitz of New York's Mount Sinai Medical Center concluded: 'None of the studies published to date demonstrates an effect on the outcome of pregnancy in most low-risk women.'[11]

In fact, some studies show that, with ultrasound, you are more likely to lose your baby. A study from Queen Charlotte's and Chelsea Hospital in London found that women having doppler ultrasound were more likely to lose their babies than those who received only standard neonatal care (17 deaths to 7).[12] It can increase the risk of miscarriage,[13] even among women exposed to occupational sonography for more than 10 hours a week.[14]

It has been shown to trigger premature birth, doubling the rate in at-risk women given weekly scans.[15] The evidence is fairly conclusive that ultrasound doesn't do any good in normal pregnancies. But does subjecting an embryo to ultrasound at a delicate stage of development do any lasting harm? New studies have emerged showing that ultrasound scanning may indeed cause subtle brain damage. According to a Norwegian study of 2,000 babies, performed by the National Centre for Foetal Medicine in Trondheim, those subjected to routine ultrasound scanning were 30 per cent more likely to be left-handed than those who weren't scanned.[16] This predilection for left-handedness appears to show up only in boys. In a later analysis of 177,000 Swedish men, those whose mothers had scans were 32 per cent more likely to be left-handed.[17] In Britain, the rate of left-handedness has more than doubled – from 5 per cent in the

1920s to 11 per cent today. Neurologists believe that slight brain damage can cause right-handed people to become left-handed.

Evidence from Australia demonstrates that frequent scans also appear to restrict growth.[18] Exposure to ultrasound also causes delayed speech, according to Canadian research. Professor James Campbell, an ear, nose and throat surgeon in Alberta, Canada, compared a group of 72 children who had speech problems with a similar group with no such difficulties. He found that most of those with delayed speech had been exposed to ultrasound in the womb, whereas most of those with normal speech had not. 'The possibility of subtle microscopic changes in developing neural tissue exposed to ultrasound waves has to be considered,' he concluded.[19]

These findings are particularly alarming given that the women in the study had only one scan apiece. Most pregnancies in Britain and North America involve at least two scans, and others many more, whether or not there is even a whiff of a problem.

Animals have exhibited delayed neuromuscular development, altered emotional behaviour and lowered birthweight with exposure at the equivalent of current diagnostic levels.[20] Rodents exposed to high-intensity ultrasound have also had low birthweights and nerve damage.[21]

Children who'd been exposed to ultrasound in the womb had a higher incidence of dyslexia, according to one study.[22] Mothers whose babies were scanned show a 90 per cent increase in foetal activity,[23] the effect of which on their future development is anyone's guess. Ultrasound also exposes the foetus to a loud noise of 100 decibels, similar to the highest notes on a piano – as loud as an underground train arriving at a station.[24]

Work performed in the laboratory may provide some clues as to how scanning could cause damage. We know that sonography produces biological effects in two ways: heat and cavitation (the production of bubbles which expand and contract with the sound waves). We also know that ultrasound causes shock waves in liquid, but we don't know if it does so in human tissue – or for that matter, amniotic fluid. Finally, we don't know whether the effects are cumulative – that is, if they increase with multiple exposure or duration. This is an important issue now that doctors routinely order multiple scans. It also may have a bearing on electronic foetal monitoring, which employs ultrasound (although at one-thousandth of a scan's peak intensity) to monitor the baby's heartbeat during labour and delivery, often by being aimed at one spot for 24 hours.

An analysis of *in vitro* studies shows that ultrasound has produced cell damage and changes in DNA. The most widely quoted studies are those of radiologist Doreen Liebeskind at New York's Albert Einstein College of Medicine. After exposing cells in suspension to low-intensity pulsed ultrasound for 30 seconds, she observed changes in cell appearances and motility, DNA, abnormal cell growth and chromosomes, some of which were passed on to succeeding cell generations. In a documentary made of Dr Liebeskind's results, the film showed normal cells with rounded edges more or less moving in tandem. After exposure to ultrasound, the cells became 'frenetic and distorted', and entangled with one another, wrote Doris Haire, president of the American Foundation of Maternal and Child Health, one of America's best-briefed and most vociferous critics of routine ultrasound use.[25] Robert Bases, chief of Radiology at Albert Einstein College, reviewing what he termed the 'bewildering array of ultrasound bioeffects described in over 700 publications since 1950', said Dr Liebeskind's results had been confirmed by four independent laboratories.[26]

Dr Liebeskind herself theorizes that these cell changes may affect the developing brain. 'There may be some subtle or delayed effect on neuron interconnection or some type of effect that is not readily apparent until later,' she says.[27] Dr Liebeskind and others believe the *in vitro* studies can help to pinpoint the subtle effects on humans that epidemiologists should be looking for. 'I'd look for possible behavioural changes – in reflexes, IQ, attention span,' she wrote.[28]

The International Childbirth Education Association (ICEA) has maintained that ultrasound is most likely to affect development (behavioural and neurological), blood cells, the immune system and a child's genetic make-up – a view that has been borne out by the recent evidence about weight and development in exposed children.[29] Ultrasound has also been shown to affect many parts of the mother's body. A British study demonstrated that ovarian ultrasound can trigger premature ovulation in the mother.[30] There also have been published reports showing ultrasound's potential to damage maternal erythrocytes (mature red blood cells) and raise chorionic gonadotropin levels (the hormone which helps to maintain the pregnancy).[31] Again, we're not really sure what this means, and whether a woman is more likely to miscarry after ultrasound exposure.

Despite the assurances of the UK's Royal College of Obstetricians and Gynaecologists, every major American government agency has insisted that ultrasound not be used routinely on pregnant women. The FDA, the American Medical Association, the US National Institute of Child Health and Human Development, a top epidemiologist for the Centers for Disease Control and Prevention, the ACOG and the Bureau of Radiological Health have all cautioned doctors to use ultrasound only when indicated (say, to investigate unexplained vaginal bleeding) – a caution that has got thrown to the winds. They also specify that there is still no research proving this diagnostic test is safe. The Bureau of Radiological Health, for instance, has stated: 'Although the body of current evidence does not indicate that diagnostic ultrasound represents an acute risk to human health, it is insufficient to justify an unqualified acceptance of safety.'[32]

Besides the safety issue, there are considerable questions about accuracy. There is a significant chance that your scan will indicate a problem when there isn't one, or fail to pick up a problem actually there. One study found a 'high rate' of false-positives; 17 per cent of the pregnant women scanned were shown to have small-for-dates babies, when only 6 per cent actually did – an error rate of nearly one out of three.[33] Another study from Harvard showed that among 3,100 scans, 18 babies were erroneously labelled abnormal, and 17 foetuses with problems were missed.[34]

Yet a third Swiss study pooling the results of all ultrasound studies concluded that 2.4 per 1,000 women will be given a false diagnosis of a malformed foetus. This high error rate has chilling repercussions for families who decide to opt for late-term abortions after a scan shows that their child has spina bifida.[35] In fact, the Swiss researchers concluded that the negligible benefits of ultrasound scanning (which don't improve the outcome of pregnancy) aren't worth exposing pregnant women to the 'risk of false diagnosis' of malformations.

In one of the largest studies on ultrasound to date (33,000 babies), ultrasound picked up only about half of the 725 babies with birth defects. Some 175 foetuses were given a false-positive result – labelled abnormal when they were healthy.[36] A Swedish study found that ultrasound picked up only a third of babies born with serious defects[37] and, in another study, only a third of growth-retarded babies were correctly diagnosed before birth. Some 2 per cent were wrongly identified as such, even though their mothers had had nearly five scans apiece.[38]

False-positives have increased 12-fold as ultrasound is increasingly used in an attempt to pick up subtle defects or conditions in late pregnancy.[39] This technology even wildly overdiagnoses *placenta praevia* (potentially fatal low-lying placenta in late pregnancy), one of its main indications; in one study, 250 women were identified as having the condition when it was only actually present in four.[40]

At one point, the British press was filled with stories of women who may have aborted healthy babies due to inaccurate scans. In one, Jacqui James of Brierley Hill in the West Midlands, a 24-year-old mother of two, was told scans done at Birmingham Maternity Hospital during her 27th week of pregnancy showed that her third baby was not growing properly and likely to have brain damage. After a family discussion, she decided she had no choice but to have an abortion. Because she was more than six months pregnant, the 'abortion' was done by caesarean section. However, the baby girl, which survived the operation for 45 minutes, was later found to be perfectly healthy.[41]

THE NEW DOWN'S TEST

Ultrasound scans are now used to predict Down's syndrome. A nuchal scan measures the depth of the dark fluid-filled space at the back of the baby's neck at 10–13 weeks of pregnancy. If the space is thicker than usual, your baby may be at risk of Down's.

However, the nuchal scan throws up false-positives, signalling Down's when it isn't. For instance, in a study of more than 96,000 pregnancies, the scan was only 80 per cent accurate, even among women at high risk of a Down's baby. According to one large-scale study, 87,000 women would have to be scanned to find one accurate diagnosis.[42] But of course the biggest risk of all in false-positives is that they open up the door to more invasive tests such as amniocentesis, which carry their own substantial risks. Ultimately, more healthy babies could be lost through amniocentesis than Down's babies be detected.

Considering its extremely poor track record of accuracy, ultrasound may not even be useful very late in pregnancy to help confirm the position of the baby. The only rationale for scanning most uneventful pregnancies is to satisfy our curiosity, to try to get a little closer to the mystery of life.

FOETAL MONITORING DURING LABOUR

When labour commences and you go to hospital to have your baby, chances are that doctors will want to strap you into an electronic foetal monitor to routinely monitor the foetal heart rate. However reassuring, this exercise appears to make no difference to the health of either you or your baby, according to British research. Interpretation of the read-outs varies widely among practitioners. What foetal monitoring does do, however, is increase the likelihood of obstetrical intervention. Women given EFM have more than a 5 per cent higher likelihood of a forceps-type delivery and a greater chance of having a caesarean than those who employ a Doppler (handheld) ultrasound device, according to British research.[43]

The *New England Journal of Medicine* reluctantly concluded, after examining seven major studies, that this form of ultrasound provides no benefits to newborns, even premature ones. In reviewing the data, the Journal accepted that the study was the final proof that foetal monitoring is ineffective in decreasing the chances of a stillbirth, a low Apgar score or neurological problems in high-risk infants. It only increases the chances of a woman having a caesarean section.[44] This conclusion was reached following a study, carried out in several medical centres in the state of Washington, which tested the widely-held view that high-risk babies who were electronically monitored died less frequently and had better outcomes than low-risk babies monitored by simple auscultation (trumpet stethoscopes) or other sonic aids. The study, which looked at premature infants in several hospitals, found that those babies monitored had no better chance of being born live than those monitored by ordinary Doppler auscultation. The final death-knell was sounded when a major California study found that the test's false-positive level – reporting a problem where there is none – is an alarming 99.8 per cent, resulting in thousands of unnecessary caesareans.[45]

Even the former head of the Oxford Perinatal Unit, Iain Chalmers, has gone on record to say that the major, properly conducted studies show that the mortality rate among technologically monitored babies was higher than that among controls.[46]

'A review of this evidence was first published eight years ago,' wrote Chalmers,[47] 'and the lack of evidence to support the use of this widely adopted form of obstetric technology has been reiterated at intervals since then.[48] For obvious reasons, it is the kind of evidence that some obstetricians would rather overlook.'

Unless you are suspected of having twins, you might be wise to avoid knee-jerk ultrasound testing, particularly before your 20th week of pregnancy when the baby is still forming.

AFP TESTS

Most of the rest of the new prenatal tests are designed to detect Down's syndrome, and new ones are devised as fast as some of the older ones seem to get discredited – this despite the fact that none of these screening tests seems to be making much difference. Despite 30,000 amniocenteses and 3,000 chorionic villus tests performed each year in the UK, less than 20 per cent of Down's syndrome babies are detected. This may have something to do with the fact that 70 per cent are born to younger mothers who don't have the tests – a fact that tends to pour cold water on the idea that Down's syndrome is solely a result of the 'tired eggs' of relatively elderly mothers.

In fact, despite medicine's attempts to protect mothers from having Down's babies, the incidence of the condition is going up. This could either be because the tests – usually amniocentesis or alpha-fetoprotein – are not detecting the condition, or because parents are choosing not to abort the babies diagnosed as suffering from the condition.

The most substantial risks you face of deformed or retarded children may result from the diagnostic tests themselves.

AFP Test

Before you go in for amnio or CVS, you're likely to have, as I did, an AFP test or a 'triple test', developed by the University of Leeds to replace advancing maternal age as the only risk factor for giving birth to a Down's syndrome baby.

AFP stands for alpha-fetoprotein (AFP), a protein produced by the foetal liver. If the baby has a spinal abnormality such as spina bifida or anencephaly, where the full brain is not developed, larger amounts of AFP than normal will be present in the amniotic fluid and the mother's blood. Low levels of AFP are considered a possible indicator of a baby with Down's syndrome. The test is given between a woman's 16th and 20th week of pregnancy.

There is no doubt that the batting average on the alpha-fetoprotein tests is appalling. After my own experience, I heard of at least three friends or acquaintances with false-positive AFP readings. Doctors accept there is a 3–4 per cent error rate of abnormally high readings on first screening, according to writer Helen Klein Ross. 'This means that of every 2,000 women tested,' she says, '100 will have an abnormal reading, but *only 1 or 2* will be carrying a foetus with this congenital defect.'[49]

Even this estimate of inaccuracy could be conservative. One study done in 1982 estimated a failure rate of 20 per cent.[50] As with many biological processes, AFP readings can change from day to day or be falsely elevated, depending on many factors: multiple pregnancies, viral hepatitis, smoking, a threatened miscarriage or even carrying a boy all can produce a false-positive, and being overweight, having insulin-dependent diabetes or just being wrong about your date of conception can produce an artificially low score[51] (some 25 per cent of all inaccurately high AFP results are due to inaccuracies about dates or a multiple pregnancy[52]). Certain races, notably Asian and black women, also seem to produce abnormally high AFP scores.[53] According to the late Dr Robert Mendelsohn, one of the first to call attention to the problems of this test in his American newsletter *The People's Doctor*, the test has false-negatives too, as evidenced in an article in *The Lancet* concerning two babies born with spinal defects whose mothers nevertheless had normal AFP readings.[54]

According to Helen Ross, the AFP test 'misses about 40 per cent of spina bifida cases, 10 per cent of anencephaly cases, and 80 per cent of foetuses with Down's syndrome. All of which makes a negative result by no means reassuring.'[55]

Twins or a miscalculation about the date of conception are two common ways that test results are thrown off. In my case, we were sure about the dates, but my daughter Caitlin turned out to be a full 10-month pregnancy, born 28 days past her estimated due date (first babies who are not induced are very often late, and my obstetrician doesn't induce labour if there is no evidence that anything is awry). As a slow grower, she probably deviated sufficiently from the norm to show up as 'abnormal'.

In other words, mostly what this test produces is a good deal of needless anxiety, which can only be dispelled by subjecting your baby to amniocentesis or ultrasound, two procedures with their own potential risks. Indeed, for anyone younger than about 39, the risk of losing a healthy baby through amniocentesis (about 1 in 100) may be greater than the risk of having a baby with Down's syndrome – if indeed age has anything to do with it.

The Triple Test

As the AFP test proved to be so inaccurate, doctors reasoned that the more markers they looked for, the more accurate the test might prove to be. The so-called 'triple test' analyses the levels of three substances in the mother's blood: unconjugated oestriol, total human chorionic gonadotrophin and AFP; low levels of oestriol, high levels of HCG and low levels of AFP are considered the first indication of the possibility that the mother is carrying a baby with Down's syndrome. These measured levels, plus the mother's age and genetic history, are thrown into some mathematical stew in order to determine her personal odds of having a Down's baby. The test is supposed to be a better marker than age alone for determining whether a woman should go on to have amniocentesis, which more accurately determines whether a child has Down's syndrome. At best, the triple test detects 70 per cent of Down's babies in women over 35, and only 50 per cent in women younger than this.[56]

All those who receive a positive triple test result must wait five or six anguished weeks before receiving the results of the recommended amnio-centesis to confirm or deny the suspicious results of the first test. If you are one of the unlucky ones who receives a false-positive, and a large percent-age now do,[57] you will needlessly undergo amniocentesis, which increases the risk of miscarriage from 3 to 4 per cent. In other words, one out of every 100 women with a false-positive triple test opting for amniocentesis may abort a normal baby.

CHORIONIC VILLUS SAMPLING

Chorionic villus sampling (CVS) was supposed to be the answer to every older mother-to-be's prayers. Although amniocentesis is well established as a test to detect Down's syndrome, you have to wait to have the test until your sixteenth week of pregnancy, then wait two or three weeks more before results are available. If the test shows an abnormality, and you do not wish to continue, you must undergo a second-trimester abortion, which entails, in effect, giving birth to a dead 20-week-old foetus, with all the physical and psychological ramifications that entails.

Then in the early seventies some medics from Sweden and the Far East figured out that you could take a tiny sample of the tissue of the 'villi', the hair-like projections of the chorion (the sac containing the embryo in the uterus, which becomes the placenta) between the 9th and 12th week of pregnancy and it would tell you the genetic typing of the foetus.

This could help to screen for Down's syndrome, as well as sickle cell anaemia, muscular dystrophy, and sex-linked abnormalities. The villus sample is taken with a needle inserted transabdominally (through the walls of the abdomen) or transcervically (through the vagina).

Lately, a number of concerns about chorionic villus sampling have finally been confirmed by several large-scale studies. The latest, conducted by the Medical Research Council, of over 3,000 women from seven different European countries, examined the results of pregnancies of women who'd had CVS against those who'd had amniocentesis.[58]

Compared with women undergoing amniocentesis, those who elect CVS were more likely to lose their babies. Only 86 per cent of the women in the CVS group had successful pregnancies, compared to 91 per cent in the amniocentesis group. This was due to a greater number of foetal deaths before 28 weeks, a higher number of terminations of supposed abnormalities, and a higher number of neonatal deaths, largely due to a higher number of premature babies born before 32 weeks.

CVS can cause massive loss of blood from the womb, which may lead to the death of the foetus. This discovery from the Erasmus University in Bilthoven, the Netherlands, counters an earlier view that the foetus could survive such a loss of blood.[59]

'The results of this trial suggest that the policy of chorionic villus sampling in the first trimester reduces the chances of a successful pregnancy outcome by 4.6 per cent,' concluded the MRC report.[60]

The study couldn't tell for sure how many of the CVS tests were false-positives because not all aborted or miscarried foetuses were tested. However, the researchers did find three false-positives, one in the CVS sample and two in the amniocentesis group, and one false-negative with CVS. Two other cases in the CVS group were thought to be false-positives.

False-positives and -negatives are potentially common because the genetic material found in the chorionic villus may not be identical to that of the foetus. In the MRC study and elsewhere, samples of the chorionic villus were found to contain abnormal chromosomes, but the babies resulting were nevertheless normal. Two doctors from Copenhagen reported such an instance; the woman went ahead and terminated what turned out to be a normal baby.[61]

In another case in Brest, France, CVS carried out on a foetus showed the chromosome linked to cystic fibrosis was present. Despite the test results, the parents decided to proceed with the pregnancy and the mother gave birth to a healthy baby girl. The doctor who reported the case estimates the chances of such a false-positive are one in six.[62]

What this means, of course, is that the chorionic membrane itself could have a defect not shared by the foetus, possibly resulting from a twin that has died and been reabsorbed. Or, it could mean that abnormal placental tissue in these early stages doesn't mean anything in the long term (the placenta of the Copenhagen case showed normal cultures on biopsy after the abortion). In other words, the entire theory upon which CVS rests – that chorionic villus will tell you about the state of the foetus – could be wrong.

Reports have now flooded in of limb abnormalities among babies whose mothers had CVS. At the Churchill Hospital in Oxford, five cases of limb-reduction defects (where arms or legs are abnormally short) occurred among nearly 300 pregnancies which had been investigated by CVS at 55 to 66 days of pregnancy.[63]

Italian researchers from Catholic University in Rome found that four of the 118 cases of 'transverse' limb reductions born between 1988 and 1990 in Italy occurred among babies born to mothers who'd had CVS.[64]

From their own data, they reckoned the risk of these deformities occurring for mothers given CVS at any point in the pregnancy was 1 in 200. This compares with an ordinary risk of 1 in 3,100 among the population at large. The risk of deformities from CVS would be even greater if other malformations besides limb reductions were considered. In one study of mothers given CVS, all 75 had produced a baby with some birth defect, from lost limbs to damaged nails.[65]

Far from being less invasive, the earlier the CVS was given, the more severe the abnormality. The greatest deformities occur among foetuses given CVS 56 days after conception.[66]

It's believed that vascular disruption or puncture of the amniotic sac might have something to do with producing the deformities. Whatever the damage results from, it's clear that the tiny villi aren't quite as dispensable as medicine once believed.

The US Centers for Disease Control and Prevention now recommends that doctors warn parents of the risk of CVS causing limb defects to their babies at least up to 76 days' (nearly 11 weeks') gestation. The CDC also warns that testing can be dangerous in foetuses older than nine weeks – assumed in the past to be the safest period.

Because of the questionable accuracy of CVS, you might have to have amniocentesis to confirm its results, thus subjecting your baby to two major insults and multiplying your risk of miscarriage. The risk of losing a baby through CVS has now been put at nearly 5 per cent. When you add amniocentesis on top of that, you start moving up to a very substantial miscarriage risk of 1 in 16.

AMNIOCENTESIS

Amniocentesis is by far the preferred test for Down's syndrome and other genetic abnormalities, and more than 30,000 amniocentesis procedures are carried out in the UK each year The procedure involves having a needle (guided by ultrasound) inserted into your abdomen and uterus and drawing out amniotic fluid. These cells are then cultured for two or three weeks and the chromosomes of the cells examined, which explains the three-week delay between the test and its results.

The risks of miscarriage are assumed to be 1 to 1.5 per 100 pregnancies, largely from damage caused by the needle or the possibility of introducing infections to the womb. In 1978, the Medical Research Council also reported a 3 per cent increase in neonatal respiratory distress and a 2.4 increase in congenital dislocations of the hip and club feet.

Because of these problems with a pregnancy that is well along, doctors reasoned that it might be safer to get in there early, while the baby is still tiny. However, far from being safer, early amniocentesis has proved to be far more dangerous. Those given the earlier procedure have nearly a 2 per cent greater incidence of miscarriage and more than a 1 per cent increase in club foot.[67]

Whether the test is given early or late, the high miscarriage rate in women given amniocentesis is worth keeping in mind if you are a woman who has delayed childbearing until you are over 35 and now are carrying a much-wanted baby.

Because of the spectre of a late-term abortion should the test prove positive, many women are opting for early amniocentesis. However, the latest information is that early amniocentesis greatly increases your risk of miscarriage. It is also slightly more likely to cause cases of club foot than does CVS, according to research at the King's College Medical School in London.[68]

In Holland, scientists considered the test so dangerous that they abandoned their study of it, considering it unethical to continue their trials into the procedure. Before this, Dutch researchers had found that eight women had miscarried after having an early amniocentesis – a number similar to the losses noted in another trial of 120 women given the test. Dr F. Vandenbussche and his colleagues from the Leiden University Hospital have warned other doctors that: 'There certainly seems no justification for the continuing unqualified advocacy of early amniocentesis on the basis of beliefs and uncontrolled observations.'[69] Another study showed that children whose mothers undergo amniocentesis reported 'significantly higher' levels of haemolytic diseases (related to red blood cell levels) than children who didn't have the test.[70]

There are also plenty of false-positives, even with this supposedly highly accurate test (there were more false results with amniocentesis than CVS in the MRC study). Anyone doubting that it can't happen to them should read the letter sent to the Spectator congratulating Dominic Lawson, after his bold refusal to have amniocentesis and even bolder defence of the joys of having the resulting Down's baby. 'You have a human being in your hands,' wrote the letter-writer, 'and that is what really matters.' He goes on:

> *This time last year my wife was pregnant, at the age of 42. The hospital called us to explain the possibility of a Down's syndrome baby at her age. Foolishly and arrogantly, we agreed to have the test. We were told that the risk of a resulting miscarriage was 1 in 200, which I considered remote.*
>
> *The long and short of it all is that we lost a healthy baby, and on 20 September 1994 at 10.45 I had the task of carrying the tiny coffin for burial. It is a day I will never forget, and I will forever blame myself for the decision to have the test.*
>
> *Please be pleased with yourself and have no regrets. Today we wish we had a Down's syndrome baby to care for and love. However, we are grateful that we have two surviving children. There must be many others who made the mistake of having the test, lost the baby and have nothing now but regrets.*[71]

Radiation and Down's Syndrome

Amid all the effort to prevent Down's syndrome, no one is asking whether we are looking in the right place. Robert Mendelsohn, who belittled the entire notion of 'tired eggs' based on age, was one of the first to warn mothers that their chances of Down's syndrome increased with the amount of accumulated exposure to x-rays, not their age per se. 'Despite overwhelming evidence that this is the case, doctors continue to tell all older women that they shouldn't have babies because their eggs may be weary, rather than determining how much radiation exposure they have had.'[72]

Mendelsohn's farsighted view about the connection between Down's syndrome and radiation has been validated. Researchers from the Freie University in Berlin discovered a direct link between Down's syndrome – which suddenly increased sixfold in the city in January 1987 – and the Chernobyl nuclear reactor accident which happened nine months earlier.[73]

These women were breathing in high levels of radiation – especially iodine-131 – for two weeks after the accident, during which time they conceived.

The researchers were able to discount the usual theory that Down's syndrome is related to the age of the mother. The average age of the mothers with Down's babies during the year of the nuclear accident was virtually identical to the average age of mothers with Down's babies the decade before, and the percentage of women over 35 with Down's babies after Chernobyl was identical to the percentage over the decade before. After making the discovery, the German researchers uncovered other studies which supported their conclusions. Incidents of Down's syndrome increased dramatically in Kerala, India and Yangjiang County, China, after women were exposed to similarly high levels of background radiation from the soil.

The study group, led by Professor Karl Sperling, accepts that its evidence 'contradicts current textbook opinion'. The age of the mother per se doesn't seem a reliable indicator of Down's syndrome, other than the fact that an older mother may have a high build-up of radiation in her system, from x-rays. They concluded that any exposure to ionizing radiation, especially around the time of conception, should be avoided.

A similar connection was made by scientists exploring the rate of Down's births and tests at nuclear plants. They examined a community in Fylde in Lancashire, and discovered that the incidence of Down's births peaked in 1958 and 1962 to 1964, when there were higher levels of nuclear fallout. The pattern was also followed in 1957, when there was a fire at the nearby Windscale – now Sellafield – nuclear power station.

Women over the age of 35 seemed most affected, again perhaps because they had already accumulated some radiation during their lifetimes and the nuclear reaction radiation sent these levels over the top.[74]

The German findings add evidence to the argument that Down's syndrome is the result of environmental factors and not simply age. In fact, a major study in 1990 discovered that Down's syndrome babies had higher levels of aluminium in their brains than did normal babies.[75]

The discovery that different racial groups have a markedly different rate of Down's syndrome offers more evidence of an environmental cause. A recent study, which tracked births in 17 states across the US between 1983 and 1990, discovered that American blacks have fewer Down's babies than any other racial group (with 7.3 per 10,000) and Hispanics fare the worse (with 11.8 per 10,000). The Down's syndrome rate also varied markedly between states, with 5.9 per 10,000 recorded in Kansas and 12.3 per 10,000 in Colorado.[76]

In a book looking at the results of over 30 years' research into Down's children, the condition appears not as daunting as medicine would have us believe. Psychologist Janet Carr has monitored a group of 54 Down's children since 1964 and found that they do not suffer from ill-health any more than a similar group of normal children. There was no significant excess of marital stress or breakdown in parents of Down's children, and no adverse effects on siblings. In fact, virtually all the families simply loved their Down's members, and wouldn't have dreamt of ending their lives.[77]

GETTING FIT BEFORE CONCEIVING

For any woman worried about producing a normal baby, it may make most sense to get yourself healthy *before* conceiving, rather than relying on a batch of tests with questionable records of safety and effectiveness. There is plenty of evidence showing a relationship between deformities at birth and low zinc, magnesium and selenium levels in the mother.[78] Foresight, the Association for Preconceptual Care, advocates that parents follow wholefood low-allergy diets, cut down on drinking and sort out vitamin/mineral deficiencies and excess levels of toxic metal accumulation in the body before attempting to conceive. In a recent study, 89 per cent of a group of 418 couples went on to give birth to healthy babies after following the Foresight diet and supplement programme. In the study groups, no baby was born before 36 weeks and none was lighter than 2.4kg (5lb 5oz). There were also no miscarriages, perinatal deaths, malformations or babies requiring admission to special care. Of the 418 couples, 75 per cent had either previous infertility problems, miscarriages or stillbirths; many were over 40.

Once you are pregnant, consider seeing an older or holistic gynaecologist or midwife, trained before the days of ultrasound. Most important information (such as multiple births or the baby's position) can be ascertained by a skilled pair of hands. A fetoscope or stethoscope is the safest way to listen to the baby's heartbeat. And remember, you can take all the videos you want of your babies – *after* they are born. Perhaps, too, there is some comfort to be found in the fact that, in 40 per cent of Down's cases, nature takes its course and the foetus does not survive to full term.

If you do have a Down's baby, investigate the nutritional programme that is helping many Down's children lead normal lives and attend mainstream schools.[79]

4

Catching It Early

SCREENING FOR CANCER

Doctors tend to visualize many diseases as a little army that starts small, enlisting, at most, a soldier or two. If they can locate and flush out the enemy when it's only two or three strong, they figure they can get in there early with their nuclear warfare and win the war, even before it gets going. The best way to root out these errant cells, they've convinced us, is with a screening test.

Because cancers can grow before you get ill or exhibit symptoms, they have been the main target of catch-it-early warfare. For all of us who dread the frightening randomness of 'silent' killers such as cancer, which are reaching epidemic proportions, this is a highly comforting notion. Doctors have managed to convince us that we can escape death just by having a simple annual screening test.

So persuasive is the catch-it-early argument that medicine has also managed to convince governments to spend millions of pounds putting into effect mass screening programmes. At the moment, women are the primary targets of these annual tests, mainly for cervical and breast cancer, although there has been talk of ovarian cancer screening, and prostate and bowel cancer screening programmes for men. Cervical screening and mammography have been in place for years in the US, and more recently Britain followed on with wholesale breast and cervical cancer campaigns, screening three-quarters of eligible groups.[1]

Despite all the money being poured into massive screening campaigns, no screening programmes anywhere are making the slightest impact on cancer mortality. In fact, because of their inordinately high potential for false-positive readings, screening may only be increasing the number of patients mutilated through unnecessary drug treatment or surgery.

Even *The Lancet* once admitted in a no-holds-barred editorial that despite 'all the media hype, the triumphalism of the profession in published research, and the almost weekly miracle breakthroughs trumpeted by the cancer charities' the number of women dying from breast cancer refuses to go down. 'Let us stop complaining that screening ought to work if only we tried harder and ask why this approach is so disappointing.'[2] One recent estimate is that mammography is 10 times more likely to pick up a benign cancer – leading to unnecessary treatment and surgery – as it is to prevent one single cancer death.[3]

SMEAR TESTS

The most widespread screening test of all is the Pap smear, so called after a fellow named Dr George Papanicolaou who first developed it. In 1941, Papanicolaou and a colleague published a study demonstrating that malignant changes in the cervix could be diagnosed by examining cells taken from the vagina.[4]

This simple, relatively painless test involves scraping a small sample of tissue from the neck of the womb, smearing it onto a slide (hence the name), applying a fixative and sending the slide to a lab for analysis to see if any unusual cells are present. If the result shows any sort of abnormality, you are referred for further diagnostic tests, which usually include a direct examination of the cervix (a colposcopy) or a biopsy and even treatment for cancer.

It was first adopted in various Western countries after publication of results from the pilot screening programme in British Columbia showed that it was having an impact on lowering mortality rates. After seeing the British Columbia results, doctors began enthusing that the Pap smear would sound the death knell for cervical cancer.[5]

Under Britain's current screening programme, some three million smears are performed every year at an estimated cost, if doctors, nurses and lab time are figured into the total, of at least £10 to £30 per woman screened.[6] In the US, with one out of every eight women developing breast cancer, women's groups are demanding action on all women's cancers, including cervical cancer.

In response, the Centers for Disease Control and Prevention released the National Strategic Plan for the Early Detection and Control of Breast and Cervical Cancers (NSP), a collaborative programme between the Food and Drug Association, the National Cancer Institute, and the CDC. This promises to hot up the screening programme, increasing the number of women and the frequency with which they are screened for these diseases.

Although there hasn't been an overall national government policy in the UK until relatively recently, most doctors in the UK regard cervical cancer screening as part of standard good practice, recommending that all women between the ages of 20 and 65 repeat the test every three to five years. *The Lancet* even recently recommended that the screening be extended to women over 65, now considered a high-risk group.[7]

Under National Health Service regulations, there is now more intense pressure on women to take the test with greater frequency as the fee per test becomes part of a doctor's bread-and-butter work. Doctors in Britain get bonus pay only if more than 50 per cent of the women on their lists receive the tests, and triple the bonus pay if 80 per cent take it. But who would quarrel with the benefits of a simple, painless, risk-free test that promises to eradicate a common killer of women?

Nobody, if it actually worked. *The problem is there is no convincing evidence anywhere to suggest that it does.* Professor James McCormick of the Department of Public Health at Dublin's Trinity College, an expert on mass screening tests, who studied much of the available medical literature on the subject, once declared: 'There is no clear evidence that this screening is beneficial, and it may well be doing more harm than good.'[8] By harm he means that many thousands of women are being subjected to risky treatments that could affect fertility for a condition they do not have or which could revert to normal.

First of all, it's hard not to think, once you examine the figures, that medicine has backed the wrong horse. Cervical cancer is not the massive killer it's often made out to be. Although some 2,000 women die from cervical cancer every year in the UK, that represents less than one-sixth of the number of women who contract breast cancer. In *The Health Scandal*, author Dr Vernon Coleman says that cervical cancer doesn't even make the top 10 causes of death among women, falling behind breast, lung, colon, stomach, ovarian, even pancreatic cancers.[9] And only 1.6 of every 1,000 women with abnormal smears go on to develop cancer.[10]

The smear test has also never been proven to save lives in any country where it has been introduced. In fact, every study shows that it is making virtually no impact. The only area in Canada where screening has been universally adopted is British Columbia; nevertheless, the death rate of cervical cancer there matches the death rate for the rest of the country.[11] Mortality rates from cervical cancer may have fallen in British Columbia, but they also fell in other parts of Canada without organized screening programmes.[12]

In the UK, the death rate from cervical cancer fell *before* the test was introduced and has stubbornly remained at the 2,000 figure (although several years ago, the government announced that the annual figure has dipped to 1,700). There is also no evidence to support the common contention that things would be worse but for the test. Dr McCormick and his colleague, the late Petr Skrabanek, say that the blind enthusiasm for cervical screening 'has produced a climate in which it has been impossible to mount controlled trials'.[13] Twenty years ago, Dr Herbert Green, a New Zealand doctor who had the temerity to dispute many dearly held assumptions about cervical cancer, was even found guilty of disgraceful misconduct for conducting a trial to see whether cancer is inevitable after an abnormal screening test.[14]

In the UK and the US, mass screening programmes like the National Cervical Screening programme have been launched without a consistent nationwide policy about when or whom to screen or how to follow up abnormalities.

Several years ago, an official study confirmed that cervical screening isn't doing any good, since death rates from cervical cancer haven't varied in two decades, despite virtually universal screening. These findings are based on monitoring nearly a quarter of a million women in Bristol over 20 years. In 1992, the death rate was similar to that of 1975, when continuous screening was introduced.[15]

If screening has managed to put a slight dent in the death rate nationally (and there is no hard evidence that screening is behind the rate's dipping from 2,000 to 1,700), it comes at an unacceptable cost, says Dr McCormick. Many thousands of women are given false-positives and unnecessarily treated and possibly even left infertile or with terrible side-effects. During every area-wide screening in the Bristol area, 15,000 women were told they were at risk of cancer, and more than 5,500 investigated and treated for mild abnormalities which never would have progressed to cancer.

Between 1988 and 1993, nearly 226,000 women were screened, and abnormalities were supposedly found in more than 15,000 – or about one out of every 15 women. This figure is absurdly high compared with the actual rate of cervical cancer, which kills one woman in 10,000. The Bristol level of false-positives (where a 'discovery' of cancer turns out to be false) demonstrates to what extent cervical screening is simply causing unnecessary worry in healthy women.[16]

Over the years, the smear test's reputation has been stained by a number of catastrophic errors. At Kent and Canterbury Hospital, for instance, more than 90,000 smears taken between 1990 and 1995 had to be rechecked, after eight women died following mistakes in reporting results. The problem, according to Britain's National Institute for Clinical Excellence (NICE), is that the test is still appallingly inaccurate.

NICE estimates that up to 13 per cent of smear tests are false-positives and 20 per cent are false-negatives, where women with possible problems will have a test result come back as normal. In other words, out of 1,000 women screened, two women who could have cancer will be given the all clear. Other research has estimated a false negative rate of up to 60 per cent.[17]

In the US, the Centers for Disease Control and Prevention recently warned against annual Pap smear testing because of the high rate of false-positives, particularly for low-grade abnormalities, which result in potentially damaging treatment for symptoms which might have gone away if left alone.[18] Even if screening were better set up in the UK and the US, the problem lies with the very medical foundation on which the test is based. *Mounting evidence suggests that the smear campaign may be based on a faulty assumption: that abnormal, or 'precancerous', cells on the cervix lead to cancer.* This assumption has been inferred from two facts: 1) that cervical cancer progresses slowly and, 2) if caught early enough, can be cured.

There are four categories of abnormal lesions, or 'cervical interstitial neoplasia': CIN I, II, III, and cancer. What we don't know is whether the early lesions – those in the CIN I and II categories – will go on to develop cancer, or even what to do about them. In one study examining the accuracy of cytology (cell) screening, some 10 per cent of women screened had cervical abnormalities, 'most of which', notes Professor McCormick, 'would not progress to cancer'.[19]

Medicine also doesn't really understand the usual progression of this kind of cancer, a fact they have tacitly begun to admit. Some cervical cancers appear to regress if left alone, while others progress so rapidly that the three-to-five year gap recommended by most screening programmes would fail to pick them up in time. On this fragile foundation, women with an abnormal smear are frightened and stigmatized by the term 'precancerous' when no one knows whether it is appropriate or not.

This very situation happened to Anna. After her smear test came up positive, the 25-year-old spent months worrying that she had cancer. She also felt deeply embarrassed by the test results, as though it were a public comment on her sex life, since cervical cancer is known to occur among women who are highly promiscuous. In the end, she discovered that she had suffered all her distress for nothing. Follow-up tests some months later proved the first test was wrong.

One study in 1988 showed that nearly half of smears with mild abnormalities reverted to normal within two years. None of the patients developed invasive cancer during long-term follow-up.[20] Similar results occurred in a study in northeast Scotland, demonstrating that there is no steady progression from mild to moderate to severe abnormality of cells.[21]

A Canadian study showed that simple inflammation of the cervix may throw up an abnormal smear. Of 411 women examined by researchers at the Memorial University of Newfoundland, in St John's, Newfoundland, the smear tests of nearly a third were shown to have inflammatory changes, nearly half of whom were shown to have some sort of infection. Ironically, even here the test was unreliable: half of the remaining women with normal smear tests also had an infection.[22]

Besides this confusion over the significance of various results, the test is so inaccurate as to be virtually pointless. There is no guarantee that a Pap smear will pick up the fact that you have cancer, and a fair likelihood that you will be told you have an abnormality that doesn't actually exist. In one study, the authors admit to false-negative rates of between 7 and 60 per cent.[23]

In another report, one in every five cervical cancer deaths was due to poor management or misdiagnosis by doctors. In one in every seven of these cases, the smear tests had been read as normal. Re-analysis of the slides showed that early abnormalities had in fact been present, but were missed.

Interpretation of the results varies wildly, depending on who is looking at the slides. You could even get a different interpretation from the same person looking at the same slide on separate occasions. This is particularly so, says Professor McCormick, with the minor changes that give rise to most reported abnormalities.[24]

A report from the National Audit Office, 'Cervical and Breast Screening in England', found a wide disparity in interpretations of findings and a lack of benchmarks against which to compare results. The audit found that in some areas of England, nearly a fifth of all smears were classified as abnormal, compared with 3 per cent in other areas.[25] This lack of any standards is responsible for many false diagnoses of cancer.

In Scotland, some 20,000 tests done under the screening programme at the Inverclyde Royal Hospital had to be re-examined after evidence that the doctor doing the analysis may have misread the results. On a preliminary re-examination, 40 out of 1,000 smears taken since 1988 were found to be 'inadequate' and to require a repeat test.[26]

The Scottish debacle is only the latest in a series of such incidents in the UK. In 1987, in Liverpool, 45,000 tests were re-examined and 911 found to have been wrongly diagnosed. In 1988, in Manchester, a batch of 3,000 tests passed as clear were re-analysed and 60 found to be suspect.

Large numbers of smears are also technically not up to scratch. Dr Chandra Grubb, head of the Department of Cytology at the Royal Free and University College Hospital in London, estimates that some 10 per cent of all smears sent to cytology departments are useless, and a further 40 per cent are of limited usefulness because doctors haven't taken the smear correctly or have taken it from the wrong site.[27] With this kind of terrible batting average, the likelihood is that screening not only isn't going to pick up your cancer, but could set you on the road to potentially risky treatments when you don't need them.

The conventional treatment for early 'precancerous' lesions employs a colposcopy (a magnifying glass with a light) and biopsy (exploratory surgery), diathermy (burning the abnormal cells) or cytotherapy (which employs a freezing probe to freeze the outlaw cells). These procedures can all cause haemorrhage or permanently damage the cervix, resulting in an 'incompetent' or narrowed cervix, and thus affect a woman's chances of carrying a baby to term.

Dr Robert Mendelsohn liked to tell the story of a colleague of his whose wife received a positive reading. She went ahead with a cone biopsy, which caused such excessive bleeding that she had to have an emergency hysterectomy, during which she almost died from the anaesthesia. All because of a test that might have been wrong in the first place.[28]

One of our readers, a young woman in her early twenties, had been diagnosed as having stage 2–3 abnormal cells, and was scheduled for an operation to have them frozen or burned out. At the eleventh hour, she decided to have a second smear test at another laboratory. Her new test showed that the first test was wrong; her problem turned out to be a simple infection.

Individual doctors also differ widely in their views of how to treat abnormalities. The British National Audit Office report showed that many doctors opt for radical treatment such as cervical conization for cases of mild abnormalities, which would eventually resolve themselves without intervention.[29]

Some reports demonstrate that getting in there early and aggressively treating cervical abnormalities doesn't do any good, anyway. In one recent study, referring women with mildly abnormal smear test results for the more invasive examination produced no more favourable outcome than adopting a policy of watchful waiting. Referring women for a colposcopy exam, often with a biopsy, or simply giving them a repeat smear test after several months produced identical results: 1.6 per 1,000 cases developed into cervical cancer. This means 2,500 women were sent for colposcopy – with its inherent risks of causing infertility – to save one case of cancer.[30]

Because of the high rate of false-positives, some countries like the US and Switzerland have now introduced a new technology called 'liquid-based cytology screening' (LBC), also known as 'monolayer cytology'. The specimen is collected by a special spatula, the head of which is rinsed into or broken off into a vial of preservative, so that the entire sample is immediately preserved in liquid.

The UK's own pilot studies showed that LBC produces more accurate results, with only 1.6 samples considered 'inadequate', or unable to be read, compared to more than 9 per cent of traditional Pap smear slides.

Nevertheless, there is some evidence that the LBC test is even less reliable and more likely to give false-positive and false-negative results than the conventional variety: 87 per cent, compared with 91 per cent for ordinary Pap smears.[31]

This questionable batting average has not deterred the UK government. In October 2003, it announced that LBC would be 'rolled out' over the next five years, with the intention of replacing the conventional Pap smear test, at a cost of some £10 million.

The National Co-ordinating Network now specifically recommends that women with minor cell abnormalities – 'borderline or mildly dyskarotic smears' – adopt a path of surveillance – that is, have the smear test repeated six months later. The women should only be referred for colposcopy if the smear continues to show abnormality. At very least, according to the US CDC, waiting an interval of three years (or five years, if you are over 50) won't affect mortality rates. If you do get a positive reading, insist on a repeat smear from another lab before going down the more invasive route of biopsies and worse.

MAMMOGRAMS

Mammography – an x-ray of the breast designed to pick up early malignancies – is the other screening test being stepped up sharply. Breast cancer, the biggest lady-killer after lung cancer, claims the lives of an estimated 40,000 American women every year;[32] some 33,000 new cases are diagnosed every year in the UK – double the incidence of the 1950s. As cases continue to spiral upward (one in nine women contract it in the US, and one in twelve in the UK), the pressure is on for women, particularly those over 40, to have regular screenings, and mammography has become a huge growth industry.

Despite decades of enormous government resource and a massive money-spinner aimed at efforts to improve early detection and local treatment, the bottom line is that the level of breast cancer mortality has remained constant.

Breast cancer deaths in England and Wales fell by 12 per cent in the 1990s. Nevertheless, health officials who ascribe this sudden drop to their extensive mammogram screening programmes have no reason to be self-congratulatory. New research has discovered no evidence to link the two, although screening has helped detect more cases earlier. The National Cancer Registration Bureau believes the fall may be more likely associated with the increasing use of the drug tamoxifen, which slows cancer growth, than with any screening. Since nationwide screening was introduced in 1988, recorded incidence of the disease in the 50–64-year age group rose by 25 per cent.[33] Furthermore, the fall in mortality began in 1985, but the first NHS screening units were not working until three years later, and Great Britain as a whole wasn't sufficiently covered until 1990. As Royal Marsden Hospital breast cancer specialist Michael Baum writes, claiming that any part of the drop in mortality is due to the screening programme is 'intellectually dishonest'.[34]

After the publication of a Swedish meta-analysis some years ago, which pooled results from five studies conducted over five to 13 years on some 300,000 women, most members of the medical establishment have adopted as gospel its results: that for women 50 and over, regular screening can reduce breast cancer mortality by 30 per cent.[35] It is also generally agreed that no studies have shown a benefit for women younger than 50.[36] In the UK, the government offers mammography to women aged 50–64, and invites them to participate every three years.

This '30-per-cent risk reduction' has been adopted as a mantra by the medical profession. It has provided a justification of sorts to screen many groups, such as women under 50, where benefits of screening have never been shown. Despite all medical evidence to the contrary, the American Cancer Society and the American College of Radiology have carried on urging all women over 40 – which of course includes this limbo group between the ages of 40 and 49 – to have annual mammograms.[37]

But even among the over-fifties, there is no conclusive evidence that mammographic screening is doing any good. In the much-quoted Swedish study, the researchers came up with their figure by pooling all the results of three bands of age groups – the 40–49-year-olds, 50–69-year-olds and 70–74-year-olds – into an overview. The study showed a positive benefit (29 per cent reduction in mortality) among the women in their fifties, but none among the women in their forties or those in their seventies.

However, when you actually examine the science behind these statistics, this is the only study to show clear benefit, even among the 50-year-olds. The 30 per cent improved survival figure being bandied about derives from several articles which examined *all* the studies of screening and attempted to pool the results. Although most studies didn't show a clear benefit, the article concluded that those that were most scientific, or 'randomized' (that is, women assigned randomly to either screening groups or controls) all proved to be of benefit.[38]

However, Dublin's Dr McCormick and his late colleague Petr Skrabanek, both scourges of unproven medical practice, have pointed out that three of the four of those trials considered most scientific 'failed to reach statistically significant benefit for women aged 50 and over'.[39] These included two studies of an aggregate of 80,000 women, which were dismissed as 'too small' by one set of screening proponents.[40] In other words, to reach their favourable statistics, academics have combined entirely different types of scientific studies – those that set out with several groups of women to see what happens to them over time, versus analysing what has already happened to several groups of women – in an attempt to make the insignificant advantages of screening appear significant. In fact, two of the best breast cancer centres in the UK failed to lower deaths significantly using annual clinical exams and every-other-year mammograms.[41]

It's also wise to keep in mind what this 30 per cent supposed reduction in mortality actually translates into. At best, it may prevent or postpone one cancer death for between 7,000 and 63,000 women invited for screening every year.[42]

More recently, researchers from the University of British Columbia in Vancouver studied all the trials since the early ones that claimed a 30 per cent reduction in deaths from breast cancer in women over 50. There has been far less publicity, the Canadian researchers point out, about all the studies that have been done since those early days, showing that mammography does no good for anyone in any age group, but does great harm through false-positives and get-in-there-early intervention. They attacked mammography and indeed recommended that they be junked altogether after discovering that only one in 14 women with a positive mammogram result indicating breast cancer will actually have the condition.

'Since the benefit achieved is marginal, the harm caused is substantial, and the costs incurred are enormous, we suggest that public funding for breast cancer screening in any age group is not justifiable,' these epidemiologists concluded.[43]

In another Canadian study, when six trials of breast cancer screening were analysed, only one in 14 women with a positive mammography result indicating breast cancer actually had the condition. As with cervical cancer, this means that many women are going through needless worry and treatment on the basis of an inaccurate test.[44]

The latest evidence concurs that regular mammograms offers no survival advantage among any age group under 60.[45] In 2002, after studying all the most recent science, a committee of US cancer experts called the The Physician Data Query board (PDQ) concluded there is insufficient evidence to show that mammograms actually prevent deaths.[46] More than one-third of mammograms give false readings overall, two-thirds false-positives,[47] and the test is accurate less than half the time and only in the second half of a woman's menstrual cycle.[48]

The rationale for screening has always been that the earlier you catch it, the smaller the tumour will be, and hence the greater your chances of beating the disease. However, this rationale doesn't take into account that cancer doesn't always metastasize at the same rate. Breast cancer isn't a tidy disease that progresses in the same way for every woman; sometimes it spreads throughout the body, other times it advances in the breast alone. Much of our treatment doesn't influence the outcome in any case.[49]

One reason may be that mammograms actually increase mortality rates. Among the under-fifties, more women die from breast cancer among screened groups than among those not given mammograms. The Canadian National Breast Cancer Screening Trial (NBSS), published in 1993, which screened 50,000 women between the ages of 40 and 49, showed that more tumours were detected in the screened group, but not only were no lives saved, but a third more women died from breast cancer in the group first offered screening.[50] Similar results occurred in three Swedish studies[51] and also in those conducted in New York.[52] One of the Swedish studies, conducted in Malmo, showed nearly a *third* more cases of breast cancer in women under 55 given mammograms over 10 years.[53] Even when you adjust results and allow that cancers among women aged 51–69 – the so-called 'high-risk group' – have been detected, screened women have nearly a 2 per cent higher incidence of breast cancer than controls.[54]

That more younger screened women die may reflect the fact that mammography is indiscriminant, picking up many cancers which would do no harm if left alone. The scattergun nature of the technology has several implications. This ability to pick up any sort of tumour falsely increases the incidence of breast cancer by a quarter to a half.[55] Adding all these benign tumours, which of course don't lead to death, into the cancer data also has the effect of making it look like more people in the screened population survive because of early detection.

By picking up all and several tumours of every variety, mammograms also could be falsely inflating the incidence of breast cancer by as much as one half.[56]

The third effect of regular mammograms is that they lead to massive, unnecessary treatment because benign tumours are often mistaken for malignant ones. In one study of over a thousand women undertaken by Harvard Medical School, only a quarter of the women whose mammograms had recorded some abnormality were actually found to have malignant tumours. Other radiology departments referring patients to the Harvard Center had an even worse batting average – getting it right only one-sixth of the time. And of course an inappropriately strong mammography report, which might include statements such as 'malignancy cannot be excluded', raises the anxiety level of the patient and referring physician and often ends up with the woman on the operating table.[57]

Routine screening is undoubtedly responsible for the huge increase in the aggressive treatment of ductal carcinoma in situ (DCIS) – some 40,000 cases in the US alone.

Since the advent of screening, the incidence of DCIS has sky-rocketed, from 2.4 per 100,000 women in 1973 to 15.8 cases per 100,000 in 1992.[58] Although many women being diagnosed with DCIS are undergoing radical mastectomies, this abnormality, or 'pre-cancer' is 'not a synonym for other forms of cancer', says Professor McCormick. Not only do many experts misunderstand DCIS, but most cases of this condition, says McCormick, would not do a woman any harm.[59]

Up until now, only relatively high doses of radiation have been associated with an increased risk of breast cancer. However, new evidence demonstrates that even moderate strengths of strong x-rays raise the risk of breast cancer five or six times in women who carry a certain gene, occurring in about 1 per cent of the population – or in at least one million American women. In 1975, Dr C. Bailar II, editor in chief of the *Journal of the National Cancer Institute*, concluded that accumulated x-ray doses in excess of 100 rads over 10 to 15 years may induce cancer of the breast.[60] A single-view mammogram offers the average breast a dose of about 200 millirads (0.2 rad).[61]

However, women with the ataxia-telangiectasia gene, says Dr Michael Swift, chief of medical genetics at North Carolina University, have an unusual sensitivity to radiation and could develop cancer after exposure to 'appallingly low' doses. He estimates that, in the US, between 5,000 and 10,000 of the 180,000 breast cancer cases diagnosed each year could be prevented if women with the gene were not exposed to the radiation from mammograms.[62]

Just four breast films (the usual pictures for one mammogram session) expose you to 1 rad (radiation absorbed dose) – about 1,000 times more than that of a chest x-ray. Each rad increases the risk of a premenopausal woman's cancer risk by 1 per cent, so that women screened for over a decade would have raised their cancer risk by 10 per cent.

Besides a genetic susceptibility, the physical trauma caused by the force of mammograms could be a factor in spreading cancer. At the moment, mammograms use 200 newtons of compression, the equivalent of 20 1kg bags of sugar per breast. Some of the modern foot-pedal operated machines are designed to exert one-third again as much force – the equivalent of your breast being squashed by 30 bags of sugar.[63] The force is thought to be necessary in order to get the best quality of image while keeping the radiation dose to a minimum.[64] A number of researchers believe that compression during mammography can rupture cysts and disseminate cancer cells.[65] This phenomenon has been observed in animal studies; if a tumour is manipulated, it can increase the rate of its spread to other parts of the body by up to 80 per cent.[66]

Many biopsies to investigate a suspicious lump found on mammography have their own set of problems. In this standard procedure, a thick needle is inserted into the breast under local anaesthetic to remove a small piece of tissue. This is then examined for cancerous cells. In one study of women undergoing biopsy, a quarter had problems afterward with the wound left by the needle such as infection or bleeding. Nine patients reported a new breast lump (all benign) developing under the biopsy scar between one to seven years after surgery. Eight patients continued to have pain in the area where the biopsy had been taken up to six years after the operation, and seven reported unsightly scars.[67]

Fine-needle aspiration, which can be done on an outpatient basis, has been served up as the less invasive alternative when a lump has been found; in this instance, a fine needle with a syringe is inserted in the breast to draw out a specimen of the lump's contents. However, doctors have been known to puncture the lung during this procedure, causing pneumothorax (in which air enters the chest, causing the lung to collapse). In 74,000 fine-needle aspirations of the breast, this occurred in about 133 patients (0.18 per cent).[68]

The experience in many countries suggests that mammograms also have a high rate of inaccuracy. In Canada, during the first four years of the eight-year trial on breast cancer screening, nearly three-quarters of test results were unacceptable. Only in the last two years of the trial were more than half the tests up to the required standard.[69]

As for women under 50, another Canadian study showed that some 87 per cent of so-called cancer cases detected by mammograms were false alarms.[70]

The high level of false-positives is partly due to poor standards in equipment. A third of women's clinics in the US were not accredited, as of early 1994. The FDA admitted that many of them were inaccurately reporting mammograms and that some women were receiving doses of radiation that were far too high.[71] Just how poor the standards are was revealed by a 1989 survey of a cross-section of mammography units carried out by the Department of Health in Michigan. One-third of the units studied routinely exceeded the various standards of radiation exposure.[72]

The US aimed to correct this problem with the Mammography Quality Standards Act, passed in October 1992, which was to establish quality-control standards and a certification system for the more than 10,000 medical facilities that perform and interpret mammograms. These quality-control standards relate to the training and education of personnel, the equipment and the dosage used, among other criteria. Doctors would also have to have continuing education in reading mammograms and be expected to interpret an average of 40 mammograms a month.

As of October 1994, every facility performing mammograms had to obtain a certificate or provisional certificate to continue to operate legally.

However, although setting standards has undoubtedly improved some of the appalling mistakes made in the past, it may do nothing to improve the inherent imprecision of the technology itself. Even mammograms of the best quality can be misread by highly experienced radiologists. In one study carried out by Yale University, 10 seasoned radiologists, with 12 years' experience in reading mammograms, each given the same 150 good-quality mammograms, differed in their interpretation a third of the time. In a quarter of cases they also radically disagreed over how the patients should be managed (such as whether they should have follow-up mammograms or exploratory surgery). Even among the 27 patients later definitely diagnosed as having breast cancer, the radiologists varied widely in their diagnosis. Nearly a third of cancers were wrongly categorized. One radiologist did not detect a cancer that was clearly visible, while another thought it was developing on the breast opposite the one where it actually was.[73]

Even if regular screening doesn't spread or cause cancer, its dubious benefits may not be worth the pain reported by a third of women undergoing the screening.[74] Helen, from Westcliff on Sea, now in her early fifties, has suffered with lumpy breasts and severe mastitis for 20 years.

She's had several routine 'horizontal' mammograms and a fine-needle aspiration of a cyst she found 12 years ago. Then, in 1991, she had another mammogram. 'This time I had to stand upright and each breast was squashed vertically against the machine. The pain was excruciating. Tears welled up in my eyes and I could hardly stop myself from shrieking. The pain lasted in both breasts for three or four days before gradually subsiding,' she says.

SCREENING FOR OVARIAN CANCER

Today, most US gynaecologists routinely screen for ovarian cancer. This widespread screening was prompted by the highly publicized death in 1989 of the actress and comedienne Gilda Radner at the age of 42 from ovarian cancer. Screening involves ultrasound, pelvic examinations, and analysis of the blood.

However, this flurry of activity among doctors is against the express recommendations of the American government. The National Institutes of Health (NIH) has recommended *against* routine screening, declaring that it is inaccurate and even dangerous.[75]

The NIH said that these tests are so unreliable that surgeons have unnecessarily operated on many women who don't have the disease. Even if doctors do get it right, by the time the cancer shows up it's too late. And in only a quarter of cases is ovarian cancer detected at a stage early enough for effective treatment.[76]

PROSTATE CANCER

With cancer of the prostate, the grape-size gland between the rectum and scrotum, medicine has been pushing to adopt routine screening of the over-fifties for the second major killer of older men. The three screening techniques include prostate-specific antigen test(PSA), transrectal ultrasound (TRUS), and digital rectal examination (DRE). However, an analysis by the Toronto Hospital in Ontario, Canada, concludes that high inaccuracy associated with these methods can also do more harm than good. The main risk is unnecessary surgery, which causes widespread incontinence and impotence in a third of cases.[77] Furthermore, no evidence exists to show that men given a prostatectomy will survive any longer than those left alone and undergoing 'watchful waiting'.

The biggest problem occurs with the PSA test, which examines the amount of a certain protein in the blood, thought to correlate with the degree of prostate cancer present. However, the prostate-specific antigen has proved indiscriminate and highly inaccurate: a recent review of the data concluded that two-thirds of men with elevated PSA levels don't have prostate cancer.[78]

The problem lies with the test itself, which cannot distinguish between benign and cancerous tumours, and also with its interpretation, as doctors still disagree over what constitutes a level indicative of cancer. Newer tests are claimed to provide more accuracy, particularly when tied in with a patient's age, but to date, the research shows that the test is worse than useless.

One study discovered that 366 men given the 'all clear' with a PSA test went on to develop prostate cancer, while raised values – which indicate the presence of the cancer – were found in just 47 per cent of men who in fact had prostate cancer.[79] Other research from Harvard Medical School found that the PSA tests fail to diagnose prostate cancer correctly in 82 per cent of cases.[80] Even when a biopsy is thrown in with the PSA test, only 40 per cent of prostate cancer gets detected.[81]

Recently it has been discovered that the PSA can give false readings if the man has ejaculated in the previous two days. Men over 40 have very high PSA levels immediately after ejaculating, and though these start to fall significantly only six hours later, it takes 48 hours or more for the levels to normalize.[82]

As with mammography, screening for prostate cancer may actually increases your chances of dying. The European Institute of Oncology in Milan found that more men who undergo PSA screening die from prostate cancer than those who aren't screened.[83]

SCREENING AGAINST SCREENING

So how can you protect yourself against cancer, or – perhaps more importantly – against the screening tests themselves? Unless you have various risk factors in your family or yourself, there is no good scientific reason why you should engage in regular screening of any sort if you are healthy and have no symptoms. Professor McCormick says the most important early warning for cervical cancer (early enough in most cases for treatment) may be a persistent vaginal discharge or any sort of inter-menstrual bleeding, for instance, after coitus. The likelihood of cervical cancer increases with a woman's number of sexual partners, whether she smokes, takes the Pill or other prescribed hormones, whether she's had any sexually transmitted disease or began her sexual life early. If you don't fall into any of these categories, be wary of your doctor pressurizing you into taking the test, particularly as he now stands to benefit financially from it.

If you do have to have a cervical exam, you might wish to insist on a visual examination of the cervix. In a study of 45,000 women in Delhi, India, where cytological screening is not available, visual exams picked up nearly three-quarters of the cancers found among the sample group, by means of cervical erosions which bled when touched, small growths or, in general, a suspicious-looking cervix.[84]

As for mammograms, medicine in general has downplayed the importance of regular physical examination of breasts as a diagnostic tool. An advisor to Britain's chief medical officer admitted that 'more than 90 per cent of breast tumours are found by the women themselves'.[85] In fact, a seven-year study of 33,000 women showed that self-examination could reduce breast cancer deaths by up to one-fifth. Although some lumps detected by mammogram aren't palpable (able to be felt with the hand or fingers alone), the reverse is true as well. Indeed, one researcher believes that routine screening lulls you into a false sense of security, so that you tend to ignore warning signs such as suspicious lumps.[86]

If you don't want a mammogram, make sure to opt for a regular programme of self-examination (your doctor can teach you how to do it) and breast examination by your doctor. If he is unwilling or has limited experience of physical examinations, you might ask to be referred to a clinic where these are routinely carried out, or find another doctor. New research shows that regular self-examination and yearly exams by a trained health professional offer more accurate prediction of cancer than mammograms.[87] If you do decide to have a mammogram, shop around. Make sure the equipment is specially designed for mammography and therefore able to give the best image with the least radiation, and ask a lot of questions about the number taken each week, as well as when the machine was last inspected. (Machines should be tested at least once a year.)

If a lump is found, either through mammography or self-examination, you need to establish whether or not it is malignant. Some harmless cysts can be identified as such through a physical examination. If your doctor tells you it's a cyst but still suggests sending you for a biopsy, find out if it's really necessary. A benign lump often changes with your cycle, becoming more tender before a period; a cancerous one won't.

If you do produce a lump, you might wish to consider ultrasound, which may be safer (for all but foetal cells). Although the technology is vastly improving and will probably eventually develop into a good tool, there are still some problems with accuracy. The success of ultrasound largely depends on the skill of the operator, as images can be hard to read and are open to misinterpretation. In particular, operators worry about visualizing 'artefacts' – that is, a ghosted image of something that isn't there – or mistaking something quite normal for something sinister, confusing a normal structure for an abnormality. This all adds up to the fact that you should only have a test performed with highly trained operators who are well skilled in all the latest equipment and equally well trained in distinguishing real from phantom images. With breast examinations, the most commonly used equipment is 'real time' high-resolution ultrasonography – which means you see on screen exactly what the transducer is picking up at that moment. According to one study of 100 women with at least one breast nodule, the overall rate of accuracy of ultrasound was 74.8 per cent. This, of course, means that the diagnosis was wrong in one out of four cases. In 10 cases the ultrasound diagnosed benign breast cysts as cancerous, and also missed one breast cyst and one abscess altogether.[88]

According to Professor William Lees, Director of Radiology at UCL Hospitals Trust in London, the best ultrasound should have Doppler as part of the system and use the two types in tandem, which will boost an operator's confidence about the accuracy of his diagnosis.

Colour Doppler ultrasound measures the flow of blood, which in malignant tumours tends to be abnormal. In one study, the overall accuracy for detecting breast tumours was 82 per cent.[89]

Nevertheless, the technology appears to be improving; presently the colour method is used by comparing a colour spectrum analysis compared with surrounding tissue; in cancerous tumours, the colour is typically more intense with sharp margins. In one study among 70 patients, this method missed only a single tumour.[90]

Professor Lees believes that a skilled operator combining both methods should approach an accuracy rate of 85 per cent.

At the end of the day, ultrasound seems to have a similar batting average to mammograms. In one review of 80 patients with both benign and malignant lesions, mammograms picked up five cancers missed by ultrasound, but ultrasound discovered nine cancers missed by mammograms. In yet another study, ultrasound picked up four cancers that weren't yet palpable.[91]

The newest and safest possibility is thermography (measuring the heat of the body's skin cells – cancer cells are hotter).

No matter what the technology, the most important questions you should ask concern the expertise of the operator. Always opt for someone highly experienced, particularly in breast scans. Don't be shy about asking his accuracy rate or if there have been any serious cases he has missed. Also ask about the state of the equipment – how new it is, how accurate, and when it was last serviced.

For breast cancers, the best prevention of all is to avoid the birth control Pill, HRT and all other prescribed hormones, which have proven cancer risks, chemicals such as parabens, to breastfeed your babies for as long as possible, to eat a wholefood, unprocessed diet rich in fresh organic fruits and vegetables and essential fatty acids (EFAs) and to avoid pesticides and dairy products, which have been implicated in breast cancer. As for ovarian cancer, only those women over age 50 in high-risk groups – those whose relatives have contracted ovarian cancer, have no children, are from North European stock or have histories of breast, colon or endometrial cancers – should be regularly monitored. However, if your test comes up positive, it's important that you have the results confirmed by other methods before consenting to surgery.

With prostate cancer, your best odds appear to be avoiding the test, unless you have symptoms. If you do get cancer, consider maintaining a watchful wait-and-see attitude and use other forms of therapy, such as hormonal treatment, rather than rushing into surgery, particularly if you are over 70. Prostate cancer is, in the main, a slow-growing form of cancer, and you're much more likely to die with it than from it. According to autopsy studies, a third of men in the European Union have prostate cancer, but only 1 per cent will die from it before something else claims their lives.[92]

PART III

PREVENTION

5

Crazy about Cholesterol:
Medicine's Red Herring

Despite what appears to be a reasonable track record for killing off people once they get ill, modern medicine promotes the view that doctors have enough understanding of your body to prevent illness even before it has begun. Increasingly doctors have turned their hand to what they like to call 'preventive' medicine – that is, dispensing 'just-in-case' medicine to you and your loved ones while you're still healthy, to stop disease before it starts. Throughout medical history, preventive medicine has been responsible for a number of alarming medical notions – such as routinely x-raying pregnant women to measure their pelvic size, which contributed to an increase in childhood leukaemia, or giving them diethylstilbestrol to 'prevent' miscarriage, which also caused cancer and infertility among an entire generation of children. The problem with such an approach is that the pre-emptive strike almost always causes even more illness than the disease it is meant to prevent. For the drug companies, this is nothing so much as an unexpected bonus. The industry continually creates its own markets by setting off new health epidemics, which pave the way for yet more new bestselling miracle drugs – a renewal process akin to eating continually from your own hand.

THE CHOLESTEROL FALLACY

Increasingly, doctors have come to believe that preventive medicine is a matter of identifying certain risk factors in lifestyles that increase a person's chances of coming down with a disease. In the 1950s it was Dr Ancel Keys, director of the Laboratory of Physiological Hygiene at the University of Minnesota, who first postulated that high-fat food was the cause of heart attacks. Dr Keys produced a chart that showed a correlation between total intake of fat and fatal heart disease in six countries. His limited data was seized upon by medicine, which first hypothesized that high dietary intake of fat caused a high level of cholesterol in the blood, which in turn furred up arteries and set up a chain of events which eventually led to a heart attack or stroke. According to this reasoning, cardiovascular disease could largely be prevented by lowering blood cholesterol levels, either by drugs or by limiting fat intake.

This single hypothesis spawned an entire food and medical industry devoted to screening for high blood cholesterol and lowering it through drugs and processed, low-fat foods. Most of the population of the Western world has now become conditioned to obsess over fat, and millions of patients in the US and the UK have been bullied onto long-term medication.

In fact, cholesterol-lowering may be one of the biggest red herrings of the century. The extraordinary fact remains that no one has even been able to *prove* a cause-and-effect relationship between cholesterol or high-fat diet and heart disease. *Indeed, the amazing fact of it is, most patients with heart disease have normal cholesterol levels.*[1]

After 60 years of this 'preventive' medicine, evidence is emerging that cholesterol-lowering drugs and extremely low-cholesterol diets might actually *increase* your chances of dying. Many of the regimes recommended by medicine may, in fact, be among the main culprits in causing heart disease. Nor has any cholesterol-lowering drug been proved over time to be capable of lowering overall mortality rates; in many cases, the number of heart attacks may have dropped, but deaths from other heart problems have risen, as have overall deaths caused by other factors.

Since Keys' first simple correlation, more stringent studies have proved that cholesterol may not even be the main cause of heart disease. One study involving nearly 20,000 men and women from Copenhagen demonstrated that only those with cholesterol blood levels in the top 5 per cent were at risk of developing heart disease.[2]

In the 1950s, Keys himself went on to organize the massive Seven Countries Study, examining the lifestyles of 16 local populations of seven Western countries including the US to determine causes of coronary heart disease.[3] But after collating their data, gleaned over 25 years, the researchers had to conclude that risk factors were a complex mix of factors, including cholesterol, smoking, high blood-pressure and overall diet. The importance of diet was suggested by the marked difference in levels of heart disease in different countries. No simple correlation was found between fat intake and heart attacks.[4]

Many populations with high levels of heart disease don't have correspondingly high levels of fat in their diets. For instance, a group of Dutch researchers travelled to Minsk (Belarus), an area unusually high in heart disease, and took fatty tissue samples from a group of men and women who'd been hospitalized for minor problems. After analysing the fat samples, the researchers could find no evidence that the Minsk sample contained unusually high levels of saturated fats or unusually low levels of essential fatty acids (EFAs), both considered risk factors for heart disease. They concluded that dietary fat probably wasn't the major cause of heart disease in that area.[5]

In one of the largest-ever studies of heart disease and lifestyle, in Framingham, Massachusetts, a large part of the population has been studied for nearly half a century to determine risk factors for heart disease and atherosclerosis. Nevertheless, no association has been made between high cholesterol levels and men after middle age – the time when men are supposed to be most at risk. Women with high cholesterol have died at the same rate as those with low cholesterol levels. Although more people with high cholesterol have died than those with low cholesterol, deaths have been from all causes, not simply heart disease. Indeed, the only connection made between total cholesterol levels and heart attack risk has been made in males from their low 30s to their early 60s.[6]

A major California study discovered that neither high nor low cholesterol levels seem to have any bearing on any of the major illnesses, including heart disease and cancer. Researchers from the University of Southern

California, who analysed about 2,000 deaths among a group of 7,000 middle-aged men, all of Japanese descent, concluded that early deaths were caused by other risk factors, but never cholesterol on its own.[7]

Even in elderly patients, who would logically seem most at risk, science hasn't been able to link high cholesterol levels with heart disease. A large batch of patients over 70 were followed for four years. A high cholesterol level (over 240 milligrams per decilitre) didn't put them at a greater risk of dying from anything, including heart disease, a heart attack, or unstable angina.[8] Similar findings have resulted in Australian and New York studies in the elderly.[9]

For women, a low-fat diet may actually increase their risk of heart disease. In one group of 15,000 Scottish women, those with higher levels of cholesterol than men were shown to be less likely to die from heart disease than men with the highest levels. Lowering a woman's cholesterol levels also seems to lower her levels of high-density lipoprotein, the good form of cholesterol that actually protects against heart disease.[10]

This kind of conflicting data suggests that high cholesterol may simply be a marker of something gone awry in the body, but that the real cause of heart disease lies elsewhere. It has even been shown that cholesterol does not cause initial injury to arteries, but only accumulates in the blood or in arteries months after something else has caused the injury.[11]

The latest evidence shows that a high cholesterol level may be protective in the elderly. Dutch scientists studied medical records of over 700 old people. Those with the highest cholesterol counts avoided cancer and infectious diseases and lived longest.[12]

Since the cholesterol hypothesis was first advanced, pharmaceutical companies have experimented with a variety of substances to lower cholesterol, achieving a modest reduction of about 10 per cent. However, in the 1980s they unleashed 'statins', which were found to inhibit the body's production of cholesterol by up to 40 per cent. Any residual scepticism among doctors about the cholesterol hypothesis was virtually swept aside in late 1994 by the publication of a single trial, the Scandinavian Simvastatin Survival Study, which appeared to vindicate cholesterol-lowering drugs, at least among those patients with a heart condition and high cholesterol levels. Dubbed the 4S study, it followed 4,444 patients ('four' was obviously the leitmotif here) with a heart condition and high cholesterol levels. After five and a half years, the group given cholesterol drugs had a 42 per cent lower rate of fatal heart attacks and a one-third reduction in heart disease over those given a placebo. (Women in the group did not enjoy the same improved survival statistics; although only a fifth of the study population were women, in the placebo group the mortality rate was half of what it was for men, suggesting, once again, that high cholesterol levels may be a meaningless indicator of future heart disease in women.)[13]

Within a week, the medical press was firmly on the cholesterol bandwagon, proclaiming, 'Simvastatin saves lives.'[14] Michael Brown and Joseph Goldstein, the 1985 Nobel prizewinners for their work on cholesterol, broke what had been a long silence over the cholesterol controversy at a 1994 meeting of the American Heart Association in Dallas, Texas, to talk of the 'landmark' results and 'definitive answer' provided by the Scandinavian study.

Hard at the heels of the 4S study was a Scottish study, the West of Scotland Coronary Prevention Study (WOSCOPS). This purported to show that, with men who had high levels of cholesterol but no history of heart disease, pravastatin, another 'statin' cholesterol-lowering drug, could prevent heart attacks by a third.[15] Other studies, including one reviewing all the other studies, concluded that pravastatin could reduce the rate of heart attacks by at least 60 per cent and could slow hardening of the arteries.[16]

Although there were many important differences between these trials, the effect on the rank and file in medicine was galvanic. The WOSCOP study was widely interpreted to mean that otherwise healthy men with high cholesterol levels could take cholesterol drugs and reduce their chances of dying of heart disease by nearly a third. All patients with higher cholesterol levels, of whatever age or sex, were being placed on cholesterol-lowering drugs for life.[17] One hospital in Dundee, which maintained statistics about the level of cholesterol-drug prescribing before and after the publications of the 4S study, found a striking increase both in the percentage of patients whose cholesterol was being measured (by a third) and in the percentage of patients being prescribed drugs (by nearly eight times).[18] Many of those receiving the drugs were elderly or female, even though the drugs hadn't really been studied in terms of either category of patient. In fact, though the 4S study showed limited benefit of cholesterol-lowering drugs for women, and though women weren't even included in WOSCOPS, more than half of all cholesterol patients now receiving the drugs in the US are women.[19]

Only a few brave dissidents have questioned the design of the 4S study and point out what they view as a number of basic flaws. For one thing, anyone with coronary heart disease was allowed into the study, whether his illness was caused by hardened arteries or not. In the treated group, there were 38 additional people who had, by the time they entered the study, already been given bypass surgery or angioplasty and who therefore were less likely to die. And 54 more smokers were in the control group, which just might have had something to do with their greater mortality rate.[20]

William Stehbens of the Wellington School of Medicine in New Zealand pointed out (and, as a pathologist, he should know) that diagnosing CHD or gauging the severity of atherosclerosis is a highly inexact science – until people die. In the 4S study, the actual difference in the death rate between the two groups from all causes was only 3.3 per cent. Finally, Stehbens notes, almost in an aside, that the control group took a placebo containing methylcellulose, which when given intravenously to rabbits causes tissue storage in arteries, a condition that sounds not dissimilar to the effect of atherosclerosis.

In the WOSCOP study, the deaths from heart disease in the control group (those not taking the drug) were higher in number than in the general population – closer to the average deaths in people 10 years or older – suggesting that particular people chosen to represent the 'average citizen' happened to be more ill than usual.[21] Furthermore, although pravastatin did reduce cholesterol levels and the number of heart attacks or death from heart attacks in the WOSCOPS, *it did not significantly save lives from other coronary disease or any other cause. A review of all the studies with pravastatin also failed to show that a reduction in heart attacks translated into a significant number of lives being saved.* Any improvements in the death rate, other than from heart attacks, were not considered 'statistically significant'.[22] And even if you tally in the survival statistics from heart attacks, overall survival over five years in the WOSCOPS trial was only increased from 96 to 97 per cent, and in the 4S trial from 87.7 to 91.3 per cent.[23]

This means that many people with no history of heart attack may be put on cholesterol-lowering drugs indefinitely for an extremely minimal gain.

A scant 15 years later, after those two studies statins have become the most popular weapon in your doctor's arsenal, and one of the biggest moneyspinning drugs of all time.

The four major studies on statins performed since have had conflicting results. For instance, the CARE (Cholesterol and Recurrent Events) trial, which involved several American, Canadian and British university hospitals, tried out pravastatin to lower cholesterol in patients who'd already suffered a heart attack. However, after five years, not only wasn't there much difference between the treated and untreated groups in terms of fatal heart attacks, but a few more had died from other causes in the pravastatin group. There was, however, a lower incidence of stroke and non-fatal heart attacks.[24]

Then, the Air Force/Texas Coronary Atherosclerosis Prevent Study (AFCAPS/TexCAPS) was set up to determine whether statins could prevent heart attacks in some 6,000 men and women with normal cholesterol levels. After five years, although fewer people had heart attacks or angina in the treated group (3.5 per cent as against 5.5 per cent in the untreated group), the statins made no difference to overall mortality. Virtually the same percentage died in both groups.[25]

Most recently, the Australian Long-term Intervention with Pravastatin in Ischemic Disease) study (LIPID) trial, set up by the National Health and Medical Research Council Clinical Trials Centre at the University of Sydney, included patients with both high and low levels of cholesterol who'd suffered previous heart disease.

After six years, the rates of death and heart disease were significantly lower in the treatment group than in the control group.[26] But the most impressive results to date were compiled by the Heart Protection Study (HPS) in Oxford, which examined the effect of giving 20,000 people at high risk of coronary heart disease statins over five years.

The HPS study concluded that routine use of cholesterol-lowering drugs in patients at high risk of vascular disease can reduce the incidence of heart attack and strokes by a third.[27]

According to the investigators, five years of statin treatment can prevent heart attacks, strokes or other major vascular events in one in 10 people who have had a heart attack, in eight in 100 people with angina or some other sign of coronary heart disease, in seven in 100 people who have ever had a stroke, and in seven in 100 people with diabetes.

Speaking before the American Heart Association's Scientific Sessions 2001 in late November, Rory Collins, co-director of Oxford University's Clinical Trial Service Unit and lead investigator of HPS, declared statins as the 'new aspirin'. Collins said his evidence moved statins outside the sideshow arena of cholesterol-lowering medication, placing them firmly into the centre ring of preventive treatment for heart and vascular disease.

If an extra 20 million high-risk people around the world had statin treatment, he estimated, it would save about 50,000 lives each year. That translates into about 1,000 lives saved a week.

THE ALL-PURPOSE DRUG

Probably because so many drugs have such horrendous side-effects, once a drug has been shown to do any good at all, doctors seize upon it as an all-purpose product, and begin to throw it at other, unrelated diseases in the hope that it will work. With these kinds of initially promising studies, statins soon came to be looked upon as a magic bullet for all the diseases of old age. Doctors began to hand them out for everything from osteoporosis to senile dementia, solely on the basis of the theory, proposed by several doctors, that statins could help treat osteoporosis in women,[28] reduce the risks of stroke in patients with heart disease[29] and benefit heart patients, because the drug could help new blood vessels to grow.[30]

Time has shown these assumptions to be flawed. For instance, one large-scale study of more than 80,000 patients by Southampton General Hospital showed that the fracture rate of long-term statin users was actually *greater* than in non-users in anything less than high doses, where the effect was marginal.[31]

Whatever the beneficial effect of statins on lowering mortality, lowering cholesterol has nothing whatever to do with it.

As many critics point out, statins have worked just as well in young people and women – populations where high cholesterol has never been shown to be linked to a heart attack. It didn't seem to matter whether cholesterol was lowered a great deal or just a little. Statins also protect against strokes, which are not caused by high cholesterol levels. The life-saving elements may have more to due with another mechanism – perhaps their effect on smooth muscle cells inside the arterial walls or their effect on inhibiting the production of thromboxane, which causes blood to clot.[32]

But even allowing for this, the actual beneficial effect is quite small. Although a reduction in the 'relative risk' (the chances of getting the disease) is large, the actual percentage of lives saved is tiny, especially among healthy people; in the AFCAPS/TexCAPS trial, for instance, only 0.12 per cent fewer people died in the group taking the statin drugs. Any small advantage of statin drugs must be set against the risks of taking the drug as a 'prescription for life'.

Dr Thomas Newman of the University of California at San Francisco, who has written extensively on US medical policy concerning cholesterol, has examined epidemiological data suggesting that these drugs are less beneficial to women, the elderly and younger men (in both of the big cholesterol studies, the subjects were all middle-aged men).[33] There may even be a slightly increased rate of death among women on cholesterol-lowering drugs.[34] But in any case, doctors don't agree about whether women should lower their cholesterol. Earlier evidence has shown that a woman's risk of developing a heart condition isn't lessened even if cholesterol levels are lowered through diet. There is no evidence linking high cholesterol levels in women with heart conditions in later life.[35]

Some researchers also have noted that slightly more people died from all causes in the 4S study. Although this number wasn't considered significant, we need more studies of the drugs to determine if cholesterol-lowering drugs could be responsible for increasing deaths from other causes.[36] So far, we do know that a low blood cholesterol concentration can cause haemorrhagic stroke.[37]

NOT-SO-WONDER DRUGS

Although statins have always been regarded as some of the safest drugs around, mounting evidence is tallying a long list of side-effects. One of the first to be recognized is myopathy, or muscle weakness, and its more severe form, rhabdomyolysis, where severely weakened muscles release toxic muscle-cell components into the bloodstream, which eventually can cause kidney failure and other potentially fatal conditions. A recent review found simvastatin to be the worst culprit.[38]

Although muscle weakness was already recognized as a side-effect with statins, it was considered a rare occurrence preceding acute liver failure. One of the drugs, called cerivastatin, has been taken off the market because of the number of patients who have developed myopathy while on the drug.[39]

Mick, aged 50, took statins for 10 years to bring down his high cholesterol count. For the last four of them he'd suffered a number of problems, including extreme muscle stiffness, back pain that extended round to the front of his chest under the rib cage, pins and needles in his arms and hands and also numbness and weakness, to the point where he was unable to pick up objects. He discussed these problems with four doctors, all of whom told Mick that his problems were not related to the drug.

When his leg muscles became so stiff that he had trouble walking, his partner suggested he take a break from the statin he was taking. After one month there was a slight improvement; after three months the improvement was remarkable, Mick says. He could even play squash – after being told by his physiotherapist that he would never play again.

Other side-effects include leg pain, oedema (water-retention), myalgia, sinusitis, insomnia and impotence; erection dysfunction can appear as soon as two days after starting treatment.[40]

Other serious problems include pneumonia, liver toxicity, pancreatitis and fatal ulcerative colitis. The drug has also been found to enter the brain, lowering the cholesterol within brain cells, which likely accounts for such side-effects as depression, sleep problems and memory loss.

Statins also affect nerves. They can cause a polyneuropathy (or peripheral neuropathy), characterized by weakness, numbness, pain and tingling in the hands and feet.[41] One large Danish study showed that, of 166 cases of so-called idiopathic polyneuropathy, more than half were definitely or probably linked to statins.[42]

Although they've made a goodly number of people rich, what statins have singularly *failed* to do is solve the problem of heart disease. Although they seem to have some beneficial properties, these effects are modest compared to the growing evidence indicating their role in causing heart failure.

One of the few doctors brave enough to point the finger at statins is Dr Peter Lansjoen, a cardiologist from Tyler, Texas. Lansjoen has put together astonishing evidence that statins block coenzyme Q10, which is essential for the smooth running of the muscles of the heart. When this enzyme is deficient over the long term it can cause serious problems with heart rhythm and, eventually, heart failure.

According to Lansjoen, during his 17 years of practice as a cardiologist he has seen a 'frightening increase' in heart failure after statin usage. Currently he sees two or three new cases of what he calls 'statin cardiomy-opathy' (where the heart loses its ability to pump blood efficiently) every week. It is well known that patients taking statins lose coenzyme Q10 according to the dosage. The drugs block production of both cholesterol and CoQ10 by inhibiting the enzyme precursor of not only cholesterol, but also of CoQ10.

CoQ10 helps in chemical reactions, particularly those involving cellu-lar energy production, and helps make cell membranes stronger against oxygen damage. It is abundant in the heart largely because of the huge energy requirements of those cells.

Studies have shown that a deficiency of CoQ10 is linked with heart failure[43] and impaired heart function.[44]

Out of 15 published studies, nine have confirmed that statins can significantly lower CoQ10 levels.[45]

Critics believe that widespread statin use has caused a surge in cases of statin cardiomyopathy, or disturbance of heart rhythm, leading to irregular heartbeats. Drug manufacturers tacitly acknowledge this effect in the several drug formulations that offer a statin combined with CoQ10.

Another problem with blocking CoQ10 is that it interferes with the brain's performance, causing memory loss and muddled thinking. In an elderly person, this kind of side-effect is almost invariably passed off as age-related dementia, requiring yet another coterie of wonder drugs.

Heart failure has surged to epidemic proportions in Western countries during the 15 years of statin use. In the US alone, 4.8 million Americans are diagnosed with the condition, and half of them will die within five years. This represents a doubling of cases and a fourfold increase in heart-disease-related deaths in the US.

A Violent End

The biggest problem with cholesterol lowering is that patients on cholesterol-lowering programmes may be more likely to die from other causes. In the early nineties a number of large-scale studies began appearing which showed that patients on cholesterol diets or drugs were more likely to die from violent deaths, including suicide, than those eating what they wanted.[46] This bizarre connection was dismissed as a quirk – until it was confirmed by a number of subsequent international studies.

Research from Italy has confirmed that low cholesterol levels indeed tend to make people suicidal. Researchers from Corso studied the blood levels of 300 people who'd attempted suicide, against an identical number who hadn't ever tried to harm themselves. In virtually all cases, the suicide group had lower levels of cholesterol close to the time they tried to kill themselves.[47]

Cholesterol drugs, or even a very low-fat diet, may contribute to a decrease in serotonin, a brain hormone which normally keeps harmful impulses, such as aggressive behaviour, in check. In animal studies, mice with lowered cholesterol levels also showed a decrease in the number of serotonin receptors in their brains.[48] One effect of the new class of selective serotonin re-uptake inhibitor (SSRI) anti-depressants, such as fluoxetine (Prozac), is to block serotonin from reaching certain cells in the nervous system. Numerous instances of violent or suicidal tendencies have been reported among patients taking these drugs. One study in a geriatric unit in Italy found that among older people, the risk of depression was highest among those with the lowest blood concentration.[49]

Researchers from the University of California at San Diego have their own theory about the link between low cholesterol and violent death. The California researchers found that depression was three times more common in those with low blood cholesterol than in those with higher levels in those over 70. What's more, they also found that the extent of depression correlated with the level of cholesterol: the lower the cholesterol, the more depressed the patient.[50] This problem may only occur in older people, since there has never been any evidence of a relationship among younger people between violence and drugs taken to control cholesterol levels. We do have some evidence that people on weight-loss programmes have significantly reduced levels of tryptophan in their blood. Women also placed on very low-fat diets have lower levels of tryptophan and a significant change in their levels of serotonin.[51] Tryptophan, an essential amino acid, is what serotonin is mainly derived from, and we get tryptophan from certain foods, mainly proteins, and dietary supplements. When the diets of several countries are compared, those with low trypto-phan intake have a higher rate of suicide. We also have evidence that patients suffering from severe depression have low levels of tryptophan, and get worse if they are put on low-tryptophan diets. As their depression improves, so do their levels of tryptophan.[52]

Other evidence has shown a greater risk of suicide, the higher the level of cholesterol,[53] and one overview trial failed to find an association.[54] However, the answer may lie in changes in our diet over the last century, which have altered the ratio of the two classes of essential fatty acids, with a decrease in omega-3 fatty acids, such as are found in fatty fish and flaxseed oil. When this ratio is altered (as it would be for either a high- or low-fat diet), patients have been shown to have increased levels of depres-sion.[55]

Whatever the association, it's obvious that medicine doesn't yet under-stand the delicate interrelation of hormonal messages that the brain receives, nor the dietary requirements necessary to sustain them. By some well-intended fiddling here and there, it could be creating a good deal more havoc than the very worst Western diet.

The latest suspicion is that cholesterol-lowering drugs may cause cancer with long-term use. Cholesterol policy expert Dr Thomas Newman of the University of California at San Francisco, and his colleague Dr Stephen Hulley, analysed the data published in the American drug reference bible, the *Physician's Desk Reference*, plus population studies of cancer and cholesterol levels and clinical trials of cholesterol lowering to discover a definite link between some of the popular cholesterol-lowering drugs and a risk of cancer. Tests carried out on rodents clearly show the carcinogenic effects of the drugs, especially if taken over the long term. Drs Newman and Hulley suggest that the levels of statin cholesterol-lowering drugs being taken by humans are close to the levels that have proved carcinogenic in these experimental animals.[56] In Britain, gemfi-brozil, marketed as Lopid, has been linked to tumour growth in mice and rats, but only when the animals have been given 10 times the recommended dose per day. Although other drugs have been shown to cause cancer in animals without posing a threat to humans, Newman and Hulley argue that the human exposure to cholesterol-lowering drugs is much closer to the dose that causes cancer in rodents. The UK's drugs reference guide, the *ABPI Data Sheet Compendium*, reports a 'significant increase' in liver cancer in rats given the overdose. Since approval, several cholesterol-lowering drugs have been associated with lung, thyroid, testis and lymph node cancers.[57]

The scientists note that the drugs were approved by the US Food and Drug Administration on the basis of less than 10 years' clinical trials. The full effects of the drugs may not become clear for 30 years, particularly as many people are now being encouraged to take the drugs for many decades.

The carcinogenic potential of two of the drugs, lovastatin and gemfibrozil, were discussed in a drugs advisory committee meeting of the FDA. The drug manufacturer representative of lovastatin 'downplayed the importance of the studies', the California researchers maintain. The data were also prepared in milligrams per kilogram of body weight, which may have confused the committee.

Even though they approved the drug, the FDA committee appears to have had reservations. Their original recommendation was that gemfibrozil should be used as a drug of last resort, only after exercise, diet and weight control have failed to lower cholesterol levels. The popularity of the drug since then suggests it has been far more widely used than the committee wanted.

In the CARE study there was a significant increase in breast cancer among those taking statins.[58]

DIETS FOR HEART DISEASE

There are dietary measures which have been shown to reverse heart disease, but they are more complex than those which simply lower fat. To determine whether comprehensive lifestyle changes might affect coronary atherosclerosis, a group of patients embarked on a low-fat vegetarian diet, stopped smoking, trained in stress management and engaged in a moderate exercise. They were compared with another group with similar clogged arteries who did not undergo the special lifestyle modifications. After a year, the vegetarian group's coronary arteries had widened by 3 per cent, while the control group's had narrowed by 4 per cent. In all, 82 per cent of the experimental group had shown improvement, demonstrating that a comprehensive lifestyle change could reverse even severe coronary athero-sclerosis without drugs after only one year.[59] A more recent study measuring coronary arteries with a special CT scanning showed that disease was reversed in 99 per cent of patients over five years.[60]

In another study, patients given a cholesterol-lowering diet alone also were able to reverse coronary artery disease – nearly as much as those given a diet and drugs.[61] And women runners were found to have higher levels of high-density lipoprotein (HDL – the 'good' cholesterol needed by our bodies which appears to protect against heart disease), the more they exercised.[62] Giving up smoking, which appears to exacerbate the vascular abnormalities of people with high blood cholesterol, is possibly one of the most meaningful lifestyle changes you can make.[63]

But perhaps the most interesting connection occurs between 'good' and 'bad' carbohydrates. London researchers from Hammersmith Hospital have discovered that eating carbohydrates with a high glycaemic index (a number is assigned to foods based on how they affect blood sugar levels) decreases levels of HDL (high-density lipoprotein) cholesterol, the 'good' cholesterol which protects against cardiovascular disease.[64] Dr Michel Montignac, one of the pioneers of the low-GI diet, has found that the cholesterol levels of many of his patients normalize once they follow a diet with lower GI carbohydrates.[65]

Margarine and Other Plastic Food

Patients on low-fat diets often consume specially processed low-fat foods, which may themselves contribute to disease. Most processed and low-fat foods are deficient in essential fatty acids; the usual effect of consuming them is to set up an imbalance in our bodies, which lowers the 'good' cholesterol and increases the 'bad' cholesterol.[66]

One of the most dangerous of these low-fat foods appears to be margarine, made from hydrogenated oils. This is performed by heating up the oil to a high temperature and sending hydrogen through it.

Hydrogenation began after 1912, so that polyunsaturated fats could compete with butter and lard. During hydrogenation, trans fatty acids are produced; these artificial unsaturated fatty acids have a different molecular structure to those found in the tissues of humans and other mammals. This production process, used in the manufacture of margarine, creates 'trans isomers' of fatty acids, which resemble the chemical configuration of saturated fat.[67]

The amounts of trans fatty acids (TFAs) in processed foods can range from 5 per cent to 75 per cent of the total fat; neither US nor British law requires manufacturers to state the amount of hydrogenated fat in a product, only whether or not it is present at all.[68] TFAs can have a 'disastrous' effect on your body's ability to use essential fatty acids, says nutritional expert Dr Leo Galland, author of *Superimmunity for Kids* (E. P. Dutton). They are even worse when heated, turning into something akin to the polymers in plastic.

Hydrogenated fats are in fast foods such as chips and doughnuts, and in the vegetable oils contained in shortenings and biscuits. They account for up to 10 per cent of the content of some margarines. Other manufacturers, like Van den Berghs, the makers of Flora, have now removed hydrogenation entirely.

George V. Mann, a doctor from Nashville, Tennessee who has researched and written widely on the subject, argues that lipo-protein receptors in cells are impaired by TFAs. Since this impairment prevents the body from processing cholesterol-bearing low-density lipoproteins, the cells crank up their rate of synthesizing cholesterol, eventually leading to high levels in the blood. We know from numerous studies that blood cholesterol quickly increases in people fed TFAs.[69] Another study, this one by Harvard Medical School, of 85,000 women over eight years found that those eating margarine had an *increased* risk of coronary heart disease.

The more TFAs you eat (and are stored in body fat), the greater your apparent risk of heart disease. One Welsh study showed a strong association between TFA content in body fat and death from heart disease.[70]

Partially hydrogenated vegetable oils have not only failed to provide the expected benefits as a substitute for highly saturated fats but have 'contributed to the occurrence of coronary heart disease', the Harvard researchers concluded.[71]

Dr Mary Enig, formerly of the Department of Chemistry and Biochemistry at the University of Maryland, who analysed the trans fatty acid content of some 600 foods, reckons that Americans eat between 11 and 28 grams of trans fatty acids a day – or one-fifth of their total intake of fat. To give you some idea of how this happens, one large portion of chips cooked in partially hydrogenated oil contains 8 grams of trans fatty acids, as does 60 g of imitation cheese.[72] The Harvard study reckons that TFAs could account for 6 per cent of all deaths from heart disease, or 30,000 deaths a year in the US alone. And of course heart disease rates are high in northern European countries, where consumption of TFAs is high, and low in the Mediterranean countries, where the main dietary fat is olive oil and TFA intake is low.

An epidemic of heart disease can be directly linked to the introduction of partially hydrogenated fats in food, with the first major outbreak recorded in 1920. Before the First World War, when cheese and butter were staples of the diet, death from coronary thrombosis was rare. None the less, researchers consistently linked heart disease to animal fats, found in butter, giving margarine manufacturers the opportunity to claim their products were better for your heart.

The influential EURAMIC study, which covered eight European countries and Israel, suggested there is no conclusive evidence to show that margarine is linked to heart problems. But it did warn that there could be some connection in countries where there is a very high margarine intake.

The EURAMIC study based its findings on two groups of men – one with a serious heart condition and another without any history of heart problems. They discovered that both groups had similar levels of trans fatty acids in their tissues.[73]

There may also be another issue here. In Dr George V. Mann's studies of the African Maasai, young men consistently had low cholesterol concentrations, even though their diets were high in saturated fats, mainly from milk and beef. Dr Mann concluded that the Maasai, who got about 4–7 g a day of TFAs from cow's milk, were below the threshold at which the body's ability to metabolize fat starts to be impaired. In the US, the average daily intake of TFAs is 12–20 g daily. Or it may well be that the story is even more complicated than this. The Maasai could be protected because they eat their own native whole foods – albeit those containing saturated fats – and not the adulterated ones consumed by most people in the West.

THE TROUBLE WITH TODAY'S FOOD

The main reason that medicine is so befuddled about this entire cholesterol business is its insistence upon searching for – and isolating – a single, dietary risk factor. There is also great (and misplaced) interest in a piecemeal approach to nutrition – in the particular micronutrients which combat this or that disease. In taking this approach, medicine blinds itself to a couple of obvious differences between Westerners and all the more 'primitive' populations with low heart disease, including cultures such as the Eskimos, who thrive on a high-fat diet.

Numerous studies show that when more primitive populations begin to consume a Western diet, they start dying of heart attacks. But the main difference between what they're eating and what we're eating is not meat nor fats but *whole foods*. The culprit appears to be the large-scale adulterating, or 'dismembering', of everything we put in our mouths. This includes the massive addition of refined sugar, which increases blood fats and lowers the strength of the immune system.

In examining current 20th-century Western diets, Dr Stephen Davies, who pioneered nutritional medicine in Britain, points out that people haven't changed much over 40,000 years – but, at least here in the West, our diet has.[74] He quotes S. Boyd Eaton and Melvin Konner, writing about paleolithic nutrition in the *New England Journal of Medicine*: 'Even the development of agriculture 10,000 years ago has apparently had a minimal effect on our genes. Certain haemaglobinopathies and retention of intestinal lactase into adulthood are "recent" genetic evolutionary trends, but few other examples are known.'[75]

In other words, the business of food might be modern and industrial, but our stomachs are still in the hunting-and-gathering stage. At that time, we consumed 21 per cent of our total dietary energy from fats, 34 per cent from protein, and 45.7 g of fibre (with cholesterol intake a whopping 591 mg, compared to the usual recommendations these days of 300 mg). Today, the average UK male takes in 14.1 per cent of his dietary energy from protein and 37.6 per cent from fats, with only 390 mg of cholesterol and 24.9 g of fibre.

By modern-day dietary standards, cavemen should have been dropping like flies. But clearly fat is a very small part of the story. 'Intensive livestock farming of pigs and chickens in particular, where the animals are kept indoors in overcrowded conditions, is associated with nutrient deficiencies of these animals,' writes Stephen Davies. 'Food processing and refining techniques further compromise nutrient content, as do intensive farming techniques which result in soil demineralization. Agrichemicals and other environmental pollutants find their way in to the food chain, and further disrupt the nutrient value of the foods and stress our detoxification … mechanisms.'[76]

What Stephen Davies is saying is that many degenerative illnesses such as coronary heart disease could be, in large part, the failure of our bodies to catch up with the 20th century's virtual revolution in what constitutes 'food'. In other words, the culprit isn't necessarily cholesterol or any other single food, but the very means we now employ to grow, collect, sell and prepare what appears on the table. Think of the extraordinary demands placed on each of us by the wholesale stripping of vital nutrients from our food and the inclusion of thousands of strange new elements into our diets.

Today's meat business makes liberal use of steroids, antibiotics, tranquillizers and beta-blockers. Agrichemicals currently employ pesticides, herbicides, rodenticides, fungicides and nitrate fertilizers. Current food processing refines wheat and sugar, which reduces their trace mineral and vitamin content, as do current storage methods, food irradiation, and the addition of some 4,000 food additives, colourings, sweeteners, texture modifiers and preservatives.

Native Nutrition

Because most dietary recommendations are faddish, your safest bet is to follow some of the basic dietary principles shared by many healthy native populations. In his book *Native Nutrition: Eating According to Ancestral Wisdom* (Healing Arts Press), naturopath Ronald F. Schmid, examines studies of native populations by Dr Weston Price and Dr Francis M. Pottenger:

Eskimos of Alaska, the Swiss of the Loetschental Valley, Native Americans, Africans, and South Sea islanders. All these populations, which lived on fresh fruits and vegetables, grains, wild game and fish or healthy, free-roaming animals and, in some cases, fresh, unprocessed dairy products, were or are impressive for their strong, healthy bodies, straight perfect teeth and freedom from the degenerative diseases plaguing us nowadays in the West.

Although their diets varied enormously (the African Maasai mainly eat meat, milk and blood, while the traditional Maori of New Zealand eat fish, kelp and roots), they share certain basic similarities. According to American dietary expert Dr Annemarie Colbin in her excellent book *Food and Healing* (Ballantine), all these native diets have in common food that is fresh (or preserved naturally, whether smoked, dried or pickled); it is grown locally and organically, in season; and it is cooked by traditional methods.

Whenever possible, eat fresh whole foods and eschew packaged and processed foods, anything that has been added to, refined, enriched or in some way interfered with. This would include most processed baked goods, canned sauces, commercial peanut butter, sweets, 'cheese' foods, crisps and corn chips. Especially steer clear of anything such as margarines whose labels list non-foods such as partially hydrogenated vegetable oils. There is no health reason to cut out or limit eggs (so long as they are free-range), which are an excellent source of protein. Otherwise, eat a wide variety of foods, sort out your food allergies beforehand, and cut down on animal fats as the centrepiece of your meals. In general, most European oils are less refined than those produced in the US. In fact, the safest course is to cook with extra virgin olive oil that is still made by traditional methods.

Stay Connected

A little-known study of Japanese immigrants living in the US and the effect of this move on their risk of heart attacks sheds light on the importance of emotional connection in preventing heart disease. Earlier studies of native populations who move to America show that healthy people start developing heart disease as soon as they emigrate to the US. The assumption has always been that the killer is the American diet.

What this British study suggests, however, is that the cause of heart disease is the American *lifestyle*, more than its food. Those Japanese who kept their traditional cultural ways had far less heart disease, even on a diet of American fries and Burger King. The Japanese who were more prone to develop heart disease might have strictly adhered to the Japanese low-fat diet, but they bought the American way of life, lock, stock and barrel. They'd given up their community life, which was rich in connections, shared goals and values, for an upwardly-mobile, success-orientated and ultimately isolated life.[77]

This accords with another study of Roseto, an Italian-American community in Pennsylvania. Roseto had virtually no heart disease despite a high-fat diet and high rate of smoking among its citizenry – until the community abandoned its closeknit, traditional ways in favour of the modern-day 'every man for himself'.[78] Studies have shown that people who are lonely and isolated socially are two to three times more likely to die from heart disease, even with a perfect diet, than those who eat all the wrong things but stay close and connected to others.[79]

Heart disease may be primarily a spiritual issue, a crisis of isolation, of unresolved pain. To die of heart disease is literally to die of a broken heart.

This, of course, presents much more of a challenge for us in attempting to fend off heart disease. Instead of simply moderating our diet, we have also to examine our lives. Most of all, in order to live free of heart disease, it seems now vital for us to connect.

6

Vaccination:
Knee-jerk Jabs

Josie McNally thought she was doing right by her baby son, William. He was a healthy, normal, happy 13-month-old and she wanted to make sure to keep him that way. When her doctor recommended that he come in for his routine measles/mumps/rubella (MMR) jab to protect against these dangerous diseases, Josie thought nothing of it; William had sailed through his infant jabs and, besides, the doctor knew best.

Ten days after William's shot, something turned horribly wrong. William began convulsing and Josie and her husband had to rush him by ambulance to hospital. When Josie suggested her son might be reacting to the vaccination, the doctor shook his head. The fit coming after the shot could be nothing more than coincidence; it probably wouldn't recur. The hospital consultant agreed; the shot appeared to have nothing to do with it.

But the fits didn't stop, and before long William became gripped by seizures, sometimes 40 a day. He also developed a rare immune-system reaction. Now 13 years old, he's diagnosed as epileptic, continues to have convulsions uncontrollable by medication, and has the developmental age of a 14-month-old baby – as if his developmental clock stopped on the day he was vaccinated. And not long after he was given it, the vaccine William had was withdrawn. Nevertheless, to this day no one in the medical profession will officially acknowledge the vaccine had anything to do with it. The McNally family has been given no financial assistance by any government body for the considerable medical bills they will face during William's lifetime.

Most doctors fervently believe that vaccines are one of medical science's greatest success stories, responsible for wiping out many deadly infectious diseases. In fact, lurking inside most doctors is an altruist who likes to think that the eradication of disease is not only possible but just around the corner. Every so often, the World Health Organization will announce an actual date when it fully expects that diseases such as polio, measles or diphtheria will be wiped off the planet for ever.

The ardency of this faith has emboldened the profession to produce ever more shots to combat not only major killers such as polio but also a number of the mostly benign co-passengers of childhood, such as measles, mumps and chickenpox. Counting all multiple boosters in the entire suggested schedule, American children can receive some 34 vaccinations by the time they go to school, most in the first year of life; Britain, with its tuberculosis vaccine offered at birth but no hepatitis B or chickenpox vaccine, ends up with a slightly more modest 25. The US government and the World Health Organization have even sponsored the development of what they imagine will turn out to be a genetically-engineered, time-released 'Holy Grail', a supervaccine containing the raw DNA of up to 40 different diseases at one go, which will be squirted into a newborn's mouth at birth and send out booster doses at timed intervals throughout an individual's life.[1] There have been vaccines being worked on for asthma, earaches and respiratory diseases, AIDS, cancer, and even to prevent pregnancy.

It is with vaccines that the brave-new-world technocrats of medicine have lost all reason about disease and its prevention. So steadfast is this faith in the rightness of their cause that it prevents doctors from acknowledging clear factual evidence demonstrating the dangers and ineffectiveness of certain vaccines, or even cases of a disease in children who have been vaccinated against it. It also turns otherwise reasonable doctors or scientists into bullies and hysterics, shouting down dissenters, using emotional blackmail to bully parents into submission and resorting to emotive appeals, rather than common sense or fact, to argue their point of view. To launch its countrywide campaign to vaccinate school-age children against measles and rubella, the British government once ran stark, emotive black-and-white television adverts suggesting that measles strikes fatally and at random. In the US, parents have been threatened with the withholding of welfare payments if they fail to give their kids the live triple measles/mumps/rubella vaccine. Chicago health authorities once tried to give vaccination a bit of street cred by employing loudspeaker sales pitches mixed in with salsa music to encourage mothers in Hispanic neighbourhoods to bring their children in to get their shots.

In one UK campaign to inoculate all British children from 5 to 16 with the measles/rubella jab, parents were given flimsy pamphlets with virtually no mention of the side-effects long accepted by international governmental bodies. Doctors and health authorities badgered parents who'd decided against the jab with letters and phone calls to try and change their mind. And all sorts of medical experts were confidently announcing publicly that this campaign would undoubtedly eradicate measles from these shores for all time.

Britain's Department of Health pressed ahead with one of the most ambitious immunization campaigns ever seen in an industrialized country, informing parents that side-effects to booster jabs are very unlikely, having been 'carefully studied by looking at large numbers of children in the United States'.[2] In fact, the evidence on which this claim was based was rather more meagre. Before the campaign they received a fax from the US American National Immunization Program officials explaining that the only evidence that boosters were safer was based on questionnaires sent to college students receiving the shots. Medical scientists consider this type of study a highly unreliable and unscientific measure of safety and effectiveness. The real safety of reactions or boosters jabs was not yet known as the trial testing had not yet been completed.

What's worse, the UK's Public Health Laboratory Service completed a study before the campaign began, demonstrating that children given the measles/mumps/rubella jab were three times more likely to suffer from convulsions than those who didn't receive it. Two-thirds of the cases of seizures were due to the measles component alone. The study also found that the MMR vaccine caused five times the number of cases of a rare blood disorder over that expected. This study was never mentioned during the campaign, but was only published in the medical literature, and not until four months after the campaign was completed.[3]

More recently, the British government rushed through a brand-new, as yet untested vaccine for meningitis C, offering it to every child and college student in Britain on the basis of short-term tests, lasting at most a few weeks. Although a fifth of the children in one of the British tests was ill,[4] this material was never made available to parents consenting to expose their children to the jab.

Because vaccines represent the very epitome of modern medicine – the triumph of science over nature – scientific trials are most subject to medical spin-doctoring in order to paint a positive face on a negative result, ignoring any results they don't wish to hear. In America, the US government requested that the National Academy of Science review all the medical literature and report fully on what were the known and proven dangers, if any, of the various childhood vaccines. In two separate reports the NAS's Institute of Medicine, which gathered together leading paediatricians and medical scientists for the task, concluded that all nine vaccines had the potential to do serious harm. Although these conclusions were eventually included in lengthy fact sheets given to parents prior to their children's vaccinations, the National Commission on Childhood Vaccines pushed to have them edited, on the grounds that they 'confuse' parents.

In Britain, the Department of Health commissioned a report on the whooping cough vaccine by Professor Gordon Stewart, formerly of the Department of Community Medicine at the University of Glasgow and an advisor to the World Health Organization, who has long studied the vaccine. When his studies showed the risks of the vaccine outweighed the benefits, the DHSS referred the report to the Committee on the Safety of Medicines, which chose not to act on it.[5]

In this zealous climate, amid the rush to 'conquer' every possible disease, in which entire reputations rest on defending vaccination at all costs, no one is pausing to examine the possible long-term effects of pumping up to 12 or more different antigens into the immature immune systems of a generation of babies under 15 months. Including the meningitis C vaccine on the standard schedule of infant vaccinations now increases to six the number of vaccines given simultaneously to infants at two months of age.

Epidemiologists have never investigated whether there is an upper limit to the number of jabs a baby can tolerate, after which all sorts of subtle damage – asthma, learning disabilities, hyperactivity or chronic earache, for instance – come into play. *In fact, nobody has done any long-term safety studies at all.* 'We only hear about the encephalitis and the deaths,' says Dr J. Anthony Morris, formerly a director of virology at the Food and Drug Administration and the National Institutes of Health. 'But there is an entire spectrum of reactions between fever and death, and it's all those things in between that never get reported.'[6]

At the heart of the logic behind vaccination is the theory of herd immunity – that is, if enough people get vaccinated against a certain disease, it will eventually disappear. Besides an element of wishful thinking in the face of highly complex organisms such as viruses, which constantly mutate and change, the problem with this line of reasoning, of course, is its tyrannical approach: eliminating a disease is more important, in the eyes of medicine, than your child's health, which might be damaged from a vaccine, or your right to decide what is best for your family. Decide against vaccination for your child and you are considered not only an irresponsible parent but an irresponsible citizen of your community and even the world. In Britain, vaccinating your child is often a requirement for staying on your GP's list (he is paid a bonus of nearly £3,000 at this writing if 90 per cent of the children under two on his books get done. If only 70 per cent are vaccinated, that bonus shrinks to £910; any smaller percentage means he gets only a fraction of the total amount.). In the US, in the wake of the Clinton Administration's Childhood Vaccine Act it is now even more difficult for parents to get exempted from vaccinating their children.

But in Britain we still have a modicum of choice. In many countries all children are obliged to be vaccinated in order to get into school – a policy, particularly in places such as the US, that would seem to fly in the face of a number of constitutional freedoms. In this hysterical climate, the government and the medical community have made it their right to insist on administering a substance to a minor which it cannot guarantee is safe – a right no one has yet attempted to challenge in court.

A BLUNT INSTRUMENT

Vaccination is a blunt and highly imperfect instrument. The main problem isn't so much that vaccines don't work, but that they work haphazardly.

The premise of vaccination rests on the assumption that injecting an individual with weakened live or killed virus will 'trick' his body into developing antibodies to the disease, as it does when it contracts an illness naturally. But medicine doesn't really know whether vaccines work for any length of time. All that the usual scientific studies can demonstrate (as they are only conducted over the short term) is that vaccines may create antibodies in the blood. What may happen is that a number of vaccines are capable of measurably raising antibodies to a particular infectious illness, but only for a short period of time. Or even if they do raise antibodies indefinitely, this may have nothing to do with protecting an individual from contracting the disease over the long (or even the short) term. In fact, having antibodies in the blood may not be the only way the body recognizes and defends itself from disease. For instance, large numbers of people who have had illnesses such as diphtheria never produce antibodies to the disease.

In one report, for instance, measles antibodies were found in the blood of only one of seven vaccinated children who'd gone on to develop measles – they hadn't developed antibodies from either the shot or the disease itself.[7] And lately, the Public Health Laboratory in London has discovered that a quarter of blood donors between 20 and 29 had insufficient immunity to diphtheria, even though most would have been vaccinated as babies. This percentage doubled among the 50-to-59 age group.[8]

Live vaccines are made from live pathogens that are attenuated (weakened) so that they won't cause symptoms of the full disease when administered. This is accomplished supposedly by sending these pathogens through a rather mystifying process called 'serial passage', in which the viral strain is passed through up to 50 animal cells on the assumption that this will weaken them.

Not only the process but also the cells selected appear a bizarre and arbitrary choice. The polio vaccine has been passed through monkey kidney cells, the measles vaccine through chick embryo cells, rubella virus through rabbit or duck cells, and yellow fever through mice and chick embryo cells. Human cells have also been used: rubella was once grown on the tissue of aborted foetuses, and hepatitis B at one time was made from the blood of homosexual men who'd had the disease. Of course, this passage through animal and human cells invites infection or contamination with other substances, as happened with contaminated polio vaccines.

Among the childhood vaccines, the live vaccines include the tuberculosis (BCG), measles-mumps-rubella (MMR), the oral polio vaccine and the chickenpox vaccine. Many vaccines are made with live antigens because the killed versions haven't worked. The main concern with live vaccines is that the disease the vaccine is supposedly protecting against has a small chance of reproducing and spreading in the recipient.

Killed vaccines are made of components of the disease – whole cells, toxins, synthesized molecules, for instance – that have been rendered inactive with heat, radiation or chemicals. The Salk polio jab, the diphtheria-whooping cough (pertussis)-tetanus (DPT), hepatitis B and *Haemophilus influenzae b* (Hib) meningitis are all among the most common killed vaccines.

The killed vaccine is supposed to preclude the possibility of the antigen being reproduced in the person receiving the vaccination – it is simply supposed to stimulate the circulation of antibodies to the antigen through the body. However, it's not quite as clear-cut as this – serious problems with killed vaccines have defied their supposed inability to reproduce in the recipient.

MYTH NO 1: DISEASES HAVE BEEN ELIMINATED PURELY AS A RESULT OF VACCINATION

The success of vaccination is based entirely on assumption. Because the incidence and death rate of many infectious diseases have radically declined, with improved sanitation and hygiene, housing, better nutrition and isolation procedures, at coincidentally the same time that vaccines have been introduced, medicine has assumed that vaccination is entirely responsible for the eradication of these diseases. Many medical textbooks lead off with the boast that one of medicine's great achievements is the eradication of smallpox through vaccination. However, if you actually examine the epidemiological statistics, you discover that between 1870 and 1872, 18 years after compulsory vaccination was introduced, four years after a coercive four-year effort to vaccinate all members of the population was in place (with stiff penalties for offenders), and at the point where 97.5 per cent of the population had been vaccinated, England experienced the worst smallpox epidemic of the century, which claimed more than 44,000 lives. In fact, three times as many people died from smallpox at that time as had in an earlier epidemic, when fewer people were vaccinated.

After 1871, the town of Leicester refused vaccination, largely because the high incidence of smallpox and death rates during the 1870 epidemic convinced the population it didn't work. In the next epidemic of 1892, Leicester relied solely on improved sanitation and quarantines. The town only suffered 19 cases and 1 death per 100,000 population, compared with the town of Warrington, which had six times the number of cases and 11 times the death rate of Leicester, even though 99 per cent of its population had been vaccinated.[9]

The World Health Organization has pointed out that the key to eradication of the disease in many parts of West and Central Africa was switching from mass immunization, which was not working very well, to a campaign of surveillance, containing the disease through isolation procedures.[10]

Sierra Leone's experience also demonstrates that vaccination wasn't responsible for the end of smallpox. In the late sixties, Sierra Leone had the highest rate of smallpox in the world. In January 1968 the country began its eradication campaign, and three of the four largest outbreaks were controlled by identifying and isolating cases alone, without immunization. Fifteen months later, the area recorded its last case of smallpox.[11]

Polio

More than any other, the polio vaccine is pointed to with pride by every government as definitive proof that mass vaccination programmes work. The US government is quick to note that during the plague years of polio, 20,000–30,000 cases per year occurred in America, compared to 20–30 cases a year today. Nevertheless, Dr Bernard Greenberg, head of the Department of Biostatistics at the University of North Carolina School of Public Health, has gone on record to say that cases of polio *increased* by 50 per cent between 1957 and 1958, and by 80 per cent from 1958 to 1959, after the introduction of mass immunization.[12] In five New England States – Massachusetts, Connecticut, New Hampshire, Rhode Island, and Vermont – cases of polio roughly doubled in 1954 and 1955, after the polio vaccine was introduced.[13] Nevertheless, in the midst of the polio panic of the 1950s, with the pressure on to find a magic bullet, statistics were manipulated by health authorities to give the opposite impression.

One such way was to give the old disease a new name – 'viral or aseptic meningitis' or 'cocksackie virus'. According to statistics from the Los Angeles County Health Index, for instance, in July 1955 there were 273 reported cases of polio and 50 cases of aseptic meningitis, compared with five cases of polio and 256 cases of aseptic meningitis a decade later.[14]

In the early part of the last century, over 3,000 deaths were attributed to 'chickenpox', and only some 500 to smallpox, even though authorities agree that chickenpox is only very rarely a fatal disease.[15]

Martha, from Sheffield, recently experienced this sort of fast-shuffle name-change with whooping cough:

Not long ago, after our two year old developed full-blown whooping cough, I took her to our GP, prepared to face a reprimand for neglecting to have her vaccinated. However, the doctor diagnosed asthma and prescribed Ventolin. I was so unconvinced by this diagnosis that I consulted another GP within the practice. To my amazement he insisted that whooping cough no longer exists (due to mass vaccination) and confirmed the diagnosis of asthma. I then pressed for a sputum test to prove or disprove the existence of whooping cough.

I later received a patronizing phone call, following my doctor's discussion with our local consultant microbiologist. 'They do not test for whooping cough because it does not exist', I was told. I then asked, should the condition clear up in a few weeks, presumably asthma would have been an unlikely diagnosis? To which he replied: 'We now have a new condition called viral asthma which is similar to whooping cough'. He said they see many children with this condition. He added, 'Since they stopped testing for whooping cough there have been no recorded cases in our area.'

Diseases such as polio operate cyclically. The great polio epidemics occurred in the 1910s, the 1930s and the 1950s; then cases sharply dropped off down to nearly zero. But at the height of the fifties epidemics, after the vaccine was introduced, as author Welene James says, quoting another writer, 'the vaccine took the credit instead of nature.'[16] American

125

medical critic Dr Robert Mendelsohn once noted: 'Diseases are like fashion, they come and go.'[17] Many vaccine programmes claim the credit for what is simply the tendency of illnesses to wax and wane. Far from science having anything to do with finally stamping out polio or tuberculosis, both diseases decided, a number of years ago, to take a breather and are now making a comeback – tuberculosis in many Western countries, polio in many parts of Canada, and diphtheria in Russia and the East.

Tetanus, Diphtheria and Whooping Cough

The incidence and number of deaths from diphtheria were declining long before the vaccine was introduced, as they were from tetanus, largely because of increased attention to wound hygiene.[18] Among all the soldiers of the Second World War, only 12 cases of tetanus were recorded – a third of which occurred among soldiers who were vaccinated.[19] The great decline in deaths from whooping cough (some 80 per cent) occurred *before* the vaccine was introduced.[20]

Measles

A similar pattern occurred with measles. The death rate from measles plummeted to greater than a 95 per cent decline (to .03 deaths per 100,000) 20 years before the vaccine was introduced.[21]

Nevertheless, in the late 1990s, despite the fact that the UK had the triple measles/mumps/rubella vaccine in place since 1988, and enjoyed an extraordinarily high coverage of vaccination among toddlers, cases of measles went up – by nearly one-fourth.[22]

In the 1990s, the US suffered from a steadily increasing epidemic of measles – the worst for decades – despite the fact that the measles vaccine in its various forms has been in effect since 1957, and the combined shot since 1975. Although the government targeted 1982 as the date of the virtual elimination of the disease, the Centers for Disease Control (CDC) in Atlanta reported a provisional total of 27,672 cases of measles in 1990, which represents a virtual doubling of reported cases in 1989, which were double the number of cases reported in the year before *that*.

Although the number of measles cases fell by one quarter (to 63,000) the year the vaccine was introduced, and bottomed out at 1,500 reported cases in 1983, the numbers suddenly swelled by 423 per cent at the end of the 1980s and then rose sharply, with the worst-hit areas of the US being Houston and Los Angeles County.

After the great resurgence of measles during 1989–91, cases of measles began to drop drastically. The Centers for Disease Control attributed this to the tremendous push given the measles and combined vaccines at the height of the epidemic; vaccine coverage increased from an average of 66 per cent in the years before 1985 to 78 per cent in 1991.

However, a few statistics confuse this optimistic assumption. First of all, the CDC estimates that, based on retrospective surveys of coverage, approximately 800,000 to two million babies and toddlers who hadn't got their shots should have been susceptible to measles. In reality, however, only 9,300 cases were reported among this age group in 1992. Although the average age of children catching measles dropped (from a median age of 12 in 1989, at the beginning of the epidemic, to an average afterwards of 4.9), nearly half of all reported cases were still among children over 5 – most of whom should have been protected.

The CDC admitted that the sudden drop in cases could have something to do with 'an overall decrease in the occurrence of measles in the Western Hemisphere'. It also may have something to do, they say, with the cyclical nature of the disease.

Hib Meningitis

The UK Government boasts that *Haemophilus influenzae b* (Hib) meningitis has been eliminated, largely due to the jab, introduced in the UK in 1992. This form of bacterial meningitis, caused by the *haemophilus influenzae type b* bacteria, mainly strikes preschoolers, with the peak incidence between six and 15 months of age. The jab was supposed to combat the most common cause of meningitis in children under five. Nevertheless, a pro-vaccine study group extolling the virtues of the Hib vaccine conceded that a 'substantial' fall also occurred in children who hadn't been vaccinated – from 99.3 to 68.5 per 100,000.[23] Furthermore, many of the only cases of Hib meningitis occur among those who have been vaccinated.[24]

MYTH NO 2: THE DISEASES YOU ARE VACCINATED AGAINST ARE DEADLY

Increasingly, the rationale for vaccination has shifted from control of deadly disease to control of nuisance diseases such as mumps or chicken-pox. In fact, a large number of the illnesses we now vaccinate against are no longer life-threatening in well-nourished children with healthy immune systems.

Measles

The zeal behind the various measles campaigns is founded on the belief that measles can be a life-threatening condition, and it seems to be one that is getting more dangerous by the year. When the Department of Health ran one of its major vaccine drives in 1989, Dr Norman Begg, consultant epidemiologist of the Public Health Laboratory Service, cited the then-official statistics that one in 5,000 children contracting measles will develop acute encephalitis, an inflammation of the brain, and one in 5,000 of those will develop SSPE (subacute sclerosing panencephalitis), an almost inevitably fatal progressive disease which causes hardening of the brain.[25]

Five years later, when one columnist encouraged parents to have their children re-vaccinated in the countrywide measles campaign, the percent-age of measles victims who might go on to develop encephalitis had shrunk to one in every 500. One in 10 of these would die and one in four would suffer permanent brain damage, the columnist maintained. As the campaign intensified, other newspapers had magnified the danger even further. By November it seemed that one out of every 17 cases of measles would turn into a case of encephalitis.

But the report of the journal geared specifically for the study of the fatal illness being worried over, the SSPE Registry, concluded that the measles-induced form of this disease is 'very rare', occurring in 1 per million cases.[26] This rare disease also doesn't appear to be so random. A study of people with SSPE concluded that environmental factors other than measles, such as serious head injuries or exposure to certain animals, played an important part in the onset of the disease.[27]

Measles can be a killer, but it doesn't strike as randomly as medicine would have us believe. In the US in 1990, at the height of a measles epidemic when 27,000 cases were reported, 89 died. But many deaths occurred among children of low-income families, where poor nutrition played a part, as did failure to treat complications. In Africa, where children are markedly deficient in vitamin A, measles does kill. However, as study after study demonstrates, even third-world children with adequate stores of vitamin A or those given vitamin A supplements are overwhelmingly likely to survive.[28]

Death due to measles is not common in developed countries. The year before the MMR vaccine was launched there were six such deaths in the UK, even though there were 42,165 reported cases of the disease.

Furthermore, in the five years between 1989 and 1994 there were only six deaths among children aged 0–19, even though there was a total of 59,263 cases of measles during this time – an average of one death a year. This represents an incidence of approximately one death for every 10,000 cases, which is almost half the incidence during 1979–1983, when 83 children died out of 467,732 cases of measles, or about one death for every 5,600 cases.

However, this lowered death rate doesn't have any bearing on the vaccine, according to Dr Richard Nicolson, editor of the *Bulletin of Medical Ethics*, but reflects the fact that doctors better understand how to treat measles. Since 1988 most deaths have occurred among adults although, again, there are only a handful every year. In Japan, most measles deaths have occurred in babies too young to be given the jab.

Norman Begg has written that deaths from measles are 'directly related to poor vaccine coverage'. In Italy there were only 10 deaths from measles between 1989–1991, even though they had only a 40 per cent coverage from the vaccine. In the following two years, coverage from the vaccine grew but deaths nearly tripled to 28, suggesting that vaccine coverage had absolutely no bearing on numbers of deaths.[29]

Mumps

Whatever the present party line, mumps has never been considered a global killer. The vaccine was only developed because of the rare complications of mumps: orchitis (testicular inflammation), aseptic meningitis, encephalitis and deafness. Children who get mumps usually suffer a swelling underneath the ear, headache, fever, vomiting and muscle aches. Besides the testicles, the female ovaries and breasts can also swell. Symptoms are usually gone in less than a week, although they may last for up to 10 days.

Whooping Cough

As WHO advisor Dr Stewart has written: 'The lesson of history – not just medical history – is that infectious diseases change in pattern, severity and frequency through time. Whooping cough was once a serious threat to life and health in all young children. Now it is no longer so, though it is often a distressing disease and dangerous in some infants.'[30]

During the whooping cough outbreaks of 1978–9 in Glamorgan, Glasgow and Surrey, in 'low-risk' areas – that is, areas of adequate nutrition – there were no cases of permanent brain damage or death among any children, nor among any babies (who are considered most at risk).[31]

Polio

Even polio is not the virulent mass killer it is always made out to be. Largely because of the 1950s epidemic (following four terms of the most highly publicized victim, US President Franklin D. Roosevelt), polio is popularly thought to cut down healthy young people at random. In fact, most cases of polio are harmless infections. The current statistics estimate that only 10 per cent of people exposed to polio will contract it, and only 1 per cent of those will come down with the paralytic variety – or 0.01 per cent of those exposed to the disease in the first place. Medical homoeopath and noted vaccine critic Dr Richard Moskowitz has termed the propensity of an individual to develop paralysis from this ordinarily harmless virus a 'special anatomical susceptibility'.[32]

Meningitis C

Although all British children now receive the meningitis C vaccine, rather than simply individual groups at high risk, children between five and fifteen are at virtually no risk of contracting meningitis C. In the five-year period between 1994 and 1999, before the vaccine was introduced, group C meningococcal disease killed approximately 20 babies under one, 21 babies aged one, 18 two-year-olds, approximately 15 three-year-olds, a handful of four-, five- and six-year-olds, and almost no other pre-adolescent children.

After babies are a year old they develop active immunity by being exposed to a non-pathogenic form of meningococcus.

Casualties do not pick up again until the age of 15 through 20, the so-called highest cluster. In this age category meningitis killed some 12 15-year-olds, approximately 30 16-year-olds, 12 17-year-olds, about 18 18-year-olds, about 18 19-year-olds, and 10 20-year-olds over five years. So, in total, the disease killed approximately 200 young children, or an average of 40 children a year (70 a year in 1999).

While no one wishes to denigrate the tragic loss of these lives, in strictly epidemiological terms the death rate of this form of meningitis is small potatoes. It rates well behind many accidents as conditions which account for appreciable numbers of childhood deaths. For instance, a baby is five times more likely to drown in his bathtub and 86 times more likely to die of cot death than to die from meningitis C. Six times as many children and young adults get knocked over and killed by cars than die of meningitis C. British traffic deaths of all varieties among children represent the highest fatalities among this age group in all of Europe, claiming the lives of 1,309 children and young adults every year – more than 32 times the rate of meningitis deaths.

As Heikki Peltola, professor of infectious diseases and paediatrician at the University of Helsinki and the Hospital for Children and Adolescents, comments, 'In no country is there an epidemic of this disease ... Generally speaking, the incidence of meningococcal disease is too low to indicate vaccinations for the whole population, or even children, but some risk groups and epidemics are important exceptions.' [33]

Furthermore, according to the Department of Health's own 'factsheet', group C meningococcal disease accounts for only 40 per cent of cases of meningitis contracted in Britain and elsewhere.

Although meningitis C is the major cause of meningococcal death among teenagers, the B version is far more deadly to babies and small children, representing at least two-thirds of all meningococcal deaths in this age group.

Nevertheless, says Wyeth, who developed the meningitis C vaccine, thus far producing a vaccine for the B strain has proved elusive.

Rubella

Rubella, like mumps, is a benign illness in children which appears not much worse than a case of flu. However, it can be dangerous to the developing foetus if a pregnant woman contracts the disease in the first trimester of pregnancy. In that case, her baby risks being born with congenital rubella syndrome, which can produce major birth defects including blindness, deafness and even limb defects.

Once again, medicine's solution to this small risk is to attempt to wipe out the illness altogether by vaccinating all children, male and female. Indeed, exposure to rubella may be less risky to pregnant women than first thought. In one study of 24 pregnant women who'd contracted rubella, as confirmed by a blood test, none of their babies were born with congenital defects.[34]

MYTH NO 3: VACCINES WILL PROTECT YOU AGAINST THESE DISEASES

The big argument put forth by apologists of vaccines, particularly of those vaccines known to have substantial side-effects (such as the jab for whooping cough) is that, imperfect as they may be, the benefits are worth the risk. The problem with this argument is that it assumes that vaccines actually work.

Whooping Cough

During outbreaks of whooping cough, half or more of the victims have already been fully vaccinated. Professor Stewart reported that, in a study of whooping cough cases for 1974 and 1978, and in 1974 in the US and Canada, a third to a half of all children who'd caught it had been fully vaccinated. When he studied close to 2,000 babies who'd got whooping cough, two-thirds of the time they'd caught it from their fully vaccinated siblings. To Dr Stewart's mind, 'no protection by vaccination is demonstrable in infants', despite the fact that this is the very population the vaccine aims to protect – the only lives usually threatened by a nasty but otherwise mostly benign disease.[35]

'The effect of the present vaccination programme is to leave the only high risk group, the infants, at risk of both the [side-effects of the] vaccine and the infection,' Dr Stewart concluded.[36]

In his view, the risk of a baby's contracting encephalitis with permanent brain damage as a result of whooping cough (1 in 38,000) is comparable to the risk of brain damage (1 in 25,000) after vaccination with the jab.[37]

During a nationwide American epidemic of whooping cough in 1993, a group of researchers from a children's hospital in Cincinnati, Ohio, discovered that the epidemic mainly occurred among children who had completed the full course of DPT vaccines.[38]

About 30 per cent of the children had hospital stays, although the epidemic did not claim any lives. As many of the children who contracted the disease were aged between 19 months and six years, and so would have been vaccinated relatively recently, even scientists have begun to agree that the whole-cell pertussis vaccine on offer doesn't offer long-term protection.

Doctors are fond of pointing out that when the whooping cough vaccine was discontinued in the early seventies in Britain for a time, the number of severe cases shot up. After a US documentary criticizing the DPT vaccine, the number of children being immunized fell. Health officials then claimed that cases of whooping cough rose as a result of vaccine levels falling.

But when former Food and Drug Administration virologist Dr J. Anthony Morris analysed 41 cases of so-called whooping cough, only five had true pertussis, and all those victims had been vaccinated. The same occurred in Wisconsin. Most of the patients didn't have whooping cough, but those who did had been vaccinated.[39]

In Britain, cases rose to 'almost unprecedented heights', wrote Professor Stewart, during the 1978–9 epidemic. This figure was also interpreted as having to do with the drop in vaccination following adverse publicity. But the number of cases reported increased in all age groups, even those for which a high percentage of immunization had been achieved.[40]

Even at the best of times, when the whooping cough vaccine does work, it has only been shown to be between 63 and 93 per cent effective

– an extraordinarily large potential difference.[41] The latest research from Sweden and Italy has shown that the vaccine is effective in just 48 per cent and 36 per cent of cases, respectively.[42] Despite take-up vaccination rates of 95 per cent or higher, whooping cough is resurfacing as an epidemic in many Western countries, particularly among very young babies.[43] In the US, whooping cough cases have more than trebled; in the UK, cases among children under a year old have increased by 29 per cent. This is despite the fact that the vaccine is touted as being 88 per cent effective among children 7–18 months old.[44]

The re-emergence of whooping cough in the US is hardly a new trend. After the vaccine was launched in the 1940s, cases of pertussis declined to an historic low in 1976. But, since the early 1980s, the incidence of whooping cough has increased cyclically, peaking every three to four years independently of vaccination.[45]

In November 2001, the UK Department of Health (DoH) modified its booster schedule to include another dose of the whooping cough vaccine after admitting that whooping cough is still a source of considerable illness and death among babies, who are catching whooping cough from their vaccinated older siblings or parents. This dose, given as a new 'acellular' version of the whooping cough vaccine (where the whooping cough toxin is inactivated by glutaraldehyde or hydrogen peroxide, or genetically modified – supposedly to make it safer) hasn't fared much better, either.

In Sweden, where it was tested on a group of infants, one fifth went on to develop whooping cough, even after they'd been given three shots. At best the vaccine was judged to work less than three-quarters of the time.[46] In the US, scientists working on the vaccine at the Mayo Clinic have explained that they don't really understand how much pertussin toxin is necessary to protect children; even those with high levels of antibodies in their blood seem to go on to get whooping cough.[47]

Tetanus and Diphtheria

The same seems to hold true for diphtheria and tetanus. A US-sponsored vaccine review has even concluded that the diphtheria vaccine 'is not as effective an immunizing agent as might be anticipated'.[48]

The effects of the diphtheria vaccine seem to wear off in adulthood. In London, a quarter of blood donors between the ages of 20 and 29 have been found to have insufficient immunity, while half of those between 50 and 59 have lost their immunity.[49] And in the new states of the former Soviet Union, the vaccine has not proved protective in curbing epidemics of diphtheria. More than 86 per cent of people given a combined diphtheria-tetanus jab went on to contract diphtheria a year after their first booster.[50]

As for tetanus, the US panel reviewing vaccines noted that the degree of potency of the vaccine 'can vary considerably from preparation to preparation'. The panel also concluded that, as the vaccine has been purified and made safer in order to prevent reaction to it, so its protective ability has diminished.[51]

Measles

The medical establishment has attempted to place the blame for the epidemic of measles that occurred at the end of the 20th century on clusters of the unvaccinated, particularly among poor, non-white populations – but the statistics again prove otherwise. According to the Government's own 1989 statistics, half the college-aged victims had been previously vaccinated. And between 1985 and 1986, more than three-quarters of all measles cases occurred in children who had been properly vaccinated.[52]

All that the measles vaccine has done has been to transform into adult diseases what were once exclusively the domain of children. In the pre-vaccine era, 90 per cent of all measles patients were five to nine years old. Once the measles vaccine was introduced, however, 55–64 per cent of measles patients were older than 10. The average age of patients during the measles outbreak at the University of California at Los Angeles during the recent US epidemic was 22.[53]

Significant numbers of these cases occurred among college-aged students, particularly those born between 1957 and 1967, when the vaccine was introduced. Students at many universities now have to provide proof they've recently been vaccinated before they are allowed to register for classes. A few years ago, the US government estimated that between 5 and 15 per cent of all students were susceptible.

America has tried at least four strains of the measles vaccine, and all four – including the Schwarz strain now being employed in Britain – have significant failure rates. Study after study in the medical literature points unerringly to clusters of vaccinated children who nevertheless contracted measles.

For instance, in a 1986 outbreak of measles in Corpus Christi, Texas, 99 per cent of the children had been vaccinated.[54] In 1988, 80 per cent of cases of measles occurred in children who had been properly vaccinated at the appropriate age.[55] The year before that, 60 per cent of cases occurred in those who'd been vaccinated.[56]

Even if booster shots are offered, they often don't work, either. In a group of individuals whose measles vaccination hadn't worked, only half given booster shots ended up with antibody levels raised to a level considered protective.[57]

Mumps

Mumps also has a spotty success rate. In numerous instances a large percentage of fully vaccinated children have gone on to contract the disease. For instance, in Switzerland, six years after the MMR vaccine was introduced the incidence of mumps shot up sharply, mostly among the vaccinated.[58] Similarly, in the US state of Tennessee, a large outbreak occurred among students, 98 per cent of whom had been vaccinated.[59]

Rubella

In terms of effectiveness, the rubella vaccine, usually included in the MMR triple vaccine, hasn't fared much better either. In one 1970s study at the University of Pennsylvania of adolescent girls given the vaccine, more than one-third lacked any evidence whatsoever of immunity.[60] Because viruses easily mutate, the vaccine may only protect you against one strain of a virus, and not any new ones. A more recent Italian study showed that 10 per cent of girls had been infected by a 'wild strain' of the virus, even within a few years of being given their shot.[61]

All that vaccination accomplishes is to increase the incidence of the disease. A few years after the countrywide measles and rubella vaccination campaign of 1994, where all school children between the ages of 5 and 16 received the double jab, the number of cases of rubella in Scotland climbed to a 13-year high. Most occurred in children and young adults aged between 15 and 34, who'd been given preschool jabs and whose immunity to rubella had worn off. Young women are therefore at their most susceptible to the disease at the point in their lives when they are most likely to get pregnant and expose their developing child to rubella.[62]

A similar pattern – where the illness suddenly became an adult one – occurred in Finland in 1982, following a mass immunization programme.[63] Furthermore, children with congenital rubella syndrome have born to mothers who'd received their full vaccination quota against rubella.[64]

HIB Meningitis

The Hib vaccine is pointed to as a modern medical success story and credited with a 15-fold decline in the incidence of the disease since the vaccine was introduced. Nevertheless, medical science has yet to produce a version of the Hib vaccine that actually works.

The first vaccine introduced in the US in 1985 was a 'polysaccharide', used in children over 15 months old. The vaccine soon began to lose credibility after doctors reported that children were getting meningitis right after they'd been vaccinated. One Minnesota study showed that the shot *increased* a child's risk fivefold of contracting the disease.[65]

Once the older version was discredited, several companies came up with a 'conjugate' vaccine – one that would marry the Hib portion with the tried and tested diphtheria vaccine (PRP-D), the diphtheria/pertussis/tetanus vaccine (PRP-DPT), or even the *Neisseria meningitidis* group b outer membrane protein complex (PRP-OMPC). The idea behind all this gobbledygook of initials was that attaching the new vaccine onto a substance known to produce antibodies would nudge the body to come up with an antibody to the Hib bug as well. In 1993, the US FDA approved Tetramune, a combination of the DTP vaccine and Hib vaccine.

The latest evidence shows that, far from increasing the effectiveness of the Hib jab, the addition of the diphtheria toxin actually *decreases* its effectiveness.[66]

In addition, the science on which the Hib vaccine success story is based is decidedly suspect. New evidence shows that the incidence of the disease has been widely underreported, largely due to the fact that the surveillance system which tracks the cases has declined by 23 per cent.[67] All the vaccine may have done was to turn Hib meningitis into an adult disease; the average age of victims, which used to be a year old, is now 25.[68]

'Trying to eliminate microorganisms and diseases is comparable to squeezing a balloon,' remarks naturopath Harald Gaier. 'You push in one side and it only makes the other side bulge.'

Polio

As for polio, scientists are beginning to concur that one of the central premises for giving the live vaccine isn't true. In true cases of polio, the virus lives in the intestine, creating what is ordinarily a harmless infection. Problems start if it travels to the bloodstream and makes its way to the nervous system, where it can cause paralysis. The killed virus, originally developed by Jonas Salk, is injected under the skin and is supposed to travel to the bloodstream and create antibodies there which will 'block' the virus before it reaches the nervous system. However, the killed polio shot does not give you 'gut immunity' – that is, doesn't raise antibodies in your intestines. That means that, while you won't get paralytic polio, the wild virus could live on in your gut and you could theoretically pass it on to someone else. Furthermore, the original Salk vaccine required three or more boosters every five years.

When first administered, the Salk vaccine was deemed a terrific success – until the polio-victim rate went up in the 1960s. Coming so hard on the heels of the double-digit victim rates of the fifties, this new development was greeted as proof that the Salk vaccine didn't work, particularly amid all the hysteria to find a 'cure'.

The live oral (OVP) vaccine, developed by Sabin, virtually replaced the Salk vaccine in the sixties, because it not only supposedly confers life-long immunity on its recipient, but stops him from becoming a carrier of the wild virus. And because recipients can excrete the vaccine virus for a number of weeks through the mouth and faeces, the theory is that you can pass on immunity to non-vaccinated individuals, thus raising the 'herd immunity'. *In other words, the live oral vaccine became the vaccine of choice largely so that you or your children could act as an immunizing force for other, unvaccinated individuals.*

Scientists now realize that there is little evidence that the live vaccine actually does achieve this 'back door' immunity among the unvaccinated. This was the conclusion of a scientific study group after an outbreak of polio in Taiwan, where up to 98 per cent of young children had been immunized.[69] Even the US FDA has acknowledged: 'We now know that secondary spread of vaccine virus to susceptible contacts plays very little part in population immunity.'[70]

There's also plenty of evidence that the polio vaccine fails. Many of today's outbreaks occur more among immunized than un-immunized populations. In 1961, for instance, Massachusetts had a polio outbreak, with more paralytic cases among the vaccinated than the unvaccinated.[71] Furthermore, even if the vaccine 'takes', you may not be adequately protected against a certain strain of the virus. During a major outbreak of hepatitis A infection in Glasgow, blood serum of 24 of the victims were also tested for antibodies to polio. Only one-third of the group had an acceptable level of antibodies against one strain of the virus.[72]

Tuberculosis (BCG Vaccine)

The Heaf test is used by most school districts to measure tuberculin sensitivity. Unlike most sensitivity tests, a negative result is supposed to mean that a child does not carry antibodies to the tubercle bacillus. However, the test is notoriously inaccurate; even the American Academy of Pediatrics warns its members that the test carries the possibility of false-negatives and false-positives. Furthermore, no one is really sure anymore what a positive test really means. It could mean that someone is immune to tuberculosis, or had prior infections, or it could mean that someone is simply allergic or sensitive to the test.

In one study of British school districts, where 92 per cent were using the Heaf test, most districts agreed on what to do with a 0 grade, which showed very little reaction (recommend immunization) or a grade 3 or 4, which indicated pronounced reaction (refer to a chest clinic for special evaluation before having the jab). The disparity occurred with those scoring grade 2.

Around one-third of the districts recommended no immunization, and approximately two-thirds recommended referral to a chest clinic for special examination before going ahead with the jab. Only a single district recommended immunization at this level of sensitivity to the test.[73]

Besides the lack of agreement about which groups should or should not receive the live tuberculosis vaccine, substantial doubts exist about its effectiveness. In 10 randomized controlled trials from around the world since the 1930s, the ability of the BCG vaccine to protect you has ranged from 80 per cent to 0.[74] On average, the shot only protects about two-thirds of children from TB.

The problem is that BCG vaccination can only limit the multiplication and spread of the tubercle bacteria; it cannot prevent infection in people exposed to the germ. In fact, there's increasing evidence that BCG vaccines offer greater protection against leprosy than tuberculosis, particularly in Third World countries, where TB is still rife. A huge African study of 83,000 people in Malawi concluded that half were protected against leprosy, but none had significant protection against tuberculosis.[75]

The London School of Hygiene and Tropical Medicine, which conducted a special analysis, found that the vaccine is just 22 per cent effective in Kenya and 20 per cent effective in some areas of India. Overall effectiveness ranges from 0 to 80 per cent around the world, possibly due to strain variations, genetic or nutritional differences, or environmental influences.[76]

MYTH NO 4: THE SIDE-EFFECTS OF VACCINES ARE RARE AND MOSTLY MILD

Just as there is no such thing as a safe drug, there is no such thing as a safe vaccine, and we are only beginning to come to grips with exactly how dangerous each one is. One of the most definitive and largest study of vaccines to date, conducted by the Centers for Disease Control and Prevention, the highest American government body on infectious diseases, was quietly announced to a handful of scientists with no publicity or press releases at a meeting of the Advisory Commission on Childhood Vaccines in Washington.

The low-key presentation in a small seminar on September 9, 1994 in Washington DC was at odds with the spectacular nature of the conclusions: namely, that a child's risk of seizure triples within days of receiving either the MMR or the DPT vaccines.

Using database technology, the CDC monitored the progress of 500,000 children across the US, tapping into computerized records of Health Maintenance Organizations and public insurance schemes such as Kaiser Permanente in California. In this way, the CDC was able to pull together virtually every piece of research and data on adverse reactions to the two triple vaccines. They identified 34 major side-effects to the jabs, ranging from asthma, blood disorders, infectious diseases and diabetes to neurological disorders, including meningitis, polio and hearing loss.

But it was the incidence of seizure that leaped off the graph, according to Dr Anthony Morris, who attended the meeting. The rate of seizure increased three times above the norm within the first day of a child receiving the DPT shot, and the rate rose 2.7 times within four to seven days of a child being given the MMR shot, increasing to 3.3 times within eight to 14 days.

Seizure, which covers epilepsy, convulsions and fainting, is already one of the most common conditions in childhood, affecting an estimated one in 20 children, or 5 per cent.[77] This high figure could reflect the effect of vaccination. Or the new findings could mean that vaccines will further increase that seizure rate to nearly 15 per cent, affecting something close to three in 20 children.

The effects of the DPT shot were immediate, causing the incidence of seizures to increase three times the normal within 24 hours of the jab being given, but then falling off rapidly to just 0.06 times the norm after the first day. The MMR vaccine, however, had a far slower effect, only reaching its most dangerous period eight to 14 days after the jab was administered. The seizures were often serious, the CDC reported, with a quarter of all cases having to be treated in hospital.[78]

In measured, neutral language, the presentation concluded that the architects of the study were interested in studying the synergistic effects among antigens when combined or simultaneously administered – that is, whether the seizures are caused by individual vaccines, or whether the antigen stew of so many vaccines given at the same time is causing, in effect, immune-system melt-down. In the UK, the Public Health Laboratory Service Statistic Unit came up with strikingly similar results: the MMR jab increased seizure risk three times, while the DPT also increased seizure risk threefold, usually three days after the dose was given. The peak increase rate of seizures and meningitis due to the Urabe strain of the mumps portion of the MMR vaccine usually occurred between 15 and 35 days afterwards.[79] A later study of nearly 700,000 children on the CDC database found an even worse result. Infants between the ages of 0 and 12 months increased their risk of having a seizure by nine times on the day they received their DTP shot.[80]

The PHLS also discovered that children given the MMR were five times more likely than expected to suffer idiopathic thrombocytopenic purpura, a blood disorder often requiring blood transfusions. The risk elsewhere has been estimated at 1 in every 30,000 vaccines.[81]

Whooping Cough

As for the individual vaccines themselves, the whooping cough, or pertussis vaccine, is acknowledged as the most overtly dangerous. Of all the adverse reactions from vaccinations now reported on the American Vaccine Adverse Event Reporting System, which was set up with the Vaccine Compensation Act, a US law recognizing that vaccines cause side-effects and arranging for a system to provide compensation for the victims, the overwhelming majority are due to the DPT vaccine. Between 1991 and 2001, there were 39,275 reports of reactions from all forms of the DPT – 6,783, or nearly one sixth of which were serious, involving death, hospitalization or permanent disability.[82] Furthermore, drug companies in America, who are obliged to pay 'tax' for compensation of future vaccine victims, pay the highest rate on the DPT vaccine – a tacit acknowledgement of its position as the most dangerous of all.

Incredible as it seems, the safety of the pertussis drug was never adequately proved before being injected into millions of babies. Essentially, the vaccine as we know it today is no different from the first lots of it created in 1912. At that time, two French bacteriologists grew the pertussis bacteria in large pots, killed it with heat, preserved this stew with formaldehyde, and went ahead and injected it into hundreds of children. Unlike most vaccines, which are detoxified and purified versions of the germ in question, the pertussis vaccine still contains the 'whole cell' of the pertussis bacteria, which is why it's called a 'whole cell' or crude vaccine.[83] This means it still contains endotoxins and cell-wall substances known to be highly toxic, causing fever, interference with growth, and death in laboratory animals. Other toxins stimulate insulin production. One predisposes animals to shock and collapse; another blocks the body's recovery mechanisms.[84]

The US's new acellular vaccine, called DTaP, has been approved by the US Food and Drug Administration since 1992, and now may be offered for babies, rather than simply as a booster shot for older children. The new variety is also being tested in Europe. Doctors are hoping that the results will assuage parents' fears about the dangers of the shot.

However, recent research suggests that the acellular vaccine may be no safer than the vaccine it is meant to replace. A large US study called the Nationwide Multicenter Acellular Pertussis Trial, which compared over 2,000 children given either the acellular vaccine or the whole-cell version, found that the rate of serious adverse reactions – death, near-death, seizures, development delay and hospital stays – did not differ between the old and new vaccines.[85]

The only safety test of the original whooping cough vaccine was conducted by the British Medical Research Council, which tried out the drug on 50,000 children aged 14 months or older. The US never did do tests of its own, but has always relied on these British tests conducted in the fifties. Furthermore, the 42 babies who had convulsions within 28 days of having been given the shot were discounted and the drug assumed to be safe, even though that level of reaction translates into about one in every 1,000 children.[86]

Though the trials were designed only to demonstrate effectiveness, not safety, US and British health authorities have used them as evidence that the vaccine is safe to give to babies as young as six weeks of age. This means the drug was never tested for safety at this dosage for newborns. It also means that two-month-old babies are given the same dosage as children three or four times their size.

In its government-sponsored report, the US National Academy of Science's Institute of Medicine (IOM), which scoured the medical literature for 17 health problems that have been associated with the DTP vaccine, concluded that the vaccine can cause anaphylactic shock (a severe life-threatening allergic reaction) and extended periods of inconsolable crying or screaming, sometimes lasting 24 hours or more.[87] According to Coulter and Fisher in their seminal work *A Shot in the Dark* (Avery), 'this kind of crying, a thin, eerie, wailing sound quite different from the child's normal cry, [very much resembles] the so-called *cri encephalique* (encephalitic scream) found in some cases of encephalitis.'[88]

The IOM committee also found a link, although it was a weaker one, between the DTP vaccine and acute encephalopathy and shock, causing total collapse.[89] Encephalitis is an inflammation of the brain, often referred to as meningitis, causing a bulging and red fontanelle among infants. The American National Vaccine Information Center has amassed many reports of children who either remain brain-damaged or die after these episodes. In almost every instance, the parents themselves have had to report their child's reaction to the drug because their doctor has insisted that the reaction was unrelated to the shot.

'My grandson had his first DPT shot and oral polio at his two-month well-baby checkup,' says a grandmother from Washington. 'After the shot he started crying. The doctor gave my daughter Pediacare (a mild infant analgesic) but it did not stop the high-pitched screaming. When the baby's temperature went down to 98, the nurse told her to feed the baby. My grandson began projectile vomiting and continued the high-pitched crying. The nurse informed my daughter this was normal. The doctor told her to give my grandson more Pediacare and, hopefully, it would make him drowsy. At 3 am they both went to sleep. At 7 am my daughter awoke and found my grandson with a purple color on one side of his face, clenched fists, blood coming from his nose and mouth and no breathing. He was dead within 21 hours of his DPT shot.'

Claire from Minnesota says that after her baby daughter's first DPT jab at her two-month well-baby clinic, she showed no unusual behaviour the first two days except that she was irritable whenever her leg was moved (where the jab had been given). 'I checked her temperature every nappy change and it was fine. She started having seizures two days after the shot,' says Claire. 'Since then she's been put on every seizure medication there is and was put in a coma for two weeks and is still having seizures. She is now at home with us having 50 to 200 seizures a day. She is very severely retarded, bed-ridden, fed with a G-tube and cortically blind.'

Based on a 10-year study, the Institute of Medicine says the vaccine could trigger an acute neurological illness in children with underlying brain or metabolic abnormalities. Researchers are now concerned that children can become brain damaged or even die if they develop a severe neurological illness within a week of receiving the vaccination.[90]

The risk of this type of neurological damage has been estimated at between 1 in every 50,000 children vaccinated.[91] Although Gordon Stewart has argued that the risk to babies of death or brain damage from whooping cough itself is comparable to the risk of death or brain damage from the shot, the actual risks of the vaccine could be much worse.[92] According to the damages paid to the families of children in Britain judged to have been hurt by the whooping cough shot, the risk of damage over the years 1958–79 worked out to be 1 in 30,000 children, at least three times that for all other vaccines.[93]

Although the IOM committee concluded there wasn't enough evidence from current medical studies to show the whooping cough vaccine could definitely cause other serious damage, it didn't rule this out. The possible damage includes juvenile diabetes, learning disabilities, attention deficit disorder, infantile spasms, and sudden infant death syndrome (SIDS).

The FDA once sponsored a study at the University of California of children receiving some 15,000 doses of DTP vaccine. In that study, nine children had convulsions and nine had episodes of collapse, a frequency for each of these conditions of one per 1,750 immunizations. However, since each child receives three to five DTP shots, the true risk of damage could be more like one per 400 children.[94] In one study of 53 babies who had died of sudden infant death, 27 had received the DPT shot within a month of their death. Six deaths occurred within 24 hours, and 17 within a week of the jab being given.[95]

In testimony before the US Senate Committee in 1985, Edward Brandt Jr, the Secretary of Health at the time, estimated that every year 35,000 children suffer brain damage from this vaccine. Other estimates by the

University of California at Los Angeles are that 1,000 infants a year die from SIDS as a direct result of DPT, which represents some 10 to 15 per cent of the total number of SIDS cases in the US.[96]

In the early 1970s, Dr Archie Kalokerinos and Glenn Dettman, who were studying aboriginal children, were puzzled when the death rate of aboriginal children skyrocketed, in some places by 50 per cent. Suddenly they made the connection: the rise in the death rate coincided with intensified efforts to immunize these children, many of whom were ill or had serious vitamin deficiencies when they received their DPT shots.[97]

As a result of this and other evidence, Sweden, Germany and Japan have omitted the whooping cough vaccine from their regular vaccine schedules.

The only large-scale study of the whooping cough vaccine ever conducted discovered that one in every 875 doses of the vaccine causes convulsions, shock or collapse. Two babies in the study died as a result.[98] As for brain damage, Swedish research discovered that one in 17,000 children suffer brain damage or death.[99] In Britain, the British National Childhood Encephalopathy Study, meant to rule out dangers of the jab, showed that one in 110,000 DPT shots causes a serious neurological reaction, and that one in 310,000 shots causes brain damage or death.[100] But, again, since children receive three shots apiece, the true figures may be higher: as many as one in 30,000 children could suffer neurological reaction, and one in 100,000 children could be brain-damaged or killed.

Tetanus

As for tetanus, the Institute of Medicine's study of vaccine damage concluded that the vaccine could cause high fever, seizures, pain, nerve damage, fatal anaphylactic shock, degeneration of the nervous system, and Guillain-Barre syndrome.[101] Tetanus boosters can also cause T-lymphocyte blood count ratios to plunge temporarily to levels similar to those of AIDS victims.[102]

Another problem with this so-called 'safe' vaccine is encephalitis or damage to the nervous system or inner ear. The *Physician's Desk Reference* warns that booster doses are more likely to increase the incidence and severity of reactions, if they are given too frequently.[103] This is probably what happened to the 14-year-old son of Mary from Exmouth. He was given a tetanus injection following a dog bite. Five days later, he had his first epileptic fit at night, and has had epilepsy ever since. Mary asked her GP if there was any connection between the two, and like so many others, her fears were brushed aside and the boy's illness put down to coincidence. After all, her GP said, the tetanus vaccine is known to have no side-effects. 'It was only when my son changed GPs, a few years go, that his new doctor sent him for a brain scan to see if there were any underlying causes such as scar tissue,' she said. 'There were none.'

Measles/Mumps/Rubella (MMR) Vaccine

In the UK, until recently we were simply told by doctors and the government that the MMR vaccine has been used safely in other countries, particularly the United States, for many years. We were also told that it provides, as former health minister Edwina Currie put it in October 1988, 'life-long protection against all three infections with a single jab'.[104]

But in the US from 1991 to 2001, 23,787 adverse incidents following MMR vaccination have been reported to the American Vaccine Adverse Events Reporting System, many requiring emergency medical treatment and leading to permanent damage or death. And if, as the National Vaccine Information Center says, these figures represent only 10–15 per cent of the total number of side-effects (because of the massive number of cases that go unreported), the true figure could be far higher.[105]

British and American vaccine experts such as the Public Health Laboratory Service's Dr Begg claim that the incidence of measles-vaccine-induced encephalitis is very rare, occurring in one in 200,000 children. Symptoms include fever, headache, possible convulsions and behavioural changes. 'Most symptoms are mild,' he says, 'and the children will recover.'

However, many studies report far greater risks. In one, from Germany, 1 of every 2,500 children vaccinated had a brain complication, and 1 in every 17,650 came down with encephalitis.[106]

About one in 400 children given the jab will suffer convulsions,[107] and nearly one-fifth of young adults given measles boosters will suffer major side-effects, including fever, eye pain and the need for bed rest.[108]

New research has made a tentative connection between the measles jab and the sharp rise of Crohn's disease and colitis in children.[109]

Two versions of the drug, manufactured by Merieux and SmithKline Beecham, were withdrawn in Britain and elsewhere in the autumn of 1992 because of the risk of contracting meningitis from the Urabe strain of the mumps portion of the vaccine. The Japanese government withdrew its own version of the MMR vaccine in April 1993 after discovering a link with meningitis. A year later, the Japanese authorities revealed that one in 1,044 children vaccinated developed aseptic meningitis.[110] The government also found evidence that the vaccine can bring on mumps, which can also be transferred to other children.

The US National Academy of Sciences IOM report concluded that the measles vaccine can cause death from measles-vaccine-strain-infection, thrombocytopenia (the rare blood condition characterized by a decrease in blood platelets), fatal shock, and arthritis. The committee also said it couldn't 'rule out' that the vaccine itself could cause cases of SSPE.[111]

Immediately after receiving a measles jab during the nationwide UK campaign in 1994, Sam, a healthy, athletic 12 year old, began losing his sense of coordination and falling down. He also began having constant seizures – sometimes 15 an hour. After becoming virtually wheelchair-bound, he was eventually diagnosed as having the fatal condition SSPE. Even though his condition is a known, admittedly rare side-effect of the measles shot, his doctors refused to make the link. Instead they argued that the jab merely set off a latent disease caused by an earlier bout of measles. The problem is, insists his mother, Sam never *had* measles.

Besides running the risk of side-effects from the vaccine, your child could also contract what has become known as atypical measles, an especially vicious form of the disease which resists treatment. In a 1965 study in Cincinnati during an epidemic of measles, 54 vaccinated children went on to develop atypical measles. Many of these children were so ill with high fever and pneumonia that they had to be hospitalized.[112]

There is even some evidence that preventing children from getting the ordinary childhood diseases prevents their immune systems from adequately developing. When children get the measles vaccine, they often contract so-called 'mild measles' with an under-developed rash. One study found evidence of a relationship between lack of rash in measles and increased incidence of degenerative diseases such as cancer later in life.[113] Many practitioners have reported that cancer patients have a particularly small number of infectious diseases of childhood in their medical history.

Mumps

German authorities have discovered 27 neurological reactions to the mumps vaccine, including meningitis, febrile convulsions, encephalitis and epilepsy.[114] Of all cases of mumps encephalitis over 15 years, one-sixth were definitely caused by the vaccine.[115] Research from Canada estimated the risk of vaccine-induced mumps encephalitis at one per 100,000;[116] a Yugoslavian study concluded it was one per 1,000.[117]

As for meningitis from the mumps vaccine, the British Department of Health's recent public assurance that the risk is only 1 in 11,000 contradicts the long-known findings published in one of the leading US paediatric journals that the rate varies from 1 in 405 to 1 in 7,000 shots given.[118]

The British government ignored these warning signals about the mumps portion of the vaccine until a surveillance study by the Public Health Laboratory Service demonstrated that an unacceptably large number of children were contracting meningitis from a certain strain of the mumps vaccine.[119] In Nottingham, a cluster of cases suggested the risk could be as high as 1 in 4,000 doses; the PHLS eventually concluded the risk was 1 in every 11,000 doses.[120]

But even when the government hastily withdrew the two versions containing the Urabe mumps virus strain – a good 18 months after Canada did so – SmithKline Beecham continued producing vaccines containing that particular strain, 'so that existing immunization programmes in areas where no alternative mumps vaccine is available need not be suspended'.[121] In other words, in some parts of the world it was considered better to hand out a vaccine known to pose dangers than to expose children to an illness that is mostly benign.

After her son suffered side-effects after receiving his MMR, Jackie Fletcher formed a group called JABS (Justice, Awareness and Basic Support) for families of children damaged chiefly by the MMR vaccine. So far she has been contacted by hundreds of families whose children allegedly have sustained damage from the now-withdrawn mumps vaccine. Nevertheless, a number of cases of alleged damage being pursued in court also concern the current MMR vaccine, produced by the US drug company Merck.

Rubella

A National Academy of Science report has accepted that the rubella portion of the MMR vaccine can cause long- or short-term arthritis. One manufacturer of the triple vaccine estimated that the rubella part of the vaccine causes arthritis in up to 3 per cent of children and in up to 20 per cent of adult women who receive it. 'Symptoms [of arthritis] may persist for a matter of months or, on rare occasions, for years,' the company reports – everything from mild aches to extreme crippling.[122] Adolescent girls are considered to be at greater risk of joint and limb symptoms.

As long ago as 1970, the US Health, Education and Welfare department reported that some '26 per cent of children receiving rubella vaccination in national testing programs developed arthralgia and arthritis. Many had to seek medical attention, and some were hospitalized to test for rheumatic fever and rheumatoid arthritis.'[123]

Dr Aubrey Tingle, a paediatric immunologist at Children's Hospital in Vancouver, British Columbia, has also undertaken major research into this area. According to his own studies, 30 per cent of adults exposed to rubella vaccine suffer arthritis in two to four weeks – ranging from mild aches in the joints to severe crippling. Tingle also found the rubella virus in one-third of adult and child patients with rheumatoid arthritis.[124]

During the 1994 UK measles appeal, the Department of Health admitted in written reports to doctors that 11 per cent of first-time recipients of the rubella vaccine will get arthritis. Nevertheless, this vital fact was omitted in the pamphlet given to parents.

Polio

With the live polio virus, the main problem is that this 'attenuated' or weakened version of the vaccine virus can genetically alter in the gut, changing into its virulent form and causing paralytic polio in its recipient or those that he has recently come into contact with. Today, virtually the only cases of polio that occur in Britain or the US are caused by the vaccine, mainly among so-called contacts – grandparents, parents or siblings who are in some way susceptible to polio – but also among the recipients themselves. Scientists have also identified a new strain of vaccine polio virus caused by the vaccine in a number of countries round the world, according to the World Health Organization.[125]

Bernard Reis, an English professor at Vassar College and former graduate of Cornell University and Harvard, described as an energetic, athletic achiever, was happily married with a baby boy, whom he dutifully took to receive the vaccines mandated by law. A month after his little boy's vaccine, Reis became tired when attempting to climb a flight of stairs and came down with what he thought was flu. Two days later he collapsed on his bathroom floor and, after being rushed to hospital, was completely paralyzed, placed on an iron lung and fed intravenously. Eleven months later he returned home in a wheelchair. 'The strain of all this was too much for my marriage, which fell apart,' he writes.[126] Since then, his life has been 'hell in slow motion'. Although able to walk haltingly, he is still extremely weak from his bout with polio. He lives on Social Security in New York public housing. He has not been able to receive other government assistance or compensation.

On February 19, the first day Bob and Marjorie were to move into their new home, Bob collapsed on the sofa. The following morning he complained that he couldn't move his left arm. A few days later he was completely paralyzed. A battery of tests later, doctors finally diagnosed Bob as having paralytic polio. His daughter Chloe had received her live polio vaccine less than two months before. No doctor had warned Bob, who has Netherton's syndrome (a skin condition) that his immune system was weakened by the cortisone he takes and that he was at high risk of contracting polio from anyone vaccinated for the disease – this despite the warning to physicians on packages of the vaccine, from Lederle, the drug manufacturer. A year to the day after Bob came down with polio, he died.

There were more than 31 cases of vaccine-induced paralytic polio in the US between 1991 and 1997,[127] and at least 10 reported cases of paralytic polio caused by the live vaccine were reported every year until the advent of an inactivated version.[128] (In the UK, 13 cases have been substantiated between 1985 and 1991.[129]) The US CDC, along with German doctors from the University of Cologne, estimated the current risk for vaccine-induced polio at five per million doses of the live vaccine given, or one case for each 200,000 first doses, which are said to be the most risky.[130] As with many official statistics, this figure could be too low; if your immune system is weakened, as it is with AIDS or if you are using drugs such as steroids, the risk is multiplied 10,000 times. In Germany, most cases of paralytic polio caused by vaccines have been among children aged two years or younger – that is, the recipients themselves.

Besides polio, your child also risks poor weight gain or other paralytic diseases with the polio vaccine. Children immunized with live agents, such as the polio vaccines, have been shown to suffer 'statistically significant' reductions in their weights, compared with children of the same size who weren't vaccinated.[131] Those who were small for their ages to begin with were especially affected.

Recently, a new disease has been appearing in China, which the medical press has dubbed 'Chinese paralytic syndrome' (CPS). Although it was previously diagnosed as the paralytic condition Guillain-Barre syndrome (GBS), researchers from the Second Hospital of Hebei Medical College in the People's Republic of China studied all the cases in depth and concluded that the disease, which strikes children and young adults, was a variation of polio.

Before oral polio vaccine (OPV) was introduced in the Hebei province in 1971, illness from polio was high, but diagnoses of GBS were uncommon. Then after 1971, the incidence of polio gradually fell, but that of GBS increased about tenfold. Three rises in the incidence of polio utterly coincided with three epidemics of GBS.

According to Yan Shen and Guohua Xi from the hospital's Department of Neuropsychiatry, the evidence strongly suggests that the polio virus is responsible for the cases diagnosed as GBS. 'The widespread use of OPV may have led to [mutation of the virus], resulting in an alteration of [the disease] and/or to a change in the main epidemic type of poliovirus,' they wrote.[132]

Cases of GBS linked to the polio vaccine also occur in the UK. Emma Whitlock went to her doctor's surgery to get a routine polio and typhoid vaccination for her family's upcoming trip to Morocco. She says:

That evening I developed a temperature, with aches and pains in my arms and legs. The pains in my legs were the most severe. About two weeks later while I was out walking one of my legs 'gave out'. It felt as though my legs were both weak, and they were numb. Some time after that my legs started to feel as though they were burning.

My condition has steadily deteriorated over the years, and I am now at the stage of being able to take only a few steps before I experience the pains and a horrible numbness in my legs, which forces me to sit down. Any kind of movement gives me the same pain, even if I travel in a car.

My hands were affected, too. They now burn when I have done too much, and there is a weakness there. Besides the limb problems, I suffer earaches and a kind of deafness, plus frequent infected neck glands which only clear up with antibiotics. I also have serious problems with balance, unsteady walking and falling. I have memory loss and often stop in mid-sentence.

These effects have all had a devastating effect on my life. I am now totally house-bound. I have been resting solidly for nearly five months to try to get the burning pain to ease. Although it has eased somewhat, the pain and numbness are constant when I attempt to walk.

Doctors have now diagnosed the problem as Guillain-Barre syndrome. When I contacted someone from the Guillain-Barre Society, he told me that I was the worst case he's ever seen. My doctor now admits that this was brought on by the vaccine.

Finland, like Sweden and the Netherlands, has always preferred to use the killed IPV vaccine. However, after 10 cases of polio erupted in 1985, the government organized a mass vaccination campaign with the live vaccine. A few weeks after the campaign, the Department of Pediatrics at the University of Oulu in Finland reported a cluster of 27 cases of childhood Guillain-Barre syndrome, which also occurred in the US following mass immunization for the swine flu in the 1970s.[133] Eleven of the children had been immunized before the onset of symptoms.

Millions of children receiving the Salk vaccine in the 1950s and 1960s have been infected with another, potentially cancer-causing virus. This virus, named SV 40, was found to be a 'fellow traveller' of the polio virus. The process of killing the polio virus was not sufficient to kill SV 40. This contaminated vaccine was then handed out to many millions of children during the initial 1955 campaign, and even later.[134] When a combined DTP and polio shot was found to contain SV 40, it was discontinued.

Meanwhile, according to Dr Anthony Morris, SV 40 and similar agents have been recovered from human brain tumours 'and also precancerous conditions in the brain'. SV 40 has been shown to cause cancer in hamsters after the equivalent of 20 human years.[135] Numerous researchers have even attempted to link infected polio vaccine with the origin of AIDS.

Recently, SV40 has been found in tissue samples of victims of certain cancers, including rare childhood brain tumours.[136] Because of the risk of getting polio from the live vaccine, various governments, including that of the US, are now considering reverting to the killed form of the vaccine (IPV), particularly as the Merieux pharmaceutical company in Europe and Connaught Labs in the US have come up with an enhanced killed vaccine (or E-IPV, in science-speak) which supposedly gives you immunity against all three types of polio after two doses. But the new vaccine seems to be trading new problems for old. The killed vaccine has been linked with GBS, motor neurone weakness, encephalitis, meningitis and convulsions, according to a Danish study.[137]

THE EXCIPIENTS IN VACCINES

Besides the vaccines themselves, children can react to the *excipients*, or extra ingredients added in. A vaccine is a complex mix of live or killed viral or bacterial antigens, or foreign invaders, plus a variety of substances to help them grow, to kill impurities, to help stabilize them and to boost their antibody-producing abilities.

The three most common chemicals in vaccine production are *thimerosal*, a preservative derived from mercury, *formalin* (a 37 per cent solution of formaldehyde, the main ingredient of embalming fluid) - included to inactivate viruses and detoxify toxins – and *aluminium sulphate*, an adjuvant or vaccine-effectiveness booster which is supposed to increase the ability of a vaccine to produce antibodies. Phenol (a disinfectant and dye), ethyene glycol (the main ingredient in antifreeze), benzethonium chloride (an antiseptic) and methylparaben (a preservative and antifungal) are also often added to the pot.

The only study that has tested the use of these substances has examined their effect on animals, and discovered that seven of the most commonly used substances have the ability to produce tumours.[138] In another study examining the use of thimerosal when used in a similar way that it is used in vaccines, patients given immunoglobulin preserved with thimerosal had raised mercury levels in their bodies.[139] Ironically, Jonas Salk, who developed the killed polio vaccine, found that thimerosal actually *inhibited* the effect of the polio vaccine.

Each of these individual ingredients has been studied in other contexts and found to have many side-effects. Studies have shown that germicides like thimerosal have a negative effect on white blood cells,[140] and of course aluminium is known to be toxic in drinking water. Mercury is among one of the most toxic substances to humans (*see* Chapter 9).

A large percentage of people have or develop allergic sensitivity to thimerosal, used as a disinfectant in vaccines. One study showed that more than a third of allergic patients undergoing allergy desensitization with shots containing thimerosal developed hypersensitivity to the mercury salt.[141] This high sensitivity to thimerosal, in some cases, is due to previous exposure to the substance in vaccinations.[142] We also know that mercury salts can cause immune-suppression in animals.[143] Children who receive vaccines with thimerosal may be exposed to higher levels of mercury than are considered safe.[144]

As for formalin, 47 studies have demonstrated an association between formaldehyde exposure and cancer, including leukaemia and cancer of the brain, colon and lymphatic tissues.[145]

Since the 1940s, scientists have been experimenting with adjuvants to kickstart vaccines in working more effectively. Adjuvants work by trapping the vaccine in a pool and then drip-feeding it into the lymph nodes and spleen. Even the tetanus toxin is used as an adjuvant to boost other vaccines that don't work very well.

Certain adjuvants, such as calcium phosphate, appear to cause more reactions than aluminium hydroxide and the adjuvants in DT vaccines.[146] Oil adjuvants, used for example in the flu vaccine, have been shown to cause hypersensitivity, cysts and arthritis, and aluminium may cause not only cysts and granulomas at the injection site, but arthritis and even cancer.[147] The metals frequently used in vaccine production can settle somewhere permanently in the body; when granulomas that have developed after vaccination have been examined by special x-ray equipment, they've shown the presence of aluminium and phosphorus in the granular debris.[148] Of the few studies that have been done on aluminium in vaccines, one shows that those containing aluminium cause the most reactions.[149] Aluminium also appears to intensify allergic reactions to the whooping cough vaccine.[150]

These substances also have varying effects on the protective ability of the vaccines, some helping them to work better than others: aluminium phosphate produces more antibodies, for instance, than sterol tyrosine or calcium phosphate.[151]

However, no one is really clear which ones really work and which are safest. As a New York Academy of Sciences article once put it: 'The body of knowledge regarding mechanisms of adjuvancy or adjuvant effect could better be described as voodoo or witchcraft.'

Besides these preservatives, many other substances get thrown in the pot. For instance, the DPT vaccine combines toxoids of diphtheria and tetanus with the whole cells of pertussis bacteria. Large amounts of diphtheria and pertussis are grown in a broth. Toxoids are the poisonous products of the tetanus and diphtheria organisms. These are produced in a stew of dextrose, beef-heart infusion, sodium chloride and casein, cut with methanol, a raw alcohol, to purify it, then dissolved in a buffer.[152] The final 'ingredient' is the whole cells of the whooping cough, or pertussis bacteria. They are grown in large vats in a culture of minerals and casein, then killed by heat or thimerosal. After one or another adjuvants such as aluminium are added, this 'stew' is complete and ready for injection into a two-month-old baby.

But no one really knows the final effect of the interaction of all these chemicals and toxoids; what we *do* know is that adding formalin to crude toxins polymerizes impurities and bacterial antigens – that is, joins them together.[153] As for what that actually does to children, your guess is as good as mine.

NEW DISEASES FROM VACCINES

Besides the dangers of individual jabs, vaccination appears to be responsible for a number of new diseases.

Getting jabbed with a weakened or killed version of a virus can cause you to develop a viral 'mutant' or encourage its growth in the population at large.

It has been estimated that 3 per cent of babies born to mothers given the hepatitis B vaccine go on to develop a mutated form of hepatitis B.[154] In one study of a large group of babies born to hepatitis B-positive mothers and given a full immunization programme against hepatitis B, one in 60 became hepatitis B-positive. One in 80 of these babies showed they had a viral mutant of the vaccine. This mutant has been associated with hepatitis and active liver disease.[155] In another study, patients vaccinated with HB had a mixture of these mutants and the usual form of hepatitis B virus, as well as mild hepatitis. But those patients whose blood had the mutant on its own eventually suffered the more severe liver disease.[156]

The other problem with mutant viruses is that they often don't get detected in blood donor screening, so that this new form of hepatitis could be transmitted through donated blood. And of course the mutant may infect individuals even if they have been vaccinated.[157]

Connections have been made between the increasing prevalence of penicillin-resistant pneumococcal meningitis and universal Hib vaccination.[158]

Eradicating one strain of a virus can also encourage other forms of it to proliferate. This is precisely what's happening with the Hib meningitis vaccine. As b-type *H. influenzae* strains are being wiped out by the vaccination, mutant non-b *H. influenzae* strains are thriving.

One study looked at 408 strains of Hib meningitis. Although 94 per cent were *H. influenzae* type b, the rest were 'non-serotypable' (NST) *haemophilus influenzae* strains. The authors predicted that as more Hib vaccine was used, NST strains would cause more middle-ear infections, sinusitis, chronic bronchitis and other mostly respiratory infections.[159]

In the 1960s, when US Army recruits were given an experimental killed pneumonia vaccine, the vaccine caused unpredictable shifts in the virus type. Epidemics of disease from these mutant viruses occurred among recruits, rendering the vaccine useless and sending the scientists scurrying back to the laboratory to develop a vaccine that would knock out the mutations as well.[160]

We're also now beginning to realize that injections of any variety (including vaccinations) can increase your risk of developing polio. H. V. Wyatt of the Department of Community Medicine at the University of Leeds was one of the first to study the astonishing connection between multiple injections of any variety, particularly penicillin, given to small children and the onset of polio, particularly in developing countries where children receive more shots than those in developed countries.[161]

'Provocation polio' after a 'just-in-case' injection is now long recognized and accepted in countries such as Britain and the US. When a cluster of cases of paralytic polio occurred after a mass vaccination campaign with the live polio virus, researchers at the University of Cologne warned that DPT (diphtheria/tetanus/whooping cough) shots shouldn't be given at the same time as the live polio vaccine.[162]

H. V. Wyatt has made a career of studying different populations through this century, comparing injected drug treatment and epidemics of polio, including the injections children have been given for congenital syphilis. He concluded that multiple injections may be responsible for 25 per cent of cases of paralysis during epidemics of polio, and make children 25 per cent more susceptible to the disease during non-epidemic periods. A single injection, he found, could increase the risk of paralysis fivefold, and turn what might have been a non-paralytic attack into a paralytic one. Even the World Health Organization's expanded vaccine programme of immunization 'might provoke poliomyelitis', he concluded.[163]

Wyatt also believed that the risk might be cumulative – that is, multiple injections over time might increase the risk of contracting polio at some point in the future, as may getting jabs at close intervals.

Wyatt's thesis provides much food for thought about the origins of the great polio epidemics of this century, which may have been abetted by the introduction of widespread vaccination and penicillin. It has also been recently validated by a study in Romania, by the US Centers for Disease Control, showing that the polio vaccine, given by injection, is causing outbreaks of the disease. While the polio jab itself appeared to trigger paralysis, the children affected had been exposed to a large number of other injections of vaccines and antibiotics. The children were at particular risk of paralysis if other injections had been given less than 30 days before the polio jab.[164]

Vaccines, particularly those for measles and tuberculosis, have also been linked with the current epidemic of myalgic encephalomyelitis (ME), also known as Chronic Fatigue syndrome, particularly among children. Doris Jones of Ilford, Essex, began researching the link between vaccines and the disorder when her son Stephen developed ME at the age of 12. He'd reacted badly to the measles vaccine when given it at a year old, undergoing repeated and prolonged screaming fits. At 10, Doris Jones says, after having been very late at talking and walking, Stephen caught measles and, two years later, glandular fever. Two months after that he had another bout of measles, this time atypical, and then developed ME, which he has now had for 24 years. Mrs Jones has unearthed studies linking ME to vaccines against tetanus, measles, cholera, flu and typhoid, and more recently to hepatitis B.

Some evidence suggests that symptoms of ME are partly due to a dysfunction in the body caused by antibody responses to incomplete, dead or even latent viruses – in other words, many of the 'attenuated' or weakened versions of viruses administered in vaccines.[165]

In one group of studies, up to a sixth of young people with ME were vaccinated the month before they came down with the disease.[166] Vaccination appears to act as a trigger if you have a dormant infection or an exhausted or impaired immune system (either because of steroid treatment or a long-term viral infection), or even if you have allergies.

A trawl through the medical literature provides devastating proof that many vaccine programmes have left us far worse off than we were before. Over 30 years, the measles vaccine has caused vicious mutations of the disease, transformed it into a disease of adults and infants, and left us with inadequate immunity to pass on to our children. Plus we now have substantial numbers of children damaged by the vaccine. But this is only the merest inkling of the repercussions of our meddling. Dr Michel Odent and his London-based Primal Health Research Centre conducted a study of long-term breastfeeding. The study started out examining whether long-term breastfeeding protects against eczema and asthma. But in the course of the investigation, the researchers came up with an utterly unexpected finding:

children immunized against whooping cough were six times more likely to have asthma than those who hadn't been given the jab.[167] In virtually every category – number of sick days, cases of earaches, admittance to hospital – the unvaccinated children were healthier.

Sarah, from Romney Marsh, Kent, has a six-year-old daughter whose asthma seems related to her jabs. 'Her reaction to the first DPT shot was to scream non-stop for 12 hours, a reaction we were told was "normal",' says Sarah. 'She was hospitalized with a high fever after the MMR vaccine, after which she developed bowel problems, and then, after the DPT booster, "full-blown" asthma.' After the complete coterie of shots, she still came down with whooping cough. Sarah continues:

> We were talked into allowing her to be given two flu vaccinations. After that, she contracted one virus after another and numerous ear infections, so that she was constantly on antibiotics. At present she is taking twice the recommended maximum dose of inhaled steroids for children. We feel that inhaled steroids are also having side-effects. She has developed thinning skin, she has gained no weight at all in 18 months, and her feet have stopped growing.

MMR and Autism

The most well-known suspected side-effect concerns the possible relationship between the MMR vaccine and the development of bowel disease and autism, as first postulated by Dr Andrew Wakefield, a gastroenterologist at the Royal Free Hospital in London, highly respected for his research into viral associations with Crohn's disease and ulcerative colitis. Wakefield and his colleagues have published several papers concerning a number of children who have presented with an unusual chronic inflammation of the intestine and regressive developmental disorder or psychosis.[168]

The children had gastrointestinal problems unlike anything that Wakefield or his colleagues had ever seen. It appeared to be a new inflammatory bowel disease, bearing a resemblance to Crohn's disease and to ulcerative colitis but with its own signature symptoms – in particular, chronic swelling of the tiny lymph glands in the final section of the small intestine. Most significantly, the condition seemed to have as its co-passenger severe regressive autism, or pervasive developmental disorder (PDD).

In classic types of autism, developmental abnormalities are apparent to the trained eye from birth. But in the case of these children, the parents alleged that they had been, to all intents and purposes, developing normally until they were given the triple jab.

Of a total of 60 children who'd developed autism just after vaccination, 93 per cent exhibited these same bowel abnormalities. Around a third of them had similar swellings in the colon, and 88 per cent had chronic colitis. Other researchers have found the same abnormalities in groups of autistic children.[169]

Wakefield postulated that the attenuated strain of the measles virus promotes an immune response insufficient to control the virus. As a result, a weakened 'infection' of sorts is established in the intestines and produces increased permeability of the gut wall as well as an abnormal increase in the number of cells in the intestinal tissues. Urine tests showed that all of the children had marked vitamin B_{12} deficiencies, as seen in other gastrointestinal disorders. Since vitamin B_{12} is necessary for the normal development of the central nervous system, Wakefield speculated that the B_{12} deficiency could be a contributory factor to the autistic regression seen in these children.

Wakefield teamed up with John O'Leary, professor of pathology at Trinity College in Dublin, who had found a persistent measles virus infection in the small intestine of 24 of 25 children with this type of autism and gastrointestinal disease.[170] Others have discovered a link between 'leftover' measles virus and autism. A Japanese scientist found measles virus particles in the blood of one-third of a small sample of autistic children.[171] Yet other researchers showed that 'persistent' measles virus infection is present in many people with Crohn's disease.[172]

The most devastating evidence has come from biopsy samples taken from the intestines of 91 children with confirmed diagnoses of ILH and enterocolitis: 75–82 per cent showed evidence of measles virus in various cells of the intestine.[173]

Andrew Wakefield and Paul Shattock of the Autism Research Unit of the University of Sunderland believe that this type of late-onset regressive autism results from the action of peptides that originate outside of the body and affect neuro-transmission within the central nervous system (CNS). Wakefield and Shattock have theorized that these peptides produce effects which are basically opioid in activity, or may help to break down the opioid peptides which occur naturally within the CNS. In either case, the CNS's regulatory role, normally performed by natural opioid peptides such as the enkephalins and endorphins, would be intensified to such an extent that a large number of CNS systems would be disrupted during a critical 'window' in a child's development. Perception, cognition, emotions, mood and behaviour would all be affected, as would all the higher executive functions of the brain. These could result in the diverse symptoms that constitute autism.[174]

With the MMR vaccine, postulates Wakefield, the attenuated (weakened) strain of the measles virus promotes an immune response that is insufficient to control the virus. Consequently, an infection becomes established in the intestines and produces the abnormalities of the intestinal wall seen in these autistic children. The aberrant peptides, says Wakefield and Shattock, are derived from an incomplete breakdown of certain foods, particularly gluten from wheat and other cereals (oats, rye and barley), and casein from milk and other dairy products.

Their theory has a solid basis in research: A number of studies have shown that autistic children have increased gut permeability.[175]

To test their theory, Shattock and his team enlisted a small group of autistic children. When *L. casein* and gluten were eliminated from the diet, the children improved, primarily in their development of language and ability to concentrate. The greatest improvements were seen in the children who were most afflicted. In more than 50 per cent of cases, these children's family doctors have been impressed enough by the improvements to prescribe them gluten-free products on the NHS.

Measles in the Brain

Dr Jeff Bradstreet of Palm Bay in Florida, whose own son developed autism after his MMR jab, studied nearly 2,000 children with autistic enterocolitis and uncovered evidence of measles virus in the spinal fluid and brains of these children. According to Alexander Harris and Co., the London-based firm of solicitors which has been contacted by some 2,500 families whose children have allegedly been damaged by the vaccine, a good half of their cases involve children who were developing normally, but then became autistic right after vaccination.

Autism is by far the most common side-effect reported to Alexander Harris and Co. Similarly, hundreds of families have registered with JABS, the parent group run by Jackie Fletcher, whose own child was allegedly damaged by the triple jab. Of 1,800 JABS children allegedly damaged by the MMR, more than 40 per cent had developed regressive autism, bowel problems and epilepsy after vaccination.

Many of Alexander Harris and Co.'s clients have videotapes of their child's development from birth, month after month, demonstrating normal, healthy development up until the point of vaccination with MMR, usually at 12–15 months. By that time a child is usually walking, may have a small vocabulary, and is pointing and interacting with the rest of the family. Then suddenly, in every one of these instances, the children lost their speech and social interaction skills, and made a sudden regression into behaviour patterns considered to be within the autistic spectrum.

These include severe difficulties in communicating and in social inter-action with others, withdrawal and awkward or repetitive and obsessive movements and patterns of behaviour.

Some of Alexander Harris and Co.'s cases involve children up to the age of four, whose normal development and speech are unmistakable up until the point of vaccination. Sarah, whose father is Italian, was bilingual at three-and-a-half, and had a large vocabulary in both languages. Two weeks after her MMR jab, she was covered from head to waist with the measles rash and suffered a high temperature and drowsiness for a few days.

As soon as the episode was over she became mute, with autistic traits as well as bowel disorders and constant diarrhoea. She also developed a blood disorder which has been identified as a side-effect of the MMR vaccine. The fact that children of this age turn autistic after vaccination tends to counter the argument that the onset of autism is coincidental, since autism is usually diagnosed at a much earlier age.

Another of JABS' members is the mother of triplets, all of whom were developing normally – a fact that was documented by medical specialists who took extra care with the children because of their multiple-birth status. At 15 months, within three or four days of their MMR jab, all three children suffered a high temperature, drowsiness and loss of appetite. Soon after they all lost their speech and ability to make eye contact, and developed behaviour considered typical of autism. One of the children also partially lost his hearing – another known side-effect of the triple jab.

Epidemiological evidence has been unearthed from the more than 7,000 participants of the national 1970 British Cohort Study, in which the health records of thousands of children were recorded and studied from birth. In this study, researchers noted the children's ages at the time of the onset of a number of infectious diseases and whether the children as adults developed inflammatory bowel disease. They found that if the children had had mumps before the age of two, they were 25 times more likely to develop ulcerative colitis as adults. Similarly, if they caught both measles and mumps within less than a year of each other, they were seven times more likely to develop ulcerative colitis and four times more likely to develop Crohn's disease.[176]

A similar epidemiological study in Iceland found that children catching mumps and measles back-to-back were 11 times more likely to develop inflammatory bowel disease later in life.

Thus, the problem is not simply catching measles. It is catching mumps *before* the age of two or having measles and mumps within less than a year of each other. This may mean that it is the mumps component, and/or giving these two live viruses at the same time to children under two, that is causing the problems.

Since Dr Wakefield published his findings, both the UK Government and medical community have embarked on several million-pound campaigns to deny any association between MMR and autism. They argue that the findings were sheer coincidence, and maintain that the children received the vaccine when autism would have been recognized and diagnosed anyway. Indeed, *The Lancet* recently asked Dr Wakefield's colleagues to retract any association between their findings and the MMR vaccine, and published a new study examining the immunization schedules of children with or without autism which failed to find a link.[177]

In an attempt to staunch the haemorrhage of parents opting out of the jab as a result of Dr Wakefield's work, the British government and Public

Health Laboratory Service (as well as other governments around the world) rushed out a number of other studies supposedly demonstrating that the link between autism and the MMR vaccine doesn't exist. All, so far, are epidemiological observational studies of populations, reliant upon a passive reporting system – one of the weakest types of investigations because you cannot isolate all the variables.[178] In some instances, says Dr Wakefield, the quality of the records are 'appalling', with symptoms not even recorded.

In the midst of this campaign, Dr Ken Aitkin, an authority on autism, commissioned by the Government to allay fears about the link between the condition and the vaccine, blew the whistle on the Government's damage-limitation exercise.

Dr Aitkin, who formed part of a 37-person strong Medical Research Council panel to study evidence between the triple jab and autism, admitted that the Department of Health did not accurately put forward the conclusion reached by the MRC. 'We did not conclude that autism was not linked to MMR,' he said recently. 'The view was that there was a problem which needed to be looked at very carefully and there was not enough evidence to rule out a link.'

The latest and most damning evidence from Denmark shows that the introduction of the MMR vaccine corresponded with an eight-fold increase in cases of autism. In this study of more than half a million children, Denmark was selected because it maintains a unique computerized registry of all children born and assigns them an identifier which tracks their health and immunization statues throughout their lives.

Using data from the Danish Psychiatric Central Register, the American researchers who conducted the study, including a specialist in autism research, compared the incidence of autism preceding and following the introduction of the MMR jab. They discovered that the prevalence of autism in children between ages 5 and 9 leapt from 8.38 cases per 100,000 children before the vaccine was launched to 71.43 cases per 100,000 children in 2002. Even after adjusting for such variables as greater diagnostic awareness, the researchers concluded that cases of autism had increased by nearly five times since the vaccine was launched. Special trends in the data showed a temporal association between the introduction of the jab and the rise in autism.[179]

This study is particularly important because it re-analysed data from the largest study to date to counter the Wakefield hypothesis. That study, published in 2002, examined the same large body of children born between 1991 and 1998.[180] However, the children were only tracked until they were four years old, and autism is not generally diagnosed in Denmark until after the age of five.

If these vaccines are providing only temporary or imperfect immunity, many of our children could grow up susceptible to rubella, mumps or measles, all of which are far more serious as adult diseases. Generations of children with inadequate immunity may grow into adults with no placental immunity to pass on to their children, who could then contract measles as babies, when they would normally be protected by their mother's antibodies. In fact, one study showed that antibody levels are lower in women young enough to have been vaccinated than in older women.[181]

German measles remains a childhood disease among the self-contained Amish communities in the US. It has increasingly become a disease of adolescence and young adulthood in the rest of the United States because of the vaccination programme. Cases among the Amish community have almost always been mild, and pregnant women appear to be naturally protected.[182]

According to the latest research, contracting diseases like measles may be *good* for children. The latest research shows that African children who catch measles tend to suffer from fewer allergic conditions such as asthma, eczema and hayfever, compared with children in developed countries. Studies from Southampton General Hospital in the UK show that children given the measles vaccine more than double their risk of developing atopy, or allergic diseases.[183]

ALTERNATIVES TO IMMUNIZATION

Vitamin A and Immunization

Even for children at risk of getting serious bouts of measles, other, less drastic measures than immunization are available. When vitamin A levels are low, the outer layers of our mucous membranes become scaly and the turnover of cells decreases. The measles virus infects and damages these tissues throughout the body; blood concentrations of vitamin A, even in well-nourished children, may decrease to less than the levels usually found in malnourished children. During measles, children with marginal liver stores of vitamin A may develop an acute vitamin A deficiency, resulting in eye damage and possibly an increased risk of death from respiratory diseases and diarrhoea.

In one study, New York researchers measured vitamin A levels in 89 children younger than two years old, and compared them with a control group. Among the children with measles, the vitamin A levels of 22 per cent were low. Those with low levels were more likely to have a fever of 40°C (104°F) or higher, to have a fever for seven days or more, and to be hospitalized.[184] Other studies demonstrate that children with even a mild vitamin A deficiency were more likely to die of measles.[185]

Giving vitamin A to children with severe (that is, life-threatening) measles can lessen the complications or chances of dying from the disease.[186] D. T. Gerald Keusch of Boston's New England Medical Center, which conducted a study among preschool children in India, went on to say that vitamin A ought to be administered to children whenever there is evidence of a vitamin A deficiency or a possibility of complications from measles. In Africa, where measles is a killer, death rates were reduced by seven times among children under two given vitamin A.[187] Vitamin A is also reputed to offer protection against polio-type viruses.[188]

For any childhood disease, administer high doses of vitamin C as well as vitamin A. Research shows that levels of vitamin C in children also plummet during infectious disease.[189] In America, Dr Fred Klenner carried out extensive research on the use of very high doses of vitamin C during childhood diseases. He used doses as high as one gram every hour around the clock in school-aged children (injections of 1–2 grams, in the case of complications) and discovered that the regime dramatically shortened the life of the disease.[190] Many herbs such as Echinacea and Berberis vulgaris also have solid scientific evidence of success in combating infectious diseases.

Other Preventive Measures

Besides breastfeeding your child for as long as possible, feeding him a healthy, wholefood diet and avoiding sending him to nursery or daycare facilities too early may protect him from many childhood diseases.

Current childcare practices, specifically our tendency to institutionalize children too early, have given rise to epidemics of certain infectious diseases such as meningitis. Both the late Dr Robert Mendelsohn and his editor Vera Chatz were the first to warn of the dangers of 'warehousing' large groups of non-potty-trained babies. Mendelsohn's suspicions were soon backed up by various studies in the medical literature, showing that daycare facilities suffer an epidemic of Hib-caused meningitis. Researchers examining eight daycare centres found that the attack rate for this type of meningitis was 1,100 cases per 100,000 – up to 24 times that of the general incidence among children under four.[191]

A more recent study concluded that centres most at risk included those where workers used towels or handkerchiefs (rather than disposable tissues) to wipe children's noses, or allowed in children who had diarrhoea or who weren't yet potty trained. Ironically, the worst places were those run as commercial businesses, rather than those staffed by volunteers.[192]

If you would feel more comfortable with some sort of booster for your child's immune system, you might want to investigate the homoeopathic alternatives. There is some scientific evidence demonstrating they work.[193] Before vaccines were developed, these nosodes were used widely to prevent a wide variety of infectious diseases. According to Government statistics of the time, the use of these homoeopathic vaccines was linked with an extraordinary drop in the incidence of TB, dysentery, typhoid fever and Asiatic cholera, whooping cough, diphtheria, scarlet fever and measles.[194] In one large-scale study, more than 18,000 children were successfully protected with a homoeopathic remedy (*Menigococcinum IICH*) against meningitis, without a single side-effect.[195]

If you do decide to have your child vaccinated, weigh up each jab carefully as to the actual threat of the disease (is it more of a nuisance rather than a serious risk to his health or life?) versus the effectiveness and also the risk of the vaccine itself. Ask yourself three important questions about each one:

- How necessary is it?

- How effective is it?

- How safe is it?

If you opt for the polio vaccine, you may wish to consider requesting that your child receives the killed rather than the live variety if it isn't already offered. In some reports, polio live vaccines have been recommended only for use in developing countries during actual epidemics, or if the killed variety hasn't worked or been feasible.

If your child has already had his shots and is due for boosters, you can request that his blood antibody levels be checked before subjecting him to the risks of shots which, in some cases, have only a 50 per cent chance of working.

You might very well be better off giving your child carrot juice and a healthy diet, rather than a knee-jerk jab, or, for babies and toddlers, putting your money on the oldest immunization programme of all: good old mother's milk.

7

Hormonal Mayhem

Doctors are among the world's most uncritical enthusiasts. They are constantly on the alert for some magic bullet that can help to alleviate the mountain of pain and suffering that threatens to overwhelm them every day of their working lives. This altruistic desire to heal the sick makes them an easy target for the drug companies. With a minimum of effort, drug salespeople can convince any doctor to embrace even the most speculative of therapies.

In their reckless enthusiasm and boundless optimism, doctors are quick to embrace a new medical breakthrough first, and slow to consider whether it has any supporting evidence. Only when all the safety data is finally in – often decades after it has been prescribed for millions – does medicine realize that it has bet its money, once again, on the wrong horse.

Now that drug companies have made a clever tactical move away from claims that their products can *heal* illness to claiming that drugs can *prevent* illness in the first place, for close to 30 years medicine's favourite preventative has been hormone replacement therapy (HRT), and the most widespread 'disease' being prevented female old age. HRT has become so enshrouded in a myth of beneficence that it has been referred to more than once as 'the most important preventive medicine of the century'.

First discovered by a British chemist, HRT was widely promoted by a Manhattan gynaecologist named Robert Wilson, who did more than anyone to first popularize HRT in the 1960s by first suggesting that the menopause was an illness and women were naturally 'missing' a vital hormone at a certain age. HRT manufacturers produced promotional films showing a 50-year-old woman in front of the fire in a nightgown, bemoaning the fact that her husband was away more often these days, and possibly had become interested in a younger woman.[1]

By the 1990s, an estimated 14 million, or about a third of all post-menopausal women in the US, were on HRT. Oestrogen became the second-most prescribed drug in America and a top seller in Britain – before a single truly scientific study evaluated what on earth this drug might do to women.[2] Doctors even made HRT a feminist issue: by depriving women of HRT, medicine was belittling or ignoring their real suffering during the menopause.

The menopause results from a falling-off in the production of the female hormones oestrogen and progesterone, which affect all systems of the body but particularly regulate the rhythms of women: the monthly cycles, pregnancy and birth, and the beginning and end of reproductive capability.

As levels of oestrogen diminish (to a lower level which the body will eventually adjust to), many women experience the familiar symptoms of the menopause: hot flushes, night sweats, vaginal dryness, cervical, vaginal and uterine thinning, and lack of interest in sex.

These hormones also affect the density of bones; after the menopause, many women suffer a thinning of the bones called osteoporosis (brittle-bone disease), which can eventually result in potentially fatal fractures of the spine or hips or the 'dowager's hump' of female old age. Doctors have also postulated that a lack of oestrogen is also behind the sharp rise in heart disease in women over 50, as women still producing oestrogen don't suffer the heart disease levels of their male counterparts.

HRT employs 'natural' oestrogens (in most cases from the urine of pregnant mares), and more recently artificial progesterone, or progestogen – essentially the same two hormones used in the birth control pill (although in the Pill, both are synthetic). The idea is to trick the body into thinking it is still pre-menopausal, in order to postpone, reduce or elimi-nate the symptoms of 'the change'. It is now available in tablets, a cream, an implant or a patch (the last of which gets changed about twice a week, in order to provide a continual 'drip feed' of hormone at the site).

When first developed in the 1960s, hormone replacement therapy was mainly prescribed for women with severe menopausal symptoms.

Although truly scientific studies (randomized, double-blind studies) were never conducted, the first observational reports threw up a few warning signals: oestrogen on its own could cause endometrial (womb-lining) cancer.[3]

Drug companies responded to this setback with the highly speculative theory that they should add synthetic progesterone into the mix, pointing to research showing that the same dangers didn't exist with 'opposed' therapy – where the added progestogen would hold the unbridled oestrogen in check.

EARLY WARNING SIGNS

Despite this reasoning, which soon became gospel in medical circles, a batch of small studies appeared suggesting a breast cancer risk with either type of preparation; the only thing disputed was exactly how substantial the risk actually was. For instance, an analysis of 16 studies of HRT concluded that, after 15 years, the risk of getting breast cancer increased by 30 per cent in women using oestrogen-only HRT, and more than doubled in those using the combination (oestrogen and progestogen) drug. This risk increased with every year of use.[4] Many other studies showed even higher risks – 60 per cent in one analysis of 37 studies,[5] and even 80 per cent for oestrogen-only preparations, according to a Swedish trial. However, the highest risk was incurred by those using the continuous combination oestrogen-progestogen drug. Far from being protective, drugs with progestogens more than quadrupled the risk.[6]

Even the landmark Nurses' Health Study, produced by Harvard Medical School and backed by the American Cancer Society, found that the risk of breast cancer was even higher in those using the oestrogen-progestogen mix. The most startling figures of all, however, concerned longer-term use. Those using HRT for more than five years had a 46 per cent increased risk of breast cancer. For women over 60, the risk leapt to 71 per cent.[7]

As for endometrial cancer, the research did not show a protective effect – quite the reverse. Oestrogen alone increased the risk from 3 to 20 times; but adding progestogen could increase your risk of getting endometrial cancer to up to 80 per cent over those who didn't take HRT.[8]

Even though these studies were small, from the moment they were published the usual risk-benefit equation used in all drug therapy just didn't stack up. As you don't actually have a disease to weigh up against a cancer risk (HRT is given to healthy women suffering symptoms during a normal physiological process), the life-threatening risk of the drug outweighed its relatively meagre benefits. Developing cancer wasn't a fair trade-off for getting rid of hot flushes and night sweats.

To rebalance the risk vs benefits, drug companies alighted upon the idea of pitching the drug as the equivalent of the female fountain of youth. HRT began being sold as an all-purpose cure-all of the bugbears of old age for all women, not just the 40 per cent who have menopausal symptoms. Doctors began to speak of HRT not simply as a curative of a collection of annoying but relatively benign symptoms, but as a preventative of all the major diseases of life after 50: heart disease, osteoporosis, stroke and even senile dementia.

This kind of statistical trade-off is often used to justify a dangerous drug in medicine. Something that can kill you by causing cancer doesn't look so bad if it can be shown to prevent diseases that you are at an even higher risk of developing. With HRT, so the argument went, the risk of breast cancer from the drug was far less than the natural risk that postmenopausal women face of developing heart disease or osteoporosis.

From the time of its launch, doctors began playing statistical games with this drug, using loosely assembled observational studies to infer a host of these future protective benefits. In time, the proclaimed benefits grew ever more outlandish. Besides curing Alzheimer's disease and strokes, HRT was even tried out in the treatment of women with inflammatory bowel disease.[9]

For many years, doctors were able to dismiss the cancer risks of HRT as speculative and unproven, largely because most studies were small and only case-controlled or observational (that is, researchers simply selected groups of women – one group on HRT and another not on HRT – and observed them over time, to see which group was healthier – a type of study not considered particularly scientific). All that was disputed was exactly how great the risk actually was. The party line that was adopted was that, sure, HRT could increases your breast cancer risk, but only by a fraction. And, besides, this was a 'treatable' cancer.

John Studd of King's College Hospital in London, who remains a staunch defender of HRT, was so confident of its benefits that at one point he dismissed the need for any extra monitoring as 'illogical'.[10] Since the statistics showed that fewer women die from HRT-caused diseases than from other causes, he did not see the cancer risk as a big deal. 'There is not enough information to suggest that breast cancer risk is a valid reason to withhold oestrogen therapy,' he once wrote.[11]

In 1990 it was my prediction that future generations would look back upon HRT and other prescribed hormones such as the Pill as among the biggest medical blunders of the century. Sadly, this intuitive belief has now been vindicated. Professor Bruno Muller-Oerlinghausen, chairman of the German Commission on the Safety of Medicines – the equivalent of the British Health Minister or the head of America's Food and Drug Adminstration – recently referred to HRT as 'the new thalidomide'.

All easy dismissal of the cancer risk was swept aside with the first large-scale legitimate scientific studies into HRT. It had taken doctors 40 years to decide that HRT merited true scientific investigation, and then only after intense pressure from women's groups. The Women's Health Initiative (WHI), a major 15-year study set up by the National Institutes of Health in America to examine the most common forms of death and illness in postmenopausal women, began the first randomized double-blind placebo-controlled trial. Of some 16,000 female participants, half were randomly placed into either a group receiving Prempro (a combination therapy manufactured by Wyeth) or a placebo. In addition, 10,000 women who'd undergone a hysterectomy received oestrogen alone. The plan was for the experimental group to take the drug for eight years, to see if it did have the protective effects it had grown famous for.

After five years, the Data and Safety Monitoring Board of the WHI shocked the world by ordering the study to an abrupt halt. The figures were suddenly indisputable: women on the drug were more likely than normal to get breast cancer. In fact, not only were they more likely to get *cancer*, but more likely to get many of the diseases HRT purported to protect against: heart disease, stroke, blood clots and dementia.[12]

Although authorities in America and elsewhere reacted to the news by advising women to stop taking the pills for long-term protective benefits, many in medicine reacted as usual to negative news by fobbing off the research as 'inappropriate'. As one meeting concluded in Madiera, in the February after the disclosure of the study: 'Although it was generally agreed that the study was well designed and executed, its relevance to standard hormone therapy for clinical practice must be seriously called into question. The target population used in the WHI is not representative of the target population for whom menopausal HRT is normally considered.'[13]

By the time that the British equivalent of the WHI study, called the Million Women Study, had weighed in, the evidence was unequivocal: women were dying from HRT. This particular research, carried out by the Medical Research Council (MRC) and Cancer Research UK, tracked more than a million British women aged 50–64 from 1996–2001. The study concluded that HRT doubles the risk of breast cancer, and raises the risk of heart attacks, blood clots and strokes. According to the study's conclusion, HRT had been responsible for 20,000 cases of breast cancer over the past 10 years alone in Britain – many of them fatal.[14]

But the big surprise of the MRC study concerned which type of HRT proved the most dangerous. For years, doctors had been hammering on about the 'protective' effects of combination therapy. However, as the Million Woman study showed, it was just these combined drugs that posed the greatest risk. After five years, 1 in 166 women may get cancer; after 10 years, 1 in 50. No matter what type of HRT, or which mode of delivery – pills, patches, continuous or sequential regimes, or even tibolone (Livial), the supposedly safer alternative – your cancer risk increases after a single year of use.

Professor Muller-Oerlinghausen, went on to describe HRT as a 'national and international tragedy'. 'More women have probably died from the ... hormone therapy than damaged children were born in the wake of the thalidomide scandal,' he announced.

Most recently, a Swedish study entitled HABITS by the University of Uppsala in Sweden, which studied the effect of HRT on women with breast cancer, was halted after preliminary results showed that women with breast cancer had a higher-than-average chance of the cancer recurring if they were on HRT. This trial of 1,300 women was meant to follow its subjects for at least five years, but was stopped after just over two years when the negative results came in. The study found that three times as many women taking HRT had a recurrence of their cancer or another tumour, compared to women who'd received other treatments for the menopause. Three times as many women taking HRT had a recurrence or new breast tumour compared with women who had received other treatments to relieve symptoms of the menopause.[15]

Although doctors routinely offer HRT to survivors of breast cancer, the American Cancer Society now believes that this could change. Indeed, the US Food and Drug Association now has mandated that warnings about the various risks be carried in every prescription packet prescribed in America.

THE MYTHS EXPLODED

Something else interesting occurred with the marketing of HRT. Invariably, in medicine, your spin on the science depends upon how enthusiastically you have embraced the therapy in the past. Enthusiasts will regard as sacrosanct a small study if it puts a positive spin on a treatment, but criticize the study's design if the research shows the treatment is dangerous or ineffective. With the alleged expanded protective effect of HRT, doctors for many years ignored the fact that any studies showing a benefit were small and observational, even though they had criticized those studies showing breast-cancer risk for precisely the same reason. Other factors (diet, lifestyle, genes, socio-economics, exercise) could have accounted for what appeared to be the HRT-induced protective effect of HRT on osteoporosis and heart disease.

The heart-protective myth of HRT largely began in 1993, when a group of US epidemiologists selected 5,000 post-menopausal women from the American South and Midwest and measured their cholesterol levels and other supposed risk factors, from which they deduced these women's supposed risk of suffering from future cardiovascular disease. After comparing the results of those on HRT with those not on the drug, the researchers concluded that HRT could reduce the risk of heart disease by 42 per cent.[16]

The researchers did acknowledge that they were making a few mighty hefty assumptions. For one thing, the study wasn't randomized – that is, the participants weren't selected randomly – so there could have been what scientists term 'selection bias': only the healthiest women with a low incidence of heart disease may have been selected to take HRT. As other researchers note, women on HRT are more likely to be white, upper middle class, educated and thin – all factors which individually lessen their heart-disease risk in the first place.[17]

In the same edition of *The Lancet*, which published the study, an editorial attempted to distance itself from its conclusions. 'The authors' calculation of the overall benefit … is speculative,' said the editorial, because the study wasn't designed to tell whether HRT actually caused metabolic changes or whether they just occurred independently.[18]

And of course the entire study was based upon what may be an erroneous assumption – that a raised cholesterol level automatically leads to heart disease.

A number of other studies appeared to show that the presence of oestrogen raises the 'good' HDL cholesterol, which is believed to protect against coronary heart disease, and lowers the 'bad' LDL cholesterol. The first studies had mainly looked at the effect of oestrogen on animal arteries or on human arteries obtained during cardiac transplants. By the time the first randomized, placebo-controlled study into the effect of HRT on heart disease (called the Postmenopausal Estrogen/Progestin Interventions [PEPI] trial) was published, the alleged heart-protection benefit was virtually set in stone. PEPI emphasized the effects of lowering LDL and raising HDL cholesterol. However, what never made the headlines was the trial's discovery that progestogen increases levels of the fat triglyceride, a known risk factor for heart disease, particularly in women. This triglyceride effect could make HRT an even more dangerous option for women with diabetes.[19]

A number of researchers agree that most of the studies showing a heart benefit with HRT have been flawed. Professor Jan Vandenbroucke and his Dutch colleagues at the Department of Clinical Epidemiology, Leiden University Hospital in the Netherlands reviewed all the individual studies concerning HRT and the heart and concluded that the studies had been 'biased', unintentionally selecting inordinately healthy women who may have been at lower risk of developing heart disease in the first place. Furthermore, women with a pre-existing heart condition were included in the studies. When you remove them from the studies, the results show similar death rates in women, whether they take HRT or not.[20] The use of HRT as a universal preventive is 'unwarranted', Vandenbroucke concluded.[21]

Vandenbroucke and his colleagues also disputed the entire theory that giving 'outside' hormones will in any way protect your heart, or even that women have an increased risk in this regard. 'Data on mortality from coronary heart disease shows that there is no acceleration in coronary heart disease in women after the age of 50,' he writes. 'Even if there were plausible biological reasons why natural oestrogens would protect against coronary heart disease, it does not follow that replacing a relative deficiency has beneficial effects.'[22]

Nevertheless, the claims of a few enthusiasts had the entire medical community in thrall for many years, and the heart-protective effects of HRT were simply taken as read for more than a decade.

But PEPI too had been small – a study of only 875 women over three years. The eventual arrival of larger studies, like the Women's Health Initiative, showed that the entire claim for a cardiovascular benefit had been built upon sand.

Researchers began experimenting with HRT to treat existing heart problems. In 1998 came the first results of the Heart and Estrogen Replacement Study (or HERS; most HRT studies are saddled with the most cloying acronyms – even WISDOM has been tried out). HERS examined the affects of combination HRT on women with heart disease.

Over the more than four years of the study, the results showed that HRT did appear to reduce LDL cholesterol by 11 per cent, and HDL cholesterol by 10 per cent. However, far from being protective, HRT doubled the risk of a heart attack during the first year and caused 24 per cent more deaths (71 vs 58) due to heart disease.[23] HERS participants were followed up for two-and-a-half years more in HERS II, and the results were clear: no effect at all, positive or negative. HRT was proved to have absolutely no cardiac benefit in those taking the drug.[24]

Other studies, such as the Estrogen Replacement and Atherosclerosis study (ERA – this time, with an acronym reminiscent of feminism), discovered that HRT had no effect on halting the progression of atherosclerosis in women with established heart disease.[25]

By the time the WHI study was published, it was clear that HRT was actually *harmful* to the heart: The WHI study was halted not only for the cancer risk but also for the damage observed to the participants' cardiovascular system. Healthy women on the drug had increased cardiovascular disease – more heart attacks, more fatalities, more strokes and more thromboembolic disease.[26]

These results not only demolish any notion that HRT is heart protective, they also point up the limitation of any heart-protective programme that relies on lowering cholesterol, when much other science has demonstrated that protection from heart disease is far more complex than controlling fats in the blood.

Indeed, one study conducted by the University of California at San Diego's Department of Family and Preventive Medicine made the astonishing discovery that women's natural levels of oestrogen give them no special protection against heart disease. The women with heart disease in this study didn't have lower levels of oestrogen than those with healthy hearts; *in fact, oestrogen levels were not found to alter to any great degree after the menopause.* Cholesterol levels and blood-pressure weren't found to be major factors in heart disease, either.[27]

For many years, doctors maintained that the oestrogens of HRT don't pose the same risk of thrombosis as those oestrogens used in the Pill. The prevailing wisdom was that the same oestrogen (albeit a different dosage) placed in the contraceptive pill and acknowledged to cause cardiovascular incidents does not cause this problem when placed in a fairly similar form in hormone replacement therapy. As the *British Medical Journal* put it: 'Many doctors have been surprised to discover that a hormonal treatment they had learnt to avoid in women at risk of cardiovascular disease is now being specifically advised in this situation.'[28]

All the large-scale studies have exploded this myth, however. The HERS study and others showed a threefold increase in thrombosis among women taking HRT.[29] Other research from Oxford showed that the greatest risk was among women who'd recently been placed on HRT.[30]

Another frequent claim made about HRT, without a shred of convincing evidence, was that it reduced the risk of stroke. Far from being protective, three studies, including the Nurse's Health Study and HERS, show that HRT at least triples the risk of stroke (as does its closely related cousin, the Pill).[31] The level of risk appears to be related to the dosage. Higher doses (0.625–1.25 mg/day of oestrogen) increase the risk from three to seven times.[32] The only 'protection' from stroke occurred in the Nurse's study at low dosages of 0.3 per day.[33]

At 45, Maria, from Tyne and Wear, was put on HRT by her doctor. From the day she took her first pill, she started to bleed. Her GP told her that the drug simply 'needed to get into her system' and told her to double up on the dosage. After she did, she began passing out and her left leg turned purple.

'When I began having pains in my stomach and chest, a doctor called out on emergency told me to stop the pills immediately. Nevertheless, I continued to pass blood clots.' At this point, Maria's GP told her that she was losing so much blood because the drug was 'now leaving her body'. Once it did, he assured her, everything would return to normal.

A month later the pain had travelled up Maria's body to her arm joints. She could neither bend nor breathe, and her chest felt like it was caving in. She was then given prednisolone, a steroid, and penicillin, and began vomiting so much that nothing would stay down. After a week she had to call out her doctor because she couldn't move, but lay on the floor on a mattress in her living room.

'My left side felt paralysed, my head flopped, I couldn't see and my speech was slurred. The GP said I'd had a reaction to penicillin, but thought the steroid would counter any ill-effects. He left me lying on the floor,' said Maria. Many tests later, the medical consensus was that Maria had suffered a stroke brought on by the HRT.

Hormones may well be able to stave off temporarily some of the confusion and woolly-headedness induced by falling hormone levels, and some women do feel very well on oestrogen. Organizations such as the Amarant Trust in Britain have long maintained that HRT can prevent Alzheimer's disease. However, a 15-year study found that HRT has no effect on keeping your brain sharp. Any reduction in cognitive function has been shown to be the same, regardless of whether or not women use oestrogen.[34]

Most experts agree that the studies of women taking oestrogen show increased bone density – and the WHI Study bore that out. However, long-term studies of HRT have shown that women following the usual recommendation to take the drug for 10 years upon the start of the menopause are not protected any more from brittle-bone disease than are those women who have never taken the drug at all. An ongoing 50-year study of the residents of Framingham, Massachusetts, concluded that HRT preserves bone mass in women only while they're taking it – and only then if it is taken for at least seven years. As soon as women stop the drug, even after a decade of use, bone-mineral density catches up in its rapid decline, so that by age 75 it is virtually the same as in women who have never taken the drug. This means HRT affords virtually no protection during those decades of life when the risk of developing osteoporosis is greatest.[35]

To get round these problems, doctors have variously recommended that HRT should be taken for ever (at which point the breast cancer risks begin to mount); or begun 10 years *after* the menopause, long after a woman has experienced all the menopausal symptoms the drug is supposed to alleviate; or even that it should be given after a woman breaks her hip, which would seem to be more than a little self-defeating.[36]

At best, oestrogen seems to have only a temporary effect. Although it may decrease the rate at which old bone is torn down, formation of new bone eventually decreases in some three to five years, anyway. One large-scale review of 31 studies on osteoporosis concluded that oestrogen didn't have a 'significant benefit' in slowing the onset of osteoporosis.[37] Another found it didn't strengthen bones in women even when they had used it for 16 years.[38]

In fact, there is some evidence that oestrogens or progestogens actually *contribute* to osteoporosis. The spinal bone density of women under study has increased once the women stopped using medroxyprogesterone as a contraceptive, compared to no change among women carrying on taking the progestogen.[39]

Dr Kitty Little, an Oxford researcher, spent many years studying the effects of hormones on bone marrow. In animal experiments, Dr Little observed that one effect of the oestrogen-progestogen combinations is to distort large cells in the bone, leading to a huge increase in abnormally sticky platelets, or tiny blood clots. These can interfere with the blood supply to the trabecular bone, the spongy bone found mainly in the spinal vertebrae.[40]

In London, Biolab's medical researcher Dr John McLaren Howard has studied the levels of nutrients necessary for bone development in women with osteoporosis, particularly the enzyme alkaline phosphatase. This enzyme works with magnesium to form calcium crystals in the bone, and so is an indicator of whether new bone is being laid down. *The lowest levels of alkaline phosphatase in Dr Howard's study were found in women with osteoporosis on HRT.*[41]

A LITANY OF SIDE-EFFECTS

Without all these claimed benefits, all HRT offers is a grocery list of potentially fatal side-effects. The most popular way to take HRT is by mouth. However, via this route, women experience a number of gastrointestinal symptoms – nausea, vomiting, abdominal cramps, bloating – and may even develop jaundice.

This may be one reason why medicine came up with the skin (transdermal) patch, which bypasses the liver, resulting in higher levels of oestrogen being absorbed by the body. However, a fifth of patients experience blistering, hyperaemia (increased blood flow in the area) and discolouration of the skin using this method. Consequently, an increasing number of doctors now use oestrogen implants, which require a small outpatient operation to insert the pellets under the skin.

Oestrogen implants (and even patches) appear to create a 'tolerance' for oestrogen that some doctors warn is similar to addiction; a woman will have higher-than-normal levels of oestrogen in her bloodstream, but nevertheless complains of the return of menopausal symptoms at increasingly frequent intervals. Although these implants are supposed to last for six months, many users complain of a return of symptoms three to nine weeks later. This phenomenon – called 'tachyphylaxis,' (which means, literally, 'too much prevention') – occurred in three out of every hundred women, in a study by the Dulwich Hospital Menopause Clinic in London.[42]

After examining a number of such studies, Dr Thomas Bewley, former president of the Royal College of Psychiatrists, and Dr Susan Bewley, a gynaecologist at University College Hospital, London, concluded that this dependence 'occurs in 15 per cent of cases', largely for psychological reasons. As they explained: 'Oestrogens are psychoactive. They lift mood, can be given by injection, and their use has powerful psychological effects.'[43]

HRT proponent John Studd once wrote that women who have psychiatric problems require larger than normal oestrogen levels, anyway. 'These women may need higher levels [of oestrogen] to obtain symptomatic relief, since many were originally treated for premenstrual syndrome (PMS) or depression [during the menopause]' he wrote.[44] Elsewhere he has said that it is 'by no means rare' for patients to require an increasing dose of hormones. 'It may just mean they are addicted to feeling better', he says.[45]

It may simply be that the oestrogen-sensitive cells in the body, continually blasted with high doses of the hormone, lose the ability to respond.[46] Or it could be that early use of oestrogens, whether in HRT, to control PMT, or as included in the Pill, may set up an increased need for replacement therapy. HRT creates artificially high levels of oestrogen in the body, which could trigger a hormonal 'crash' when these levels fall even slightly, thereby exacerbating ordinary menopausal symptoms.

Ordinarily, the body's pituitary glands and ovaries work in exquisite tandem, constantly adjusting oestrogen levels to fit the body's need of the moment, like a car set on automatic, says Dr Ellen Grant, author of *Sexual Chemistry* and a long-time critic of HRT and the Pill.[47] HRT, which delivers a constant level of oestrogen, she says, is like having a car stuck in a single gear.

Another problem with oestrogen implants is endometrial stimulation – a potential cancer-causing reaction. These days, it is acknowledged that using oestrogen-only preparations on a woman who still has a womb can increase by up to 20-fold her chances of getting endometrial cancer after several years. This is because oestrogen causes rapid proliferation of endometrial cells (as it does in pregnancy). To counteract this, most women are given progestogen for 10–12 days per month, which imitates the second half of the menstrual cycle, producing withdrawal bleeding.

Endometrial stimulation in women given the implants occurs for an average of two years after they finish taking supplemental oestrogen.[48] What this means is that, in order to lower your risk of getting endometrial cancer, you have to commit yourself to taking oral progestogen for two years or more after you finish taking oestrogen.

HRT, like the Pill, was always touted as a 'protection' against ovarian cancer. But the latest discovery by the American Cancer Society is that women who stay on HRT for more than 10 years increase their risk of developing fatal ovarian cancer by 70 per cent. In the ACS study, which tracked more than 200,000 menopausal women, the risk increased the longer the women were on HRT, although most were using twice the dosage currently used today.[49]

Most pro-HRT literature concentrates on the supposed euphoria experienced by women on the drug. What it doesn't discuss is that 70 per cent of women experience a host of side-effects with oestrogen or progestogen, and that half of all women stop taking the drug after six months.

Katie from London was one such woman:

I became incredibly ill while using HRT. My symptoms included indigestion, bloating, lethargy, extreme tension and violent headaches. My heart thumped all day, particularly when I tried to move about. My chest wall tightened, with pains down my arms, almost like a heart attack. Besides symptoms of panic, I was so ill I couldn't concentrate or even watch anything on TV, particularly emotional scenes. I came off the drug nine months ago; I am not out of the woods yet, to put it mildly. My doctor won't accept that I could still be adversely affected three weeks after stopping HRT, and wants me to see a psychiatrist! On top of everything, of course, my hot flushes have returned with a vengeance – no doubt due to having been suppressed by the HRT.

Progestogens can also alter your glucose and insulin levels,[50] cause higher than normal levels of calcium in the blood, hepatitis, liver cancer (including peliosis hepatitis, a life-threatening complication), urinary tract infections,[51] jaundice, excess fluid, with or without heart failure, and virilization – such as an increase in facial hair, and deepening of the voice – which can be irreversible. HRT also exacerbates endometriosis.[52]

Hormone supplementation is also linked with increasing the severity of migraines, because it causes an overreaction in the arteries and veins.[53] Patients have reduced their incidence of headaches 10-fold when they stopped both smoking and taking hormones.[54]

185

This is in addition to all the other side-effects of oestrogen: at least a twofold increase in the risk of gall bladder disease,[55] elevated blood-pressure, enlarged and tender breasts, changes in the shape of the eyes, and depression. Progestogens in particular have been implicated in depression.[56] Taking HRT can more than than double the risk of suicide.[57]

Harriet was first prescribed HRT (Cyclo-Progynova) for severe menopausal symptoms and to prevent osteoporosis. She was told by the hospital doctor who took her x-ray, and also by her own GP, that there was no alternative and that her bones would crumble if she didn't take it.

After three weeks I felt wonderful, but during the fifth week not only did all my previous symptoms return with a vengeance, but I also experienced urinary incontinence, [and difficulties with my vision], speech, memory and motor [co-ordination]. At times my vision appeared as though I was looking through the wrong end of binoculars (everything appeared much smaller). My speech at times was an incoherent jumble; I could not remember my name or address or recognize people or objects, and there were long gaps in the day which I could not explain. Some days I could not walk unaided, and often my husband had to drag me out of bed and make me move because my body felt encased in lead. I also became severely dyslexic. I stopped taking the tablets immediately the first symptoms occurred, but my condition continued to deteriorate. My GP just did not believe me because I could only visit the surgery on 'good' days. I was told that all I needed was 'counselling'. I declined and turned to alternative therapies. Within 18 months my central nervous system was almost back to normal – walking more than 100 yards was still a problem. However, the HRT had left me with a serious intolerance to petrochemicals. Many toiletries, household cleaners, new fabrics [and] new buildings caused asthma-like attacks, bouts of severe aggression or depression, or muscle collapse, all accompanied by tissue swelling. A strict diet and nutritional supplements (including a course of intravenous vitamins and minerals) has helped to restore my immune system, and now I do not have severe attacks.

After the Million Women results were in, the German authorities did the responsible thing and told doctors that the weight of evidence is now against HRT. Treatment in Germany is now restricted to women with particularly severe symptoms and given at the lowest possible dosages for the shortest period of time. German women are abandoning the therapy in droves.

You would have thought that this was strong meat for the UK and US to follow suit. However, Gordon Duff, chairman of the Committee of Safety of Medicines, has been sanguine on the subject. In an advisory for doctors, sent the day after the study was published, he wrote that the benefits continue to outweigh the risks: 'The results of the Million Women Study do not necessitate any urgent changes to women's treatment.'[58]

SO-CALLED 'NATURAL' ALTERNATIVES

But in other quarters, now that HRT has been largely discredited, many practitioners are on the look out for natural alternatives. One of the favourites at the moment is so-called 'natural' progesterone, which is being sold as a cream and touted as the solution for being female and over 40. 'Natural' progesterone was popularized by the late Dr John Lee, with something of the fervour of religious zeal. Although Dr Lee sincerely believed that his own studies and many others demonstrated the safety and effectiveness of natural progesterone, there remains an appalling lack of evidence about it.

Although these progesterones are called 'natural' because they are derived from yams, natural progesterone is in fact made in the test tube. Our bodies produce a basic steroid skeleton, or molecular blueprint, from which all hormones are derived. This skeleton goes through a number of natural processes, governed by enzymes from different organs, to transform into individual hormones such as progesterone.

Chemists making so-called 'natural' hormones imitate this process by extracting a number of chemical processes in the test tube, tacking on extra parts of molecules here and there, to end up with a substance with more or less the same molecular structure that our bodies produce. But all such progesterones must go through this chemical processing, and all share similar side-effects. For Gestone, one licensed progesterone in the UK, side-effects include loss of vision, double vision, migraine, changes in the cervix or breast, insomnia and changes in menstrual flow or cycle, to name a few.[59]

Progesterone is sold as a 'cosmetic' in the US and imported by the UK. As such, manufacturers are not obliged to go through the safety testing required by the US Food and Drug Administration. Because there are no US regulations, any manufacturer can put in any amount of the hormone he wishes. One laboratory, which analysed 19 body creams containing progesterone sold in the US, found that the creams contained anything from less than 2 mg to 700 mg per ounce. This is worrying when you consider the minute doses required by the body to keep things ticking over. In another survey of 27 branded natural progesterone creams, 11 had less than 2 mg or progesterone in every ounce of the cream. Some had absolutely none.[60] During the menstrual cycle of the ordinary woman, progesterone blood levels range from 0.5 to 20 nanograms per ml (equivalent of one part per billion in weight). With the rub-on cream, women could be enhancing the progesterone concentration in the blood by four or five times. Furthermore, not everyone absorbs progesterone in the same way, and those spots where you've rubbed in the cream can have far higher doses than your blood levels.[61] Although the average amount absorbed is about 10 per cent of the applied dose (5 mg if you're using 50 mg of progesterone at a time), the amount of progesterone contained in the average jar is hugely variable. Research shows that even when extraordinarily high doses of the cream is rubbed on, very little of the hormone actually enters the bloodstream.[62]

Although fans of progesterone cream claim that the progesterone shows up in the saliva tests, other studies show that the high saliva results may be paradoxical and not reflect what is actually circulating in the body.[63] One such study, carried out in Australia, showed that even high doses of progesterone cream didn't increase circulating blood progesterone concentration enough to cause any changes in the endometrium, or lining of the womb. Yet other research shows that progesterone cream has no effect on vasomotor levels, mood, bone mineral density or blood levels.[64]

The common wisdom also has it that 'natural' progesterone prevents breast cancer. Proponents of rub-on progesterone point to a single study showing that when women with tumours rubbed on cream, the breasts showed a reduction in cell division associated with cancer. However, the study was tiny, including only 40 women observed for less than two weeks.[65] Another study used as evidence of the value of progesterone as a cancer fighter showed that breast cancer survivors taking 50 mg of progestins (medroxyprogesterone acetate) had half the rate of re-occurrence of disease.[66] Other research shows just the reverse, and for good reason. Some epidemiologists believe that high levels of progesterone may be a risk factor for breast cancer,[67] and progesterone is a listed carcinogen in many chemical handbooks.[68] We also know from studies of women who get breast cancer that women with the highest levels of progesterone have a more than eightfold rise in the rate of breast cancer.[69] Other studies have shown that high concentrations of progesterone in the breast increases the risk of breast cancer.[70] As one of the tasks of progesterone is to ensure that a woman's body will not reject a developing foetus, progesterone acts powerfully as an immune-system suppressant.[71]

Martha used rub-on progesterone after her first bout of breast cancer, only to have the cancer return; she sued the American medical centre which prescribed the cream to 'prevent' the recurrence. Other women have written in to say that they've been very ill on rub-on creams. 'It took us both months to sort out our hormones after discontinuing use,' wrote Sally from Detroit. 'I was also advised to take two tbsp of flax oil a day and 1 tbsp of flax seed. After doing this for four or five months, my breasts were still sore and my groin was aching.'

To reconcile much conflicting research, some proponents have put forward the argument that progesterone causes breast cancer in low doses but prevents it in high doses. American breast cancer specialist Dr David Zava, who has carried out some study of the effect of progesterone and plant hormones, suspects that: 'Progesterone at very low dose acts in synergy with estradiol to stimulate cell proliferation. Only at the higher dose does progesterone begin to down-regulate oestrogen and shut down oestrogen-regulated cell proliferation.'

Even if this were true, and it is only Zava's opinion, as he says he has been unable to fund research on this issue, no one knows the exact threshold at which a carcinogen turns into a preventative. This is precisely the same type of argument that doctors have used to distinguish between the hormones in HRT and those of the Pill. Certainly the experience of doctors with even tried-and-tested hormones like tamoxifen, used in high doses to block oestrogen-sensitive cancers, in the end cause other cancers.

Although John Lee built his platform on the claim that these creams prevent osteoporosis, there is no scientific evidence to show that progesterone protects bones,[72] and the evidence that exists shows that it actually causes the condition.[73] A number of critics have suggested that Lee's own study was not much more than a hypothesis, developed from simple observation of his patients, without proper scientific controls.[74] One study of women taking the cream for more than a year found no effect on bone density after an entire year of use.[75]

Naturopath Harald Gaier has found that his female patients using natural progesterone don't end up with much success. 'I have had women who have used protesterone creams and had bone densitometry before and after the treatment, only to find that the deterioration had carried on,' he says. 'The women who have used the cream without results don't just feel let down, they feel irate.'

The practitioners who advocate natural progesterone have no idea what, if anything is the optimum use, and women are experimenting with brands, dosages and locations on their body. As one women wrote in to a pro-progesterone website: 'I had an experience last fall when I had been using ProGest on my breasts regularly for some time, had a period, then my breasts (nipples especially), in spite of continued use of P after the period, got very sore, and hot. This worried me; I'd read about increased breast temperature being associated with breast cancer.'

She was assured that most likely the amount of progesterone that she was using was too low, and that using a high dosage (100 mg/g) would 'down-regulate' cell proliferation. In the absence of any evidence, every woman using it for whatever reason is simply experimenting on herself.

Besides natural progesterone, doctors and naturopaths have turned their attention to food and plant sources of female hormones. Phytoestrols are compounds which have a similar molecular structure to oestrogen, and their effects are comparable, although weaker, to those of oestrogen itself. The phytoestrogen family includes: isoflavones (which are found mainly in beans such as soybeans, red clover and alfalfa); lignans (in seeds, especially flaxseed, nuts and grains, such as rye and millet fruit, certain vegetables,) and coumestans (in legumes and red clover).

Encouraged by the fact that Japanese women – with their high-soya diet have phyto-oestrogen levels in their urine of up to 1,000 times higher than those of American women[76] and much lower frequency of hot flushes and other menopausal symptoms than women in the West, manufacturers have been falling over themselves to create plant estrogen products.

Nevertheless, the latest evidence shows that women may be substituting one type of hormone replacement for another. Plant oestrogens can have effects just as powerful as synthetic estrogens. For instance, Dr Zava just completed an intriguing study on the estrogen and progesterone activity of foods, herbs and spices. In his study, Zava tested the ability of more than 250 herbal extracts to bind to oestrogen and progesterone receptors in breast tumour cells. Those found to bind to oestrogen receptors – soy, licorice, red clover, thyme, turmeric, hops, and verbena – acted as tumour promoters. The herbs with the highest binding to progesterone receptors were red clover, verbena, oregano, turmeric, thyme and damiana. The highest oestrogen-binding agent were soy isoflavones, which in low doses appear to promote proliferation of breast tissue.

This is consistent with growing research showing that phytoestrogens are as potent as other types of hormone replacement for causing cancer. For instance, studies have shown that women consuming large amounts of soy have a increased rate of cell proliferation, a precursor to cancer.[77]

Genistein is now being sold over the counter in potent dosages that are virtually the equivalent of those of hormone replacement therapy, when even small doses of genistein have been shown to promote tumours growth in the breast. In one study, genistein was found to promote breast growth; the authors cautioned women with breast cancer not to consume soy.[78] Another study shows that even high dietary intake of soy for a few weeks can increase the proliferation of cells in the breast.[79]

Oestrogen found in red clover is known to have six times the oestrogenic effect of other plant-derived oestrogens:[80] sheep fed a diet of red clover have suffered from permanent infertility.[81] Other research shows that genistein, daidzein and coumoestrol can cause chromosomal abnormalities.[82] We even have evidence that red clover causes the same cell growth as oestradiol, the oestrogen used in HRT.[83]

Zava and other researchers again use the high-dose/low-dose effect argument: high doses are the type needed to suppress the growth of breast and other tumours. Even if this is true, no one knows how much becomes suppressive, how these added hormones interact with a woman's own hormone levels, which also can vary enormously or what exactly the effect of long-term high-dose supplementation with plant hormones actually can do.

ALTERNATIVES TO HORMONE REPLACEMENT THERAPY (HRT)

If you decide that all these risks aren't worth taking just to rid yourself of hot flushes, there are many alternatives. Many nutritional doctors, including those with great experience in treating women during the menopause, argue that the kind of menopause you experience, like your degree of morning sickness or PMT, simply reflects your nutritional state. They believe that a difficult menopause *is* a 'deficiency disease', but not of oestrogen. The root of the problem is deficiency in one of a number of vital micronutrients, food intolerance, or the inefficient function of certain organs.

According to Dr Ellen Grant, 'Hot flushes are not a sign of oestrogen deficiency … [but] a result of an allergic reaction.' Flushes are very similar to headaches, migraine and rises in blood-pressure.[84] John Mansfield, a British allergy specialist and author of *Arthritis: the Allergy Connection* (Thorsons) and other books, concurs that many menopausal symptoms are related to food sensitivity or candida albicans (yeast) overgrowth. 'Once we put women on an elimination diet, the severe symptoms stop.'

Most nutritional practitioners now advocate an unprocessed, wholefood diet with first-class proteins, and a sensible, individually-tailored supplement programme with high levels of magnesium (at least 500 mg daily), zinc (at least 30 mg), boron (3 mg), which helps the body make its own oestrogen; at least 10 mg manganese and 1 gm vitamin C per day, vitamin K if accelerated bone-formation is desirable, vitamin D, folic acid, at least 50–100 mg of B6 (or 50 mg pyridoxal-5-phosphate, the first metabolite of B6), essential fatty acids and at least 40 units per day of vitamin E to help ovaries maximize their output of oestrogen during the early stages of the menopause. Eat moderate amounts of plant phytoestrogens and change your diet away from red meat to include many pulses and whole grains like brown rice.

It's vital to look after your adrenal gland, the major organ involved in adaptive changes in the body. Because it has the highest concentration of vitamin C and pantothenic acid of any organ, it's wise to ensure an abundance of these two essential nutrients.

Have your practitioner make sure that your thyroid is functioning normally.

For hot flushes, try 1,000–2,000 mg a day of hesperiden–derived bioflavonoids on an empty stomach, and supplements of the amino acid beta alanine; or lachesis (30c potency), used four times a day for a few days then reducing gradually to once a day just before bedtime. An alternative homoeopathic remedy is silver nitrate (30c). For low libido, have regular sex.

To prevent osteoporosis, the solution is far more complicated than simply wolfing down glasses of milk or calcium pills, as most doctors now recommend. American researcher Dr Guy Abraham has demonstrated that most cases of osteoporosis are not caused by calcium deficiency and cannot be prevented by calcium megadosing. Instead he found that magnesium deficiency plays a key role because this mineral is necessary to activate bone enzyme alkaline phosphatase.

In his own study, Dr Abraham gave magnesium to 19 women taking HRT.[85] After eight months, the bone mineral density in the women taking the supplements had increased by 11 per cent, compared with no increase in the women taking HRT alone. Although 15 of the 19 women had bone mineral density below that considered likely to cause fractures, after a year, only half still had bones that were too thin. Bone mineral levels were still improving after two years.

In John McLaren Howard's study, besides the enzyme alkaline phosphatase, women with osteoporosis were found to be low in magnesium, zinc, manganese and vitamin C.

Regular, weight-bearing exercise has consistently been shown to stave off bone loss, even in women past the menopause, despite the usual medical claims that if you don't exercise before 40, you can't do anything to improve your bones. Regular exercise has been shown to halve your risk of hip fracture,[86] and twice-weekly high-intensity exercise has been shown to increase bone density and to improve muscle mass, strength and balance in postmenopausal women – all important points if you want to avoid fracture. Cigarette smoking accelerates the destruction of oestrogen and so hastens the onset of both the menopause and osteoporosis. If you stop smoking, you reduce your risk of hip fracture by 25 per cent.[87]

Another reason we in the West may be plagued with osteoporosis is our tendency to eat excessive amounts of protein. As calcium is needed to metabolize protein, a high-protein diet means calcium is constantly leeched from the bones. Osteoporosis is virtually unknown in places such as Africa, where the inhabitants eat far fewer proteins.[88]

Also be sure to get your digestive function checked since low stomach acid can be responsible for low absorption of calcium. You may wish to take a supplement of vitamin D_3, which increases the uptake of calcium in the diet, and small supplements of boron, which help to metabolize vitamin D_3.[89]

PART IV

TREATMENT

8

Miracle Cures

ANTIBIOTICS

I owe my life to antibiotics. In 1942, when my mother was 24, her dentist unwisely extracted a tooth while she had the flu. Within days her neck ballooned with a streptococcus infection, and she was rushed to hospital. My father, then her fiancé, wept helplessly at her bedside while priests filed past him after administering the last rites.

And then the wonder drug arrived. As a last resort, my mother was given penicillin, still in experimental use then. Within a day or two the swelling that had almost obscured her face simply melted away. My ordinarily doubting father rushed off to church and humbly knelt before the altar, convinced that he had witnessed a miracle.

In those days, antibiotics were being tested to combat deadly bacterial infections. As a result of the work of Alexander Fleming and others, penicillin began to be used gingerly during the Second World War, against such life-threatening illnesses as septicaemia, meningitis or pneumonia. There is perhaps no other family of drugs that has so revolutionized – indeed defined – modern medicine.

Nevertheless, 50 years on this century's wonder drug has become one of the most abused substances in modern medicine. What was once reserved for life-threatening illnesses such as lobar pneumonia is now routinely handed out at the surgery for athlete's foot or colds – anytime a benign infection is suspected, or even suspected of one day developing. Up until now, an unnecessary antibiotic was only thought to cause a tummy

197

upset or a reaction in the approximately 5 per cent of those truly allergic to them. But a growing body of opinion believes that repeated courses of antibiotics can so disturb a person's internal ecology that it begins a process of disease that could end in ME, diabetes, or even cancer.

With the notable exception of antibiotics (so long as they are used very judiciously), the fact is that drugs do not make you better. At your next dinner party, try playing the following game. Challenge everyone around the table to produce a single drug that can cure people of an illness, other than antibiotics. If you come up with anything, stop whatever you're doing and call me.

After many years of wracking my brain, trawling through the information on thousands of drugs on the market, I cannot think of a single category of drug besides antibiotics that will do anything more than what drug companies call 'maintenance' – that is, making the patient more comfortable with his illness, or trying to prevent the disease from getting worse, often at the risk of developing a number of other conditions potentially far worse than the one being treated.

Medical science has devised a number of amazing preparations which are capable of cleverly interrupting certain processes – depression, wakefulness, stomach acid-production, ovulation, hormone production, inflammation, pain, even the electrical signals controlling your heart. They've managed to come up with certain crude replacements for the body's delicate machinery, as insulin does for people with diabetes, or steroids for people with Addison's disease. Medicine is good at interrupting psychotic behaviour or the menstrual cycle – in effect, at blocking tab A from slotting into slot B.

What 20th-century medicine isn't very good at, though, is curing. There isn't one single drug out there besides antibiotics that is capable of clearing up even the most benign condition. In fact, since the development of the big breakthroughs in medicine – antibiotics and cortisone – in the 1940s, medicine hasn't come up with one drug that represents a major type of cure in medical science. In the main, virtually all the drugs developed supposedly to treat the big chronic diseases such as asthma, arthritis, high blood pressure, high cholesterol, eczema and the like at best alleviate some symptoms but in many instances leave millions of people far worse off than they were before.

This is because medicine, in the main, doesn't understand why we get ill. Doctors understand *how* most diseases progress in minute detail, but rarely *why* they start. Consequently, the drugs developed to treat these diseases are crude and clumsy, suppressing one or more symptoms of a disease or, in some cases, as with asthma, blocking what may be a healthy immunological defence.[1] And because medicine doesn't know how to cure anything besides some infections, many new types of preparations get pounced on as soon as they are released, as a sort of flavour of the month, and tried out on an ever-widening circle of illnesses to see if they will be the one to do the trick. Cyclosporine used to be the fad in medicine, used to treat every autoimmune disease from arthritis to lupus erythematosus to psoriasis. Originally developed to stop the body from rejecting transplant organs, it acts by lowering the immune system T-cells and brings with it a host of dangerous side-effects such as skin cancer and other types of malignancies. It's also associated with liver and kidney damage. Now the new drugs *du jour* are the statins. Although first launched to lower cholesterol, they are now being used to treat every ailment from osteoporosis to Alzheimer's disease.

Because its natural domain is waging war in an emergency setting, medicine uses this self-same weaponry against even everyday or chronic ailments. But this approach doesn't work as well on your everyday problem like haemorrhoids or PMS – and too often resembles using a sledgehammer to swat a flea.

It is nothing less than astonishing how little we know about many of the drug treatments we take for granted. Doctors freely admit they've never known exactly how aspirin works. Because they're stumbling around in the dark, they also often don't know when drug therapy is virtually useless and when to leave well enough alone.

Because of the highly sophisticated tools available to epidemiologists (the scientists who study disease in populations), doctors appear to have lost the ability to make the simple connection between giving people a drug that can, say, cause cancer, and the incidence of cancer going up. Their conspiracy of faith in medicine may be why doctors like to pretend that drugs don't have side-effects. My mailbag is full of stories from exasperated patients describing how their doctors have insisted that the obvious, demonstrable side-effects of a drug are 'coincidental'. But the statistics disprove any coincidence. In the US, some 659,000 people aged 60 and older were hospitalized in 1990 after reacting to a drug, to name just one statistic.[2] More recently, the *Journal of the American Medical Association* announced that drugs and doctors are the third-leading cause of death, responsible for a quarter of a million deaths a year in America alone.[3]

DRUG TESTING ON THE PUBLIC

In the heady world of the pharmaceutical industry, the most profitable industry in the world – where world sales have doubled in the last five years – the pressure is always intense to develop new products. New products represent nearly a fifth of all sales by drug companies, and nearly a third of all prescriptions written. In this highly competitive arena, the search is always on for the new innovative breakthrough, the new Viagra that will revolutionize treatment in a particular area and redefine the marketplace.

The simple fact is that the true nature – and dangers – of any drug are only fully understood after it has been released on the market. Drugs companies are obliged by the Committee on Review of Medicines (and in the US by the American Food and Drug Administration) to conduct animal and human studies before releasing drugs. To prove its safety, quality and efficacy, a drug has to pass through several stages before a licence to market is granted. The first stage usually involves animal testing, which is supposed to give a crude indication of the therapeutic effects and dosage; the second is an early study on healthy human volunteers to assess more accurately the required dosage; the third, the most exhaustive and expensive, involves clinical trials.

Sometimes a trial tests a new drug against a placebo, but there are no guidelines as to which kind of trial needs to take place. A test group can range from as few as 18 people to several thousand or more. This test group is shockingly low compared to the tens of thousands being unwittingly tested with a drug, once it has received a licence. Some tests are stopped early and the drug given the go-ahead if the test response seems particularly favourable, as it did with the anti-AIDS drug AZT, which was later discounted as preventive medicine in the Concorde tests after it had been handed out to thousands who were HIV-positive but still healthy as 'prevention'.[4]

In the UK, the anti-arthritis drug Opren was tested at the usual dose on only 116 people in the UK, mostly for less than three weeks. On the basis of this information, plus some trials in the US, a licence was granted in the UK (whereas the US Food and Drug Administration decided to wait for the results of further tests). As it turned out, to date over 4,000 Britons, many elderly, have contacted the Opren Action Group alleging some injury, mainly persistent increased sensitivity to light; 83 deaths have been associated with the drug. The drug was withdrawn in 1982.

Drug companies, which of course must answer to their shareholders, face enormous pressure to produce a successful trial. By the time a drug is ready to be tested on humans, it may have been researched and developed for a decade or more, costing the company as much as £150m. This none-too-subtle pressure is one factor in what is becoming a wealth of poorly performed drug testing. The US Food and Drug Administration has discovered 'serious deficiencies' in 11 per cent of all clinical trials in the US. A review in the prestigious *Science* magazine found that the conclusions reached by researchers are often flawed by the most basic errors in design and analysis. Besides failing to randomize subjects properly, the researchers often scour their data and divide it into smaller and smaller subgroups in order to come up with the desired result. They're also often guilty of removing data from their analysis or substituting misleading numbers, again in order to come up with the 'right' conclusion.[5] 'Much poor research arises because researchers feel compelled for career reasons to carry out research that they are ill equipped to perform, and nobody stops them,' wrote Douglas G. Altman, head of the Medical Statistics Laboratory of the Imperial Cancer Research Fund.[6]

DATA TORTURE

An even larger potential problem is fraud, or 'data torture', its newest euphemism. No one knows the exact extent of fraud in medical research, but approximately 40 per cent of the deans of the major US graduate schools say they know of confirmed cases of scientific misconduct occurring in their own institutions.

More than one-quarter of the scientists surveyed by the American Association for the Advancement of Sciences admitted that they had personally encountered at least two instances of research that they suspected was falsified, fabricated or plagiarized in the previous decade.[7] Because many journals don't employ a statistical 'referee' to review a paper before it is published, it is relatively easy to get a fraudulent study into print.

For 20 years, US congressional committees have been occupied with investigating the recurrent problem of fraud in research. A decade ago a shudder went through the medical community about fraud, sparked by the US lumpectomy trials, where Dr Roger Poisson of St Luc Hospital in Montreal fiddled with data and included women who blatantly should have been disqualified. When he was found out, it transpired that Dr Poisson was misguidedly acting from the best of motives; he felt that the largest number of his patients 'deserved the best treatment'. To ensure this, he fabricated a wealth of data, including information on the size of their tumours. However, his actions betray an inability, typical among many in medicine, to act as an impartial scientific judge without fear or favour: he already believed a certain course to be the best one, and manipulated his data to support his beliefs.[8]

Fraud and misconduct are so rife that even a number of rising stars in the scientific community have been implicated. Dr John Darsee, noted for his research in cardiology at Harvard Medical School, was found to have published the results of a number of studies which had never in fact taken place. Dr Stephen E. Breuning, a professor at the University of Pittsburgh, became nationally recognized for his work with the mentally retarded and for his published studies supposedly showing that mentally retarded children improved markedly when taken off certain tranquillizers. For years, Dr Breuning criss-crossed the US, expounding on his theories, until it was eventually discovered that much of his data had never existed, or his subjects ever been tested. Eventually Dr Breuning pleaded guilty to two felonies and served time in a halfway house prison. Nevertheless, even after his public exposure a number of scientific journals attempted to prevent his co-authors from publicly retracting the results of articles in which he'd been involved.[9]

Now, in the computer era, fraud may be even more difficult to detect. The fraud squad of the US Food and Drug Administration used to be able to inspect the actual raw data in paper notebooks and lab reports. But these days, digital imaging allows scientists to 'clean up' their data by means of electronic cameras, which record even the most elementary cell slides. In this digital format, the image can be changed to match whatever outcome the researcher is hoping to achieve.[10]

Even if done properly, drug tests are usually short term, demonstrating only either short-term safety or benefits. It is only after the drugs are released and studied in people like you and me (if, indeed, that happens) that drug companies get a picture of how safe or dangerous a drug really is. As Sir William Asscher, former chairman of the Committee on Safety of Medicines, put it, 'by the time a drug is licensed, we really know very little in the case of a new chemical entity about its possible risks.'[11] And both Britain and the US have a highly inadequate adverse events reporting system, reliant upon the good-will of doctors to admit to side-effects of drugs they themselves give to their patients.

Even if drugs were studied more thoroughly before being tried out on patients, most drug approaches to treating illness take the nature of a giant experiment. For all the big chronic problems – asthma, psoriasis, arthritis, eczema – drug treatment is given largely on a suck-it-and-see (or inhale-it-and-see) basis, ending up with the patient taking a medicine cupboard of drugs whose side-effects range from blindness, cancer and mental disorders to death. This sort of approach usually indicates that your doctor is hoping that, by throwing a load of drugs at a problem, it may eventually go away.

TOO MUCH OF A GOOD THING

The problem with antibiotics is a problem often seen in medicine, the philosophy of excess: if one is good, two must be twice as good, and what works in an emergency must be doubly good for your everyday ailment. Study after study in the medical literature of the last decade points to massive and incorrect over-use of antibiotics. A 1981 audit of antibiotic use in the States, published in the *Review of Infectious Diseases*, claimed that in half of all cases where antibiotics were prescribed, the medical condition didn't warrant them, or the prescribing doctor prescribed the wrong drug, the wrong dosage or the incorrect duration for taking the drug. In Britain, these prescribing habits were paralleled in two studies published in *The Wrong Kind of Medicine?* (Hodder & Stoughton) by Charles Medawar, director of the consumer organization Social Audit, which showed that antibiotic use in three British hospitals was inappropriate in about two thirds of cases.[12] In a 1999 review of 18 family practices, in nearly three quarters of cases the patients with acute respiratory tract infections (i.e. flu) left the doctor's surgery with an antibiotic prescription in their hands. Nevertheless, according to the criteria for antibiotics use set by the CDC, a prescription was uncalled for in 8 out of 10 cases.[13]

The fact is, in the overwhelming majority of cases, antibiotics are prescribed for conditions they cannot treat. In 97 per cent of cases, antibiotics are given for viral ear, nose and throat problems or for what is assumed to be cystitis but may only be thrush – conditions which, in most cases, do not respond to antibiotics.[14] In the doctor's surgery, reckons allergy specialist Dr John Mansfield, in 'three out of four instances' antibiotics are used as 'placebos': to 'cure' such things as colds. In the States, in 1983, more than half of the more than 32 million patients who saw doctors for treatment of the common cold were unnecessarily given a prescription for an antibiotic. But, as any medical student knows, viral infections (the cause of colds and flu) do not respond to antibiotics.

Besides respiratory infections, the next most common use of antibiotics (about a quarter) is for childhood middle-ear infections. Although these infections (referred to as otitis media) are usually self-resolving, the rationale has always been to use the antibiotics as a just-in-case measure – in case meningitis or mastoiditis develops. In the States, antibiotic prescriptions to children under 10 more than doubled between 1977 and 1986, and now account for around half of all antibiotic paediatric prescriptions.

This meteoric rise in prescriptions for ear infections has paralleled a similar rise in the number of cases of ear infections for children under three (more than two-thirds of all American children will suffer one or more bouts of middle ear infection). In other words, despite the wholesale attack on these infections with antibiotics, the incidence of them is rising. Except when real pain is present, there is no evidence that antibiotics do any good at all. In fact, a number of studies show that antibiotics actually just make things worse. Children not given the drug tend to have fewer recurrences, compared to those given antibiotics.[15] Other research shows that in three-quarters of cases, repeated antibiotic therapy may eliminate bacteria, but not middle-ear fluid, suggesting that bacteria isn't the source of the problem.[16]

In a shocking number of cases, the doctor himself doesn't know that penicillin won't cure a cold or flu. But in many cases your doctor hands you a prescription just to get rid of you. In the study of American family practices, doctors often claimed they felt overt or covert pressure from their patients to prescribe an antibiotic.[17] Indeed, one medical magazine published an article entitled: 'Otitis Media: Can You Stop Prescribing for the Mother?' The article, written by a GP, noted that doctors use antibiotics with ear infections, in effect, as:

> a placebo … Any mother who has sat up half the night with a crying child needs something to placate her. Any child whose excruciating earache has caused all this fuss needs a let out especially if it magically disappears as they reach the doctor's surgery.[18]

Even if a doctor believes an antibiotic is truly necessary, he usually prescribes it before he knows for sure. In most instances, the GP might take a lab sample of the suspected infection, but he'll also hand the patient a course of antibiotics to start immediately. The patient could be halfway through the course before he discovers he's taken the wrong drug, or taken it for no reason.

This makes sense in life-threatening cases where a patient might be dead in the 36 or 72 hours required to get results back from the lab, but not with more benign problems, particularly when clinical diagnoses so often are wrong. In only half of all so-called cases of cystitis, for instance, are *Escherichia coli* bacteria, the cause of true cystitis, actually present, says Professor Ian Phillips, a microbiologist at London's St Thomas' Hospital.[19]

Hospitals also tend to over-use antibiotics as a just-in-case measure for surgical patients 'in case' they develop infections during surgery. 'For instance, it's known that antibiotics are helpful during surgery of the large bowel to prevent infection,' says Phillips. 'This gets extrapolated into completely clean surgery like hysterectomies or appendectomies where there is no clear indication,' he says. Hospitals even routinely administer antibiotics to premature newborns, 'just in case' they fall prey to bacteria.

Up till now, doctors haven't worried about over-prescribing because they figured the drugs do little harm to patients other than perhaps a little tummy upset. Only 5 per cent of the population was thought to be seriously allergic to penicillin. But a glance at the *British National Formulary* reveals many potentially crippling side-effects of antibiotics: prolonged use of neomycin to treat liver disease can cause the liver to malfunction: tetracycline can permanently stain a child's teeth yellow; chloromycetin can interfere with the bone marrow's production of red blood cells; and chloramphenicol can cause irreversible, potentially fatal bone-marrow depression.

Even more worrisome, repeated courses of antibiotics appear to seriously disturb our immune systems in ways that medicine doesn't yet understand. Health writer Geoffrey Cannon, author of *Superbug* (Virgin Publishing), refers to the current use of antibiotics as the 'Domestos theory of human health – if there are bacteria present in the gut then they must be blasted out.' Allergy specialist Dr John Mansfield, who regularly treats immune system disorders such as candida albicans, believes that 'undoubtedly the most common cause is the broad-spectrum antibiotic. Three or four courses can often push a patient over the precipice into chronic illness.'

Because antibiotics wipe out good bacteria and bad, once the good bacteria in the gut are eliminated candida or one or another opportunistic yeasts or moulds in the gut can overpopulate. The toxins they send out can inhibit T-lymphocytes, the main search-and-destroy cells in the immune system. This in turn can weaken the body, Dr Mansfield says, leaving it open for more serious problems: gastrointestinal or hormonal disorders, severe allergies, psoriasis or even multiple sclerosis. Many such cases can be treated with dietary and medical management. But even if a patient is lucky enough to find a sympathetic and knowledgeable doctor, there is no guarantee that his immune system won't be permanently damaged. There are even some speculative arguments that continually stripping off the friendly bacteria and mucosa in the gut could lead to Crohn's disease and irritable bowel syndrome.

We also don't yet know the long-term effects on this generation of children, who receive many courses of antibiotics before they even reach their teens. Sally Bunday, of the Hyperactive Children's Support Group, claims her group sees a definite correlation between antibiotic use and hyperactivity among children – a relationship supported by the findings of American allergist Dr William Crook.[20] In Sally's case, her son was given four years' courses of antibiotics by their GP to cure persistent catarrh. 'And he was 5 before we had a decent night's sleep and the problem was diagnosed,' she says.

Other connections have been made between over-use of antibiotics and childhood developmental problems. A nine-month survey by the Developmental Delay Registry of 800 families in the US, most of whom have children with developmental problems, found that children who had taken more than 20 courses of antibiotics between the ages of one and 12 years were 50 per cent more likely to suffer some developmental problems, from autism to speech difficulties. Conversely, children who'd been given three or fewer courses were half as likely to have developmental problems. Nearly three-quarters of the affected children had been developing normally up until the age of one. The affected children were far more likely to have had ear infections or to have had grommets placed, which gives added credence to the antibiotics link because so many paediatricians use the drug to treat the condition.[21]

Sally Smith of Lewes, East Sussex experienced this with her child, Luke:

Our son was using about a dozen words by 17 months. Then he fell ill with a respiratory infection and was prescribed the antibiotic amoxycillin. Suddenly Luke lost his vocabulary. In fact, he did not speak again for almost eight years.

Sally attended a medical conference two years later, at which doctors reported observing children between the ages of one and two regressing, losing their speech and developing signs of withdrawal and behavioural problems after being administered antibiotics. Other evidence suggests that antibiotics can also affect hearing. Overuse in the developing countries has caused an epidemic of deafness among children. Some two-thirds of deafness has been linked with wholesale antibiotic use, which in some cases, are being sold over the counter.[22]

More worrisome, antibiotic over-use may possibly even lead to illnesses such as diabetes. Dr Lisa Landymore-Lim of Australia, while studying for her chemistry doctorate, decided to examine all patients with diabetes whose disease was diagnosed before age 23. She discovered that the more antibiotics a child was exposed to, either in the womb or at the beginning of his life, the more likely he was to develop diabetes at an early age.[23] In one of many similar cases, a six-year-old who'd ended up developing diabetes had been given amoxycillin five times before his first birthday, twice during his second year, and three more times during his third and fourth years. Besides nine other course of antibiotics, he received cephalosporin, antihistamines, a powerful anti-vomiting drug and one for gastrointestinal spasms, and Bactrim, a very potent antibiotic. This sort of revolving-door prescribing for children is becoming commonplace today.

Repeated courses of antibiotics only encourage the development of supergerms in your body which will resist treatment from the antibiotics, so that when you really need the drug, it won't work. This kind of 'transfer resistance' can also affect the population at large, as it has with gonorrhoea and staphylococcus infections. A moderate course of penicillin use to cure both these diseases easily. Now it takes two giant doses of penicillin, often in combination with another antibiotic, to do the job. In some parts of Africa and in the Philippines, penicillin won't work at all.

Resistance rates of the staph germ have been isolated in hospitals in Athens, where antibiotics are enthusiastically prescribed, and have been found to have increased in a single year by about 50 per cent to all drugs but penicillin, where resistance was already at 80 per cent.[24] In America, antibiotic effectiveness has declined in the past decade because of persistent overuse.[25] In fact, there's some evidence that children given antibiotics when they are too young become carriers of antibiotic-resistant bacteria. An Icelandic study of children under seven found that those who'd recently had antibiotics and lived in an area where antibiotics were liberally handed out were carrying antibiotic-resistant *pneumococci* germs.[26]

ASTHMA DRUGS

Despite greater diagnostic skills, better identification of the causes of the disease and ever more sophisticated drug cocktails with which to treat it, doctors and asthma associations are stymied by the fact that the epidemic incidence of asthma and asthma-related deaths continues to go up. The latest US figures compiled by the American government, which analysed data for 1982–92, show that the annual death rate for asthma in young people between the ages of 5 and 34 has increased a whopping 40 per cent, to over 5,000 deaths per year.[27]

Today, it's difficult to determine whether the disease or the 'cure' is responsible for killing off patients. Beta-agonists administered by a metered-dose inhaler, specifically albuterol (salbutamol) and fenoterol, have been associated with an increased risk of death or near death.[28] The marked rise in asthma deaths during the 1960s in many countries coincided with the introduction of high-strength isoprenaline inhalers.[29] When the inhalers were withdrawn, mortality fell to previous levels. But the problems haven't been due just to beta2-agonists. In many countries a rise in asthma deaths occurred in the 1980s, particularly in New Zealand, which two studies showed was linked to the popularity of fenoterol, a type of beta2-agonist, but also oral steroids and theophylline, another type of asthma drug.[30]

Regular inhalation of beta2-agonists has also been shown to cause 'hyper-responsiveness' – that is, excessive constriction of the bronchi,[31] and potentially fatal abnormal heartbeats, or the spread of the allergen to more remote airways, thus increasing inflammation or even causing the bronchial muscles to constrict to a fatal degree.[32]

Over time, these drugs may also make the disease worse. In one study, patients receiving fenoterol four times a day had worse outcomes after six months than those given inhaled drugs only as needed.[33] Regular use of certain beta2-agonists also causes a greater decline in lung function than does 'on-demand' use.[34] And some patients have had symptoms improve once doses of inhaled beta2-agonists were reduced.

Inhalers such as Ventolin have many established side-effects, including sudden lowering of blood-pressure, swelling around the heart, and collapse. GlaxoSmithKline, the current manufacturer of Ventolin, also warns doctors that the drug often has a 'paradoxical effect' – that is, it causes bronchospasms, the very situation it is meant to prevent![35]

Deaths from asthma are often due to very high doses of drugs from inhalers. In a recent Canadian study, asthmatics who inhaled 13 or more canisters of fenoterol in a year increased their risk of dying *90 times*. As for salbutamol, those who used 25 or more annual doses in smaller sized canisters were 40 times more likely to die.[36] Although both doses far exceed the recommended limit, asthmatics can grow very dependent on inhalers, reaching for them at the first sign of shortness of breath.

In fact, the risk of death begins to increase dramatically when only 1.4 canisters a month of inhaled beta-agonists are used, particularly among users of fenoterol.[37] The new long-lasting, high potency beta2-agonists such as salmeterol (Serevent), which control asthma symptoms for 12 hours at a puff, could also exacerbate the problem.

STEROIDS

Steroids are fast catching up with antibiotics as the most abused class of drugs in your doctor's black bag. There's no doubt that the discovery of steroids half a century ago was a major advance in medicine – a life-saver for those like the late President John F. Kennedy, who suffered from Addison's disease, a disease of the adrenal glands causing insufficient hormone production. Steroids mimic the action of the adrenal glands, the body's most powerful regulators of general metabolism. John Stirling, director of the vitamin company Biocare, credits a very short course (three injections) of steroids with jump-starting his failing adrenal system after anaphylactic shock, thereby saving his life.

The problem is, like antibiotics steroids appear to be a miracle 'cure'. Patients with crippling arthritis or asthma seem to be instantly better on steroids. The wheeze, the swelling, the pain go away. So doctors turn to steroids as the first, rather than last, line of attack for their anti-inflammatory and anti-allergic effects.

As with antibiotics, what was once reserved for the extreme emergency is now being used on the most trivial of conditions. Steroids are now handed out as readily as antibiotics, even to babies, at the first sign of inflammation of any sort. The latest drug set to replace gripe water for babies with croup is a steroid (budesonide); hydrocortisone is included in the latest over-the-counter medication for piles. Steroids make up many over-the-counter skin drugs, and are considered the drug of choice for asthma, eczema, arthritis, back problems, bowel problems such as ulcerative colitis – indeed, for any and all inflammations or allergic reactions – and new uses are still being invented.

The sole exception is Addison's disease, where steroids act as a replacement therapy to cortisone, much as insulin is given to people with diabetes.

Far from being a wonder drug 'cure all', steroids cannot cure one single condition. All they do is suppress your body's ability to express a normal response. In a few instances, this type of suppression will give the body a chance to heal itself. But more often, the effect is immediate, devastating and permanently damaging. And we are only now realizing just how quickly damage can occur. Doctors have always assumed that patients can only suffer side-effects after long-term use. However, we are lately discovering that *there is no such thing as a safe dose*. Permanent debilitating damage can occur weeks after you've begun treatment, even on low doses. A randomized, double-blind, placebo-controlled study conducted in the Netherlands showed that prednisone has a major effect on the bone mineral density of the lumbar spine. Those patients taking only 10 mg of prednisone (prednisolone in the UK) daily suffered a decrease in bone density of 8 per cent after only five months of using steroids. Once the patients were off the drugs, their bone density increased somewhat, but not to pre-treatment levels. This bone loss was considered comparable to that suffered by women who had had their ovaries removed.

The level of bone loss was similar to that reported at much higher doses of the drugs, which suggests that when it comes to dosage, more is not necessarily any more dangerous than less. The Dutch researchers concluded that 'the use of prednisone should be limited as much as possible to short periods of time'.[38]

Even low doses of inhaled steroids (400 micrograms per day) reduce bone formation.[39] Rub-on steroids have caused Cushing's syndrome in children as soon as a month after treatment has begun,[40] and inhaled steroids slow growth in children after six weeks.[41]

Although steroids are used for virtually all types of inflammatory and auto-immune illnesses, they have not been subjected to long-term scientific study to find out how or whether they work for specific conditions. Septic shock and adult respiratory distress syndrome are two conditions where steroids were widely used as treatment – until scientific trials demonstrated that they were not only of no benefit, but may actually have been doing harm.[42]

Unlike with antibiotics, steroids are *all* broad-spectrum — that is, they don't affect simply the area of the body you wish to treat, but scatter their effects through every cell: the central nervous system, cells in the bone, smooth muscle, blood, liver and a number of other organs of the body.[43] Scientists have been trying to rearrange the chemistry of cortisone to make it more specific to certain parts of the body, but so far this goal has proved elusive.[44]

Doctors seem to have a particular blind spot about these drugs, oblivious to the terrible carnage that even the manufacturers admit steroids are capable of. For 30 years we've known that steroids can routinely cause overactivity of the adrenal hormones, which produces Cushing's disease, characterized by a fat abdomen and face, a 'buffalo hump' in the back of the neck, high blood-pressure and muscle weakness. They can also cause muscle wasting, hyperglycaemia, water retention, skin atrophy, bruising, stretchmarks, insomnia, serious mood changes, symptoms of schizophrenia or manic depression ('steroid psychosis'), osteoporosis, cataracts, glaucoma, menstrual problems, impotence, loss of libido, allergic shock, recurrent thrush of the mouth, and diabetes.

The Incidence of Side-Effects

The British association GASP (Group Against Steroid Prescriptions) once polled its 15,000 members to document just how common these side-effects are. In their study, they discovered that at least 70 per cent or more of the group suffered weight gain, bruising, pain (to the back and legs — even though steroids are routinely prescribed for back pain), muscle weakness and mood swings. Two-thirds polled complained of moon face, headaches, fluid retention, slowness in healing, thinning skin and depression. A full half reported they'd developed osteoporosis, and the same percentage memory loss, sensitivity to light and loss of sex drive. A third complained of buffalo hump, stretchmarks and high blood-pressure. Almost a quarter had cataracts, and a quarter had period problems. Others complained of psychosis, damage to the immune system, angina and hair loss.

Most significantly, more than half the members had never been warned of these potential side-effects. In another survey of 104 patients, less than two-thirds recalled receiving any advice from their doctor on potential side-effects.[45]

The most worrying aspect of steroids concerns the possibility that your pituitary gland will stop producing ACTH, a hormone which regulates the adrenal glands, needed by the body during stress and to fight infections. Once you're on steroids, it can be impossible to stop.

Patients on steroids for prolonged periods can turn into steroid 'junkies' unable to withdraw from taking the drugs; when the body is flooded with extra cortisone, the adrenal glands decrease their own output – sometimes to zero.

Deaths from lack of adrenal gland function have occurred when patients have switched from oral to inhaled steroids without overlapping the drugs. Doctors now know that you must gradually withdraw steroids, so the adrenals have a chance to start making cortisone on their own again. But this process is extremely slow: for patients on long-term use, it could take up to two years for the body to produce enough adrenal hormone to respond to extra stress from an illness or an accident. Surgeons often give steroids to such patients before operations, but this means that weaning has to begin all over again.

Doctors also sometimes maintain that if you inhale or rub on steroids, you are less likely to suffer side-effects. But new evidence shows that inhaled steroids are not as harmless as previously supposed. The consensus up until now has been that beclomethasone dipropionate (BDP) of 400–800 micrograms daily is appropriate for the three- to five-year-old age group. However, a group of paediatric consultants from various hospitals in Britain showed that this dose was every bit as powerful as 200 times more of the oral variety (80–160 mg) in suppressing the adrenal and pituitary glands.[46] This dosage has also produced significant growth retardation in children.

Steroids in Children

The use of steroids in children is difficult to justify. For 30 years we've known that prolonged use for asthma and eczema retards growth in children[47] and delays puberty. Many studies of children with juvenile chronic arthritis given steroids show they suffer growth retardation.[48] Children given topical and inhaled steroids are prone to the same side-effects, such as stunted growth and adrenal suppression.[49]

Steroids may also affect a child's cognitive performance. In one study, where children on combination steroid drugs were given tests of visual retention association, the performance of children on the drugs (some six to eight hours after receiving steroid medication) was significantly worse than that of a group of non-asthmatics. Although these differences disappeared a day or so after the medication was given, they may nevertheless be constant for those children permanently on the drugs.[50]

Evidence also suggests that topical and inhaled steroids can cause cataracts and glaucoma, ordinarily only associated with oral steroids.[51]

Bone mineral density has also been found to be lower with children the longer they stay on steroids.[52] And even inhaled drugs for such diseases as asthma are found to have adverse effects on bone metabolism and adrenal function at higher dosages (more than 1,000 micrograms per day).[53] Steroids can even cause death of the mass of bone (osteonecrosis), necessitating joint replacement.[54]

Despite the so-called dramatic effects on such crippling conditions as rheumatoid arthritis, new research demonstrates that these anti-inflammatory effects appear to wear off in time, leaving sufferers worse off than before. Patients at the Royal University Hospital in Saskatchewan, Canada, taking prednisone (1 to 23 mg) for an average of 6.9 years, had similar rheumatoid arthritis symptoms (joint swelling, reduced mobility) after five years as those who'd never taken the drug. After 10 years, the condition of the group on prednisone was *worse* than the non-drug group, with increased fractures and cataracts.[55]

Medicine has even turned this state of affairs into a syndrome, called 'steroid-resistant asthma', which includes patients who don't respond to normal doses of cortisone and in whom the drug, in some cases, makes the asthma worse.

Many otherwise benign infections become life-threatening in children on steroids. In the summer of 1992, Lexie McConnell, a nine-year-old living in Oxford, was diagnosed as having toxoplasmosis. Although there was no imminent danger of the disease affecting her sight, and the illness might have resolved itself, it was affecting an area near Lexie's retina and, in the view of her doctor, ought to be treated. Her father Art explains:

Within 24 hours of commencing steroid treatment, Lexie was deeply ill with side-effects; immediately her face ballooned. We were told that she should lead a normal life, so we sent her to school, and swimming, although she was often too ill to stay. By November, she had put on an enormous amount of weight and had terrible pains, holes in her tongue and black stools, which we later found out indicated internal bleeding.

Finally, when she was in excruciating pain, we took her to the hospital. After many hours, she was eventually found to have chickenpox. The doctors also mentioned that she could have had a disseminated herpes simplex infection.

It was only then that Art and his wife learned that the drugs had basically left Lexie without an immune system and that she could die from anything, even a cold sore.

'By Saturday, she went into intensive care and lost consciousness,' says her dad. 'An hour later, she died.'

DRUGS FOR ECZEMA

With eczema – another illness doctors don't understand – physicians reach for one or another powerful drug to stamp out the inflammation, but not the problem. The drugs of choice are steroids, the immune-suppressant cyclosporine, or even oral psoralen photochemotherapy (oral PUVA), a treatment option for psoriasis which is linked with genital cancer.[56]

As with inhaled steroids, rub-on steroids have long been touted as the 'safe alternative' to systemic steroids, but there's little evidence to back this up. Increasingly, topical steroids are showing themselves to be every bit as dangerous as their orally-delivered cousins. Rub-on corticosteroids can produce an array of serious skin problems,[57] damage bones and organs,[58] and cause permanent adrenal suppression.[59] They've also been implicated in Cushing's syndrome in children, as soon as a month after treatment, and, like the oral variety, may impair the responses of the pituitary and adrenal glands, thus requiring yet more (oral) steroids during illness or trauma.[60]

Like asthmatics, children with eczema are prone to the side-effects of long-term use of steroids, such as stunted growth and adrenal disease.[61] One child covered with eczema from head to foot from 18 months of age was treated once a day from age six with a layer of betamethasone ointment over his entire body; by age 13, he was about nine-and-a-half inches smaller than average. Although he experienced some catch-up growth once the steroids were discontinued, he never recovered what was estimated to be his likely size.[62]

Even hydrocortisone cream, supposedly so mild it is often prescribed for babies, is known to have a myriad of side-effects, including thinning of the skin, especially on the face, stretchmarks, delayed healing or ulceration of wounds, suppression of the adrenal glands, and sugar in the urine.

In fact, increasing evidence is emerging to suggest that topical and inhaled steroids can cause eye damage – cataracts and glaucoma – of the kind ordinarily associated only with the use of oral steroids.[63] Cases of psychotic episodes with inhaled steroids, again assumed to be caused only by the swallowed variety, are also coming to light.[64]

ARTHRITIS DRUGS

No area offers the potential for a major money-spinner than something that will take away the pain of arthritis, a market possibly bigger than any but cholesterol-lowering and vaccination. Such is the desperation of medicine to find a breakthrough for arthritis that they were once experimenting with chemotherapy that was originally developed to combat non-Hodgkin's lymphoma – a drug so toxic that it can cause acute respiratory failure within an hour of taking it.[65]

Medical treatment for arthritis has a decided air of desperation. Doctors not only don't know how to sort out the problem but often make a hash of things, throwing a load of potentially lethal drugs at the condition and then prescribing new drugs to deal with the side-effects caused by the 'treatment'. Conventional medicine tends to take the view that there is no known cause or cure for arthritis, and so all that it can do with certainty is to alleviate your pain.

The most common front-line drug for both rheumatoid and osteoarthritis used to be aspirin at high doses. This has now been virtually replaced by the 'non-steroidal anti-inflammatory drugs', or NSAIDs as they're known in the trade. In the US there are at least 14 such drugs on the market; several years ago one of them (ibuprofen) got taken off the list of prescribed drugs and was made available over the counter. Increasingly doctors now turn to NSAIDs as a first port of call; in 1984, nearly one in seven Americans was treated with one of these drugs, a figure that is now grossly out of date as they are prescribed for everything from headaches to period pains. Arthritis offers drug companies a $10 billion industry in NSAIDs alone.

These drugs mainly work by blocking the enzyme cyclo-oxygenase, or COX, which inhibits the synthesis of prostaglandins. As prostaglandins control the inflammation in the body, blocking the enzyme involved in the production of prostaglandins will suppress inflammation. The problem is that the drugs don't just inhibit the prostaglandin that concerns your joint pain; they roadblock all formation, particularly at such high doses. Since this substance plays a major role in many other functions of the body, including normal gastrointestinal function, NSAIDs, not surprisingly, interfere with them. In the case of the gastrointestinal tract, this can result in gastric erosion, peptic-ulcer formation and perforation, major upper gastrointestinal haemorrhage, and inflammation and changes in the permeability of the intestine and lower bowel.[66]

Once you begin taking NSAIDs, you multiply by seven times your chances of being hospitalized due to gastrointestinal adverse effects.[67] These statistics could be very conservative; the US Food and Drug Administration once estimated is that 200,000 cases of gastric bleeding occur each year, with 10,000 to 20,000 deaths. In the UK, some 4,000 people die each year from taking NSAIDs – twice the number of deaths from asthma. The elderly, or those with a history of peptic ulcers, are at particular risk. The US Food and Drug Administration now places a warning on each NSAID prescription: 'Serious gastrointestinal toxicity such as bleeding, ulceration and perforation can occur at any time, with or without warning symptoms, in patients treated chronically with NSAID therapy.'

With or without warning symptoms. Because NSAIDs reduce pain, particularly at high doses, they also often mask any indication that something is wrong. For many patients, the first sign that they have an ulcer is a life-threatening complication.

Besides ulcers, even the 'safest' of NSAIDs, ibuprofen, can cause colitis; the drugs indomethacin, naproxen and a sustained release preparation of ketoprofen may cause perforations of the colon.[68] Because these drugs decrease the mucosal prostaglandins, they may cause a leaky gut, resulting in an increased susceptibility to toxins passing through – a recipe for conditions like colitis.[69]

NSAIDs can also cause blurred or diminished vision, Parkinson's disease and hair and fingernail loss; they can also damage the liver and kidneys. Doctors from several medical centres, including New York's Beth Israel and Harvard Medical School in Boston, reported seven cases of 'significant hepatitis' and one death from diclofenac sodium (Voltaren), although they didn't know whether this drug was alone in causing these problems or whether any of the others could as well.[70] Arthritis patients taking NSAIDs have had false-positive results in tests for hepatitis, indicating possible damage to the liver.[71]

NSAIDs can also increase the risk of high blood-pressure (hypertension), especially if taken in large doses. In one study, of nearly 10,000 patients in Boston, Massachusetts who'd recently started on medication to lower their blood-pressure, 41 per cent were found to have been taking NSAIDS during the previous year. These results showed that NSAIDs more than doubled a patient's odds of developing hypertension.[72]

Colitis and Crohn's disease remain mysteries to most doctors. One likely cause still unrecognized by most gastroenterologists is the link between non-steroidal anti-inflammatories and the development of these diseases, even though NSAIDs are well known to injure the mucosa of the colon and to cause ulcers. Of the 60 new cases of colitis and colon problems seen in a three-year period at the General Hospital in Jersey, 23 (or 38 per cent) had developed while the patient was taking an NSAID. None of those 23 patients had a pre-existing inflammatory bowel disease.

Although a large number of NSAIDs were implicated, diclofenac and mefanamic acid (Ponstan) were the most common culprits. The drugs had usually been taken orally, but even the rectal and intramuscular variety caused colitis within a few days of therapy.

In some instances, the colitis was mild and would rapidly improve once the drug was withdrawn and yet another drug such as sulphasalazine or mesalazine was administered. But some patients developed full-blown ulcerative colitis, requiring systemic and topical steroids, and one needed to have his colon surgically removed after developing toxic megacolon in the wake of intramuscular doses of diclofenac.[73]

For all their side-effects, NSAIDs have no advantage over simple analgesics such as aspirin or paracetamol. In one study, large (2,400-mg) and small (1,200-mg) daily doses of ibuprofen worked just about as well as high daily doses (4,000 mg) of acetaminophen in controlling pain and inflammation.[74]

COX-2 Inhibitors

Although the NSAIDs had firmly staked out the arthritis market as their own, a good number of patients with arthritis were in the situation of having to take 'chaser' drugs to alleviate the pain and side-effects caused by the drugs they were taking for their condition in the first place.

Enter the COX-2 inhibitors. Until recently these were the fair-haired boys in arthritis treatment – the 'super-aspirins', drugs that at first were widely embraced as a pain-reliever with no strings attached. Indeed, the first two to be marketed – Celebrex and Vioxx (virtually all of these drugs have an 'x' incorporated into their names, making them the weirdest drug names of all time) – became, virtually overnight, the most successful drugs in medical history, snatching this mantle from Viagra.

The side-effects of the NSAIDS have to do with their indiscriminate blockage of prostaglandin synthesis. COX-2 inhibitors are supposed to work by selectively inhibiting just one of the COX enzymes – the one involved in inflammation.

As is usually the case in modern medicine, much of the fanfare over the COX-2s has been seriously overplayed. For one thing, as the post-marketing evidence began pouring in, it appeared that COX-2 inhibitors cause the same side-effects as their predecessors. Numerous trials show that many of these drugs can cause ulcers.[75] Indeed, a Norwegian study concluded that COX-2s were actually *more* dangerous than NSAIDs and caused more side-effects.[76] Bextra (valdecoxib), among the latest of the COX-2s, was approved less than a year ago and has already been linked to many life-threatening skin conditions, such as Stevens-Johnson syndrome, as well as anaphylactic shock. Other drugs, such as Celebrex (celecoxib), have been linked to deaths from gastrointestinal ulcers and heart problems.

Studies have emerged showing that patients taking Vioxx (rofecoxib) are twice as likely to suffer a cardiovascular problem, such as a heart attack, than those given an NSAID.[77] When the Food and Drug Administration in America mandated the use of a strong warning with Vioxx, Merck decide to pull the drug off the market. At the time of writing, the FDA is carefully scrutinizing the other COX-2 drugs for similar effects.

As is so often the case with a modern 'miracle' drug, the hype was premature and the testing was inadequate. The COX-2 inhibitors are not super-aspirins – just aspirin in a more dangerous suit of clothes.

DRUGS FOR HYPERTENSION

Hypertension is another area where a mountainous concoction of drugs rarely does any good against a condition that can usually be cured with judicious diet and exercise. Doctors have ploughed through a variety of drug treatments – diuretics, beta- and calcium channel-blockers, reserpine, clonidine, methyldopa – without apparent success. A study of 2,000 patients with high blood-pressure from 13 general practices in England showed that only a little more than half of those taking drugs for hypertension had achieved what is considered even a moderately healthy level.[78] In the US, only a fifth of patients on drugs managed to reach what are considered modest blood-pressure goals (less than 140 mm Hg systolic and less than 90 mm Hg diastolic) set by the US Nutritional and Health Examination Survey.[79] As for Europe, in a survey of 12,000 patients across five countries, only a third managed to achieve the blood-pressure target set by their doctors.[80]

If there isn't much evidence that blood-pressure drugs do much good, there's plenty to show they do great harm. One particularly worrisome side-effect is hypotension – or a sudden drop in blood-pressure when one stands up – which can cause dizziness and falls.

Hypertensive drugs are also the major cause of hip fractures among senior citizens.[81] Although all varieties of blood-pressure drugs have been implicated in various disorders – depression, sexual dysfunction, tiredness and appetite disturbances – diuretics (supposedly the 'safe' blood-pressure drug) have been shown to cause an 11-fold increase in diabetes;[82] beta-blockers may be one cause of cancer deaths in elderly men;[83] ACE inhibitors can cause potentially fatal kidney damage[84] or death if given too soon after a heart attack;[85] and calcium channel-blockers have been linked to severe skin conditions such as Stevens-Johnson syndrome.[86] Doctors even use these drugs to treat women with hypertension during pregnancy, in spite of the fact that beta-blockers are thought to have a harmful effect on foetal circulation,[87] and ACE inhibitors to damage or kill the developing foetus if given during the second or third trimesters of pregnancy.[88]

Beta-blockers may even affect certain kinds of memory. A team at the University of California at Irvine divided a healthy group of volunteers into two sub-groups, giving one propranolol and the other a placebo an hour before they were shown slides which told two stories. Tests taken just before the stories were shown demonstrated that all the drug-takers were fully beta-blocked.

The first story factually told in pictures the scene of a child visiting his father's workplace with his mother. The second, however, was designed to arouse strong emotions; on the way to the workplace, the child was hit by a car and badly injured.

A week after seeing these images, when all the subjects were given a surprise memory test, both groups showed similar results when recounting the first story. However, the propranolol group had significantly worse recall of the second, emotionally charged story.[89]

Although the study examined the effect of a single dose of beta-blocker on healthy subjects, rather than on heart or migraine patients, animal studies have demonstrated that memory of emotionally charged events requires activating the beta-adrenergic systems, which of course are blocked by beta-blocking drugs.

COMBINATION HEART DRUGS

When a single drug doesn't sort out a health issue, doctors tend to throw two at the problem. 'Polypharmacy' also results from a rush of enthusiasm. Most doctors believe that if one drug does some good, two will double the benefits. This is particularly the case with the elderly, who are often prescribed up to 10 drugs to take at once. Since so few hypertensive patients who receive drug treatment achieve good blood-pressure control, medicine has come up with the idea of a hypertensive drug 'team'. Today it is a rare doctor who just relies on one drug to knock high blood-pressure on the head.

The firm favourite is to combine a thiazide diuretic (the oldest main-stay of hypertension treatment) with a beta-blocker. Of the five million people in Britain on hypertension drugs, more than a third take the diuretic/beta-blocker combo. Other combinations include diuretics with ACE-inhibitors (such as captopril), alpha-blockers (like prazosin) or angiotensin-II receptor antagonists (such as losartan). ACE-inhibitors are also paired up with calcium antagonists.

These teams came about after initial studies showed that the drugs worked in combination better than diuretics alone.[90]

Thiazide diuretics work by reducing the amount of sodium and water in the body. They are alone among the diuretics in also widening the blood vessels. (Loop-acting diuretics cause the kidneys to increase the flow of urine, thereby reducing the amount of water in your body. Potassium-sparing diuretics do what the other diuretics do, but don't cause your body to lose potassium.)

Beta-blockers work by blocking the effects of adrenaline on your body's beta receptors, slowing down the nerve impulses that travel through the heart, so that it doesn't need to work so hard for blood and oxygen. Beta-blockers also block the receptors that are responsible for heart rate and the strength of the heart's beat. ACE inhibitors inhibit angiotensin-II, a peptide that narrows blood vessels and raises blood pressure.

However, the problem with taking two drugs is the potential for multi-plying the side-effects. The UK's National Institute of Clinical Excellence (NICE), which pooled the results of seven studies on more than 70,000 patients, discovered that the diuretic/beta-blocker combination increases the risk of developing diabetes by 20 per cent. The risk is 0.2 per cent per year. Although doctors are insisting that this represents a 'minimal risk', it translates into 6,666 new cases of diabetes per year.

In a study of drug side-effects to polypharmacy, diuretics and beta-blockers in combination were listed among the eight most frequent culprits.[91] The combo drugs also cause psychiatric effects, including toxic confusional states and psychosis.[92]

These are only the latest reported side-effects of the supposedly safest hypertension drugs; 3 of every 100 patients find them so intolerable they quit taking them.[93] Other side-effects of diuretics include: dizziness on standing up (due to low blood-pressure), blood disorders, skin reactions, impotence, gout, pancreatitis, and depletion of many important nutrients such as potassium, magnesium, coenzyme Q10 and zinc. Diuretics can also lead to kidney cancer. Ironically, diuretics can be especially problematic in people with heart disease.[94] They also cause the problem they're meant to prevent: low blood-pressure can lead to potentially fatal cardiovascular problems.[95]

As for beta-blockers, they can cause dryness of the mouth, eyes and skin, wheezing, breathing difficulties or shortness of breath, slow heartbeat, sleep problems, swelling of the hands and feet, intestinal problems like diarrhoea or constipation, vomiting, back or joint pain, impotence, skin rash, sore throat, depression, memory loss, confusion and even hallucinations. They can also cause angina (pain around the heart during exertion) if you stop taking them abruptly.

Drugs for Heart Disease

The beta-blocker/calcium channel-blocker combination has also become very popular for patients with coronary artery disease. The thinking behind this is that a low dose of the two drugs will decrease the number and severity of attacks of angina more effectively than a high dose of one of the drugs alone, and with fewer side-effects. Since many factors influence the balance between the supply of oxygen to the heart and its demands, and a single drug can only counter a few of these factors, doctors have simply assumed that a second heart drug with different chemical actions might work in a complementary fashion. Because drugs for angina often cause rebound circulatory effects, which work against their effectiveness, the other assumption has been that these unwanted effects can be counteracted by a second drug.

However, these two assumptions have never stood up to scientific scrutiny. According to one review of the results of a number of controlled clinical trials, combining a calcium channel-blocker with a low-dose beta-blocker rarely has any additional benefits for angina patients, and can increase adverse reactions by up to 60 per cent.[96]

The other problem is that most doctors don't really understand how each of these drugs relieves angina on its own. Beta-blockers work by blocking the receptors in the heart from receiving impulses from chemicals released during effort, or stress. Because this action inhibits the rise in heart rate and blood-pressure during exertion, it has always been assumed that the drugs relieve angina and other symptoms of coronary artery disease by decreasing heart-oxygen demand. Because electrical impulses from the heart (which control the contraction and relaxation that occur with every beat) are channelled through calcium ions, calcium channel-blockers – which work to slow down these electrical instructions – theoretically slow down your heartbeat. They also help to dilate arteries, increasing the flow of blood and supposedly easing the work the heart has to do to pump blood through the body. Consequently, many doctors have operated on the assumption that calcium-blockers relieve areas in the body with blocked blood vessels by increasing the supply of oxygen to the heart. This notion – that beta-blockers and calcium-blockers somehow work in tandem by increasing heart oxygen supply and lowering demand – is behind the strong support among the medical community for their combined use.

However, both drugs actually alleviate angina through strikingly similar effects – including reducing the heart's oxygen consumption, limiting the rise in heart rate, redistributing the blood flow from the heart and relaxing the blood vessels.

In fact, recent observations show that the two drugs don't necessarily interact well together. Although calcium-blockers can stop the arterial constriction in the heart caused by beta-blockers, this may only occur in areas of the body with normal blood flow, and may only further reduce blood flow in those areas of the heart already under threat. By the same token, while beta-blockers may prevent the rapid heart rate induced by calcium-blockers, this may do nothing to prevent the lowered blood-pressure calcium-blockers frequently cause. Calcium-blockers may even worsen angina if blood-pressure falls markedly.

In many other ways, the two operate antagonistically. Beta-blockers can increase the lowering effect on blood-pressure of the calcium-blockers, and so increase the risk of poor blood supply to the heart. The combination can also exacerbate angina if the two drugs combine to cause rapid heart beat. Beta-blockers can also cancel out the ability of calcium-blockers to relax the blood vessels. Abnormally low blood-pressure, causing dizziness and sudden falls, worsening heart failure and conduction defects (that is, problems with electrical instructions from the brain) may occur more often during combination therapy than with single-drug therapy.[97]

American doctors have also been warned to stop prescribing the calcium-channel blocker nifedipine. The US National Heart, Lung and Blood Institute has warned doctors that short-acting nifedipine 'should be used with great caution, if at all'. The warning is based on the study of 16 scientific trials of short-acting nifedipine involving more than 8,000 patients. The risk of dying increased with the dosage; the mortality risk is 1.06 times greater than the average with dosages of between 30 and 50 mg a day, increasing to nearly three times when the daily dose is 80 mg. Another study the Institute considered showed that patients on calcium-channel blockers were 60 per cent more likely to suffer a heart attack than those taking either diuretics or beta-blockers. Nifedipine was found to be the most dangerous of the calcium-channel blockers.[98]

DRUGS FOR EPILEPSY

With such a spectacular array of drug therapy at their fingertips, doctors aren't particularly good at doing nothing – at adopting a wait-and-see attitude, to see if a condition clears up by itself. Although doctors claim to be more cautious about automatically handing out anti-convulsant drugs to children with mild blackouts and seizures, the conventional wisdom still is that, unless suppressed by drug treatment, epileptic seizures will recur, and that drug treatment can affect the course of the disease, reducing the risk of early epilepsy turning into an intractable disorder.

The problem is that epilepsy is hopelessly overdiagnosed. Experts at Birmingham Children's Hospital concluded that about half the cases of so-called juvenile epilepsy are wrongly diagnosed.[99] This is significant, as more than half of the 340,000 cases of chronic epilepsy in Britain are believed to have begun in childhood. Dr Michael Prendergast, consultant child psychiatrist at Birmingham Children's Hospital, examined 311 children referred to the hospital for suspected or diagnosed epilepsy and discovered that 138 of them (44 per cent) didn't actually have it. His results are nearly identical to those of a Scottish study by the Royal Hospital for Sick Children in Glasgow. In that study, Dr John Stephenson, the hospital's consultant paediatric neurologist, found that 47 per cent of the children referred there did not in fact have epilepsy.

Jacqui, now 36, of East Grinstead, was diagnosed as having epilepsy when she was 11 after suffering several blackouts. She was immediately placed on anti-convulsants, although the first convulsion didn't appear until *after* she'd been on the drugs. She has spent years battling the myriad of drug side-effects, including blackouts and convulsions. From 1988, when she began reducing the dosage of the drugs she was taking, her seizures have correspondingly dropped in number, from 200 to several dozen a year.

David Chadwick, professor of neurology at the Walton Centre for Neurology and Neurosurgery in Liverpool, argues that epilepsy is an umbrella term referring to a group of disorders and not a single, homogeneous disease. In some cases of epilepsy, such as 'benign rolandic epilepsy' in children, where seizures (affecting only the face, throat and arm) occur only during sleep, there is strong evidence that the seizures stop by themselves by mid-adolescence. Furthermore, the preliminary data suggesting that people are better off getting drugs as early treatment is far from 'definitive'.[100]

Among the very few longer-term studies examining which factors predicted at least a five-year seizure-free remission, one found that developing epilepsy before age 16 and having no evidence of brain damage, tonic-clonic (grand mal) seizures or spike wave abnormalities on an electroencephalogram (EEC) were all factors that tended to favour remission, whether or not drugs were given.[101] (It should be noted that David Chadwick says the situation is very different with other forms of epilepsy, such as juvenile myoclonic epilepsy, where patients who've had grand mal seizures have a high probability of relapse if the drugs are withdrawn. In this group, epilepsy drugs can be life-saving.)

It's very difficult to know whether drugs given early make any difference, because untreated epileptics are difficult to find. But those studies that have been performed suggest that drugs make virtually no difference. In one, after 20 years half the group not on drugs had gone into 'remission'. This is an equivalent percentage of those who go into remission after years of taking drugs.[102] Similarly, in a group of patients in Africa and others in Ecuador whose treatment was delayed, six-month remission rates were the same as they were in populations given early drug treatment.[103]

226

New evidence shows that children who suffer their first-ever seizure are no worse off for having any treatment delayed to see if a second seizure occurs. Delaying treatment does not reduce the chances of controlling the seizures later, nor does it affect possible remission when the child grows. The only advantage of starting immediate treatment is that it can delay the next seizure, but doctors and parents who insist on it after the very first attack will never know if it was going to be the only one.[104]

Much evidence about early treatment suggests that patients taking drugs may actually be worse off. In one study, patients with seizures after a head injury who took the epilepsy drug phenytoin had more seizures than those taking a placebo.[105] Italian research comparing patients on a drug against those on a sugar pill has put paid to the belief that the treatment group supposedly runs only half the risk of having a further seizure, when there has been no difference between the two groups in terms of remission time.[106]

Doctors really don't have enough information to encourage early treatment with certainty, particularly as all epileptic drug treatment carries a host of potentially lethal effects. In one recent study, side-effects were so serious that nearly a quarter of patients on phenobarbitone, and 11 per cent of those on carbamazepine, had to be taken off the drugs.[107] In one of the first-ever medical trials to assess the safety of anti-epilepsy drugs on children, 9 per cent of children given phenobarbitone to treat their epilepsy had to come off it because of the serious side-effects they suffered. The researchers, from King's College Hospital in London, found a similar problem with phenytoin, and at least 4 per cent of children reacted to either sodium valproate or carbamazepine.[108]

Indeed, all epileptic drugs are potentially lethal; the manufacturer of valproic acid (Epilim in the UK; Depakene or Depakote in the US) warns that patients on the drug have died from liver failure.

This is what may have happened to 12-year-old Helenor Bye, who was given Epilim – at the time thought to be a safe drug. Her mother writes:

Within months she started wasting away before my eyes. She was getting thinner and started hallucinating. Eventually her hair started to fall out. The doctor was convinced she was emotionally disturbed, and that she was enjoying the attention.

Her condition continued to deteriorate until she was just half of her normal body weight. Still, the doctor thought she was just a spoilt child, twisting round her fingers two doting parents.

After eight months, she became delirious and was rushed to hospital. She died a few days later, weighing just three stone. She had to die to prove to them she was ill.

ANTI-DEPRESSANTS

Drug treatment is also highly subject to flavour-of-the-month fads. Once doctors get enthused over a new compound which has seemingly done wonders in one area, they like to try it on every illness. Until recently, the latest wonder drug was the 'selective serotonin re-uptake inhibitor', or 5-HT drug – the active compound in Prozac.

One cause (or outcome) of depression and suicidal behaviour is believed to be low levels of the brain chemical serotonin, as happens in those with lowered cholesterol levels. Prozac (or fluoxetine, its generic name) works by increasing the availability of serotonin in the brain; this is accomplished by slowing the passage (or 're-uptake') of this neurohormone into nervous system cells. Prozac has been sold as an amazing improvement over the older 'tricyclic anti-depressants' because it is not a sedative, it does not impair thinking or physical activity, and it has fewer side-effects for more patients.

Hailed in the media in the late 1980s as the breakthrough for depression we've all been waiting for, Prozac quickly became America's best selling anti-depressive, particularly after the sell-out publication of *Listening to Prozac*, America's best-selling happy pill.

Enthusiasts are already planning to widen the uses of Prozac and its clones for overweight patients, those with cancer experiencing nausea from anticancer drugs, people with obsessive compulsions and even PMS. In addition, because there is some evidence that this kind of drug reduces dependence (unlike Valium and other benzodiazepines) by stimulating the reward mechanism in the brain, doctors are discussing the possibility of using it to help control smoking and dependence on other drugs.

The glossy press about Prozac passes lightly over the more than 100 lawsuits the manufacturer Eli Lilly faced from patients claiming that

Prozac led them to suicidal and homicidal thoughts and actions. In one case, a Prozac user killed five and wounded 12 others at his place of work. In another, a woman attacked her mother by biting her, ripping out more than 20 bite-sized pieces of flesh. Eli Lilly has now reached a settlement with the families of the victims killed and injured by Joseph Wesbecken, who went on a shooting rampage while on the drug.[109]

Although the US Food and Drug Administration cleared Prozac from this association with violence, a recent study suggested that of all types of anti-depressants, the highest number of suicides have been recorded for those patients on serotonin inhibitors.[110] SSRI drugs now come with a black-box warning about suicide risk to children.

As the Prozac generation has now discovered, the best-selling happy pill offers its own array of adverse effects on virtually every system of the body. According to Eli Lilly's own published warnings on the drug, some 10 to 15 per cent of patients in initial clinical trials reported anxiety and insomnia; 9 per cent, particularly underweight patients, report significant weight loss or anorexia. In one study, 13 per cent of patients on the drug lost more than 5 per cent of their body weight.[111] In other words, about 1 in 10 patients experiences the same symptoms from the drug that the doctor is trying to treat.

Prozac has also been known to affect nearly every system of the body, including the nervous, digestive, respiratory, cardiovascular, musculoskeletal and urogenital systems, and the skin and appendages. These side-effects include, most commonly, visual disturbances, palpitations, mania/hypomania, tremors, symptoms of flu, cardiac arhythmia, back pain, rashes, sweating, nausea, diarrhoea, abdominal pain and loss of sex drive. Less common effects include antisocial behaviour, double vision, memory loss, cataracts or glaucoma, asthma, arthritis, osteoporosis, stomach bleeding, kidney inflammation and impotence. Prozac also, albeit infrequently, can cause abnormal dreams, agitation, convulsions, delusions and euphoria.[112]

Prozac may also cause sexual dysfunction in up to a third of users. In an overlooked research paper published in the *Journal of Clinical Psychiatry* in 1992, F M Jacobsen found this sort of level of sexual problems among people taking fluoxetine. A paper published in the same journal a year later found the rate of sexual dysfunction while on the drug was as high as 75 per cent.[113]

In the attempt to keep one step ahead of the game, several drug companies have launched second-generation products such as mirtazapine (Remeron), an anti-depressant that works on the serotonin levels in the brain which appear to govern mood, but not as an SSRI. Rather, this drug is termed a 'noradrenergic and selective serotonergic antidepressant' (NaSSA).

Doctors now believe a deficiency of two chemicals in the brain – norepinephrine (noradrenaline) and serotonin – is responsible for depression. Mirtazapine is believed to work by increasing the release of both of these chemicals from nerve cells in the brain.

There are two alpha-2 'serotonergic' receptor sites on brain nerve cells, and norepinephrine and serotonin ordinarily bind to these receptors, a process not affected by SSRIs. This leads to many of the usual SSRI side-effects, such as insomnia and anxiety. NaSSAs, on the other hand, seem to selectively block the sites, thereby preventing the two chemicals from binding to the nerve cells. The supposed effect of this is to enhance the mood-elevating effects of the two chemicals as they are released from the nerve cells.

With the unique action of the NaSSAs, drug companies thought they had finally sorted the problem of how to release serotonin without causing all of the serotonin-related rebound problems.

The initial findings were impressive. The drug appeared to work as well as the older drugs, with minimal side-effects: sleepiness, a tendency to overeat and, thus, weight gain.[114] On this basis, the US Food and Drug Administration, the UK Committee on Safety of Medicines and the drugs-regulating bodies of many other countries approved the use of mirtazapine.

The ink was barely dry on these approvals when serious side-effects began to be reported. The Australian government's Adverse Drug Reactions Advisory Committee announced that it had received 253 reports of adverse reactions to mirtazapine, after half a million prescriptions had been filled. These included 16 reports of convulsions and 15 cases of potentially serious blood and bone-marrow abnormalities.[115]

The blood disorders included neutropenia (reduced numbers of neutrophilic blood leucocytes, the phagocytic [cell-ingesting] cells involved in the response to inflammation), thrombocytopenia (reduced blood platelets), lymphopenia (reduced lymphocytes) and pancytopenia (a reduction in all of the blood's cell components). Most patients developed blood symptoms fewer than two months after starting treatment.

Other adverse reactions included nightmares, hallucinations, anxiety and agitation, vomiting, myalgia/arthralgia (muscle/joint pain), skin reactions, twitching, increased weight and even liver disorders.

The drug is now on a shortlist of drugs which the Committee deems are drugs of 'current interest' – in other words, those it has its eye on for adverse effects.

In England, a study involving more than 13,000 patients taking mirtazapine found that nearly 6 per cent of patients reported drowsiness or sedation with the drug, and nearly 3 per cent suffered from lassitude and malaise during the first month of treatment. Two patients presented with blood disorders: neutropenia and agranulocytosis (a sudden severe deficiency in the number of white blood cells in the blood).[116]

Migraine

In the early 1990s, the drug companies released what appeared to be a miracle to any regular sufferer of migraines: Sumatriptan (Imitrex® or Imigran®), the first of the triptans, or selective serotonin receptor agonists, appeared to be the first drug that could abort a migraine attack before it took off in full flight. Sumatriptan, a 5-HT agonist, supposedly works by reducing the swollen blood vessels around the brain.

Sumatriptan was developed after scientists revised their thinking about what causes migraine. Dr Frank Clifford-Rose of the Charing Cross Hospital, who helped co-ordinate many of the studies of sumatriptan, says that migraine, rather than being initiated by the blood vessels in the brain itself, is now believed to be a biological disease of the nervous system, and that serotonin plays a key role. It has long been known that 5-HT can cause headaches, and experiments have shown that 5-HT is released during migraine attacks.

Unlike conventional pain medication, which simply increases your tolerance to pain temporarily, the triptans work by affecting serotonin levels (which transmit nerve signals to the brain) – ultimately stopping inflamation and blood-vessel dilation around the brain.

The drug itself is a molecular twin of serotonin (5HT) and, as such, blocks the receptors of serotonin. The action is supposed to be highly selective, causing constriction of the blood vessels in the brain without affecting the some 15 other 5-HT receptors in the body related to blood clotting, the lungs, the gastrointestinal tract and many others. Glaxo was the first pharmaceutical company to come up with a drug which was chemically related to 5-HT but had the supposed ability to carry out this type of highly selective action.

In 1991 Glaxo enthusiastically launched sumatriptan as 'a revolutionary acute therapy in migraine' after a number of studies showed highly promising results. In the early trials when drug companies produced the first fast-acting injectable variety, sumatriptan had an astonishing profile, reducing headaches from moderate to severe to mild or none in 81–86 per cent of patients.[117]

Since that time, the drug me-too industry has been busy at work, churning out many sumatriptan act-a-likes: zolmitriptan, naratriptan, rizatriptan, almotriptan, frovatriptan and eletriptan. These drugs now come as injections, as tablets and even as a nasal spray. In the wake of a great deal of the initial noisy fanfare, medicine has now begun to retrench as reports flood in demonstrating that patients taking these drugs may be trading one health problem for another. Some 5–8 per cent of patients suffer chest pains, similar to those associated with angina, largely due to the fact that the drug has proved to have a vaso-constrictive effect in places other than the brain (narrowing blood vessels and restricting blood flow, thus elevating blood-pressure). Consequently, sumatriptan has been out of bounds for anyone with a heart problem. Because this drug works on blood vessels, it has always been assumed that the chest pain had to do with the heart. But evidence now shows that the pain may start in the oesophagus (the canal from your mouth to your stomach).[118] The results of one study of patients taking sumatriptan showed no electrocardiogram changes, whereas contractions of the oesophagus were shown to increase significantly with the drug. A fifth of the patients included in this study had developed chest pain, lasting between two and 45 minutes, although there seemed to be no relation in time between the onset of the pain and the abnormal recordings of the movements of the oesophagus.

Changes in the blood have been shown in patients taking the standard therapeutic dose of sumatriptan; blood-pressure in the lungs and aorta rises by 40 per cent and 20 per cent, respectively, which could mean that chest tightness arises from the veins in the lungs or those running along the breadth of the body rather than in the oesophagus.[119] In rare cases, people on sumatriptan have experienced arterial spasms in the heart.[120] There is also a small risk of poor blood flow to the heart[121]: angiographies of patients on sumatriptan showed that the drug does indeed constrict arteries.[122] One woman with no previous history of vascular disease suffered a fatal heart attack after injecting herself with sumatriptan,[123] and at least two patients developed serious irregular heartbeat.[124] In some patients the chest pressure or pain radiates out to the left arm and head, in the manner of angina.[125]

One of the most embarrassing side-effects that has dogged this otherwise successful class of drugs are rebound headaches. In an early trial, more than a third of patients who first found relief with sumatriptan suffered recurrent rebound headaches, which the drug subsequently failed to reach.[126] Some studies show that up to half of patients have rebound headaches.

The Gothenburg Migraine Clinic in Sweden has found that over half of patients given sumatriptan by injection had recurrences of migraine within five to 10 hours after nearly every treated attack. In another study, all but one of the patients had a headache the next day.[127]

In Germany, after an average of nine months a group of patients had reached the point where they had to use the drug nearly every day to prevent their headaches from recurring. One fellow who'd only suffered from migraines once a month began getting them every morning after he'd begun taking sumatriptan.[128]

Of course, the more migraines you suffer, the greater your dependence on the drug. Glaxo denies that there is any evidence of drug dependence, and points out that the drug is only approved for short-term intermittent treatment of acute migraine attacks, and not for daily prevention.

In the Gothenburg Clinic, 70 per cent of patients experience one or more side-effects, including neck pain, chest symptoms, tiredness, tingling and a reaction at the injection site. The oral variety can also cause nausea and vomiting.

Besides this multitude of side-effects, a question mark hangs over sumatriptan's genuine effectiveness in times of need. Although as many as 90 per cent of patients have responded over three treatment courses, studies have shown that only about 50–60 per cent will respond to it during any one attack.[129] Many of the drug's side-effects suggest that the supposedly selective action is not so selective after all, affecting many other 5-HT receptor sites.

As is always the case in medicine, when the dangers of one so-called miracle drug are finally exposed, the drug companies then bring out the new 'improved' version. The latest generation of drugs – eletriptan, naratriptan and rizatriptan – were supposed to sort out the reactions associated with sumatriptan. However, the latest evidence on eletriptan shows that it can cause all the side-effects of sumatriptan,[130] including flushing, palpitations, nasal discomfort, eye irritation, visual disturbance and agitation.

However, the most worrying side-effect is the possibility of heart attack or stroke. Individual case reports have been flowing in about patients with no known risk of either condition suffering either a heart attack or stroke within hours of taking one of the triptans. In Switzerland, one woman suffered a stroke within hours of injecting herself with two doses of sumatriptan; within 30 minutes of the second injection, her headache vastly increased, she began vomiting and suffered paralysis on the left side of her body before losing consciousness. In a similar situation, in the US, a woman's headache severely worsened; a later CAT scan showed she'd suffered a cerebral haemorrhage.[131]

Other single-case reports have shown fatal heart attacks with the drug among those with no history of cardiovascular disease.[132]

A recent examination of data among migraine sufferers found no association between triptan use and stroke or heart attack.[133] Nevertheless, this was a cohort study (a simple charting and comparison of the development of a group of individuals over time), which cannot be considered definitive. Many researchers say that migraine sufferers are naturally at higher risk of stroke,[134] although that has been widely disputed elsewhere.[135] Use of triptans is contraindicated in patients with hemiplegic (one-sided) or basilar (with nausea, vertigo and possibly loss of consciousness) migraine because of concern over the potential for cerebral vasoconstriction, a tacit indication that doctors themselves believe there is an association.[136]

DRUGS FOR HYPERACTIVITY

Ritalin (methylphenidate, or MPH) is America's other miracle drug, with some six million prescriptions a year to control hyperactivity and attention deficit hyperactivity disorder (ADHD). In some American schools, one-fifth of children are on the drug.[137] In Britain, Ritalin had been largely resisted by parents in Britain until recent media attention focused on it as a drug that can 'unlock' a child's potential; prescriptions have increased by 100-fold in the last decade and trebled between 2002 and 2003, so that now 200,000 prescriptions are written for Ritalin every year.

After witnessing the Ritalin success story, many other drug companies have leapt into the ADHD market. These days, parents have an array of drugs to choose from: Adderall, Concerta, Cylert, Focalin, Metadate CD and Strattera. Ritalin now even comes as a patch, so that children don't have to worry about forgetting to take their pill.

This vast increase in prescriptions has occurred in both countries despite the fact that in many instances a child is given the drugs before it has been demonstrated that he could benefit from them. A team of researchers from the United Nations International Narcotics Control Board looked at the records of nearly 400 paediatricians who'd prescribed Ritalin, and found that half the children who'd been diagnosed with attention deficit disorder had not been given any psychological or educational testing before receiving the drug. The UN concluded that frustrated parents or educators and doctors were too ready to affix a label of ADHD to a host of behavioural difficulties.[138]

Up until recently, the view espoused by Ritalin promoters is that the drug, an amphetamine, works paradoxically as a suppressant on children by correcting biochemical imbalances in the brain. Not only is there no evidence that methylphenidate corrects these imbalances, but no evidence that Ritalin makes any lasting change. As Ciba (the manufacturer) admits, there are no long-term studies on Ritalin's safety or effectiveness.[139] Furthermore, *The American Textbook of Psychiatry* shows a 75 per cent improvement with Ritalin compared with a 40 per cent response with a placebo, suggesting that half the response to Ritalin could be purely suggestive.[140] In a study in Johannesburg assessing effectiveness, only two out of 14 children responded to the drug. Furthermore, one child showed some deterioration on the drug, while another showed marked deterioration.

It's worth remembering that this drug is a class II category controlled substance, such as barbiturates, morphine and others with a high potential for addiction or abuse. Uppers supposedly have a paradoxical effect on children, quieting them down, but often the effect is mixed. Children get subdued during the day, but stimulated at night, unable to sleep. Although Novartis, which produces Ritalin, disputes any potential for addiction, the entry for Ritalin in the US *Physician's Desk Reference* carries a warning of drug dependence and psychotic episodes: 'Careful supervision is required during drug withdrawal, since severe depression as well as the effects of chronic overactivity can be unmasked.'[141] Furthermore, recent brain scans of children on the drugs show that MPH has the same effect as cocaine – as a stimulant of the brain chemical dopamine. From the data, researchers originally theorized that children with ADHD have low dopamine levels, but they were appalled to discover the powerful effects of the 'solution'. 'The data clearly show that the notion that Ritalin is a weak stimulant is completely incorrect,' says Dr Nora Volkow, who headed up the brain scan research. 'This is a cocaine-like drug.'[142]

A well-known side-effect of cocaine and amphetamines is psychosis, and indeed toxic psychosis has been observed in children on Ritalin. According to Canadian research, more than 6 per cent of children with ADHD given methylphenidate become psychotic, experiencing paranoia and hallucinations – conditions seen only in ADHD children taking the drug.[143] Psychosis, as well as depression, have also followed withdrawal of the drug in children who have been on methylphenidate long term.[144]

Numerous cases of suicide after drug withdrawal have been reported. One study showed that children treated with stimulants alone (rather than with counselling as well as drugs) had higher arrest records and were more likely to be institutionalized.[145] Possibly due to its effect on dopamine levels, MPH has been shown to cause epilepsy-like seizures, particularly in children with an unsuspected pre-existing condition.[146] Case studies have even linked it with inflammation of the arteries of the brain, causing stroke – a well-known complication of amphetamine abuse.[147]

Methylphenidate has also been shown to suppress growth,[148] make children more prone to seizures, and cause visual disturbances, nervousness, insomnia and anorexia. Among the me-too drugs, Cylert has been linked with cases of severe liver toxicity, a number of them fatal.

Besides psychosis, this drug may cause other mental disorders. Some 10 per cent of children on methylphenidate develop Tourette's syndrome (where children have involuntary bodily and vocal tics).[149] It has even been linked with obsessive-compulsive disorder, a syndrome where children become highly anxious and engage in repeated, compulsive rituals, after less than a year of use.[150] Between 1990 and 2000, the US FDA's Division of Pharmacovigilance and Epidemiology received reports of 186 deaths and 569 hospitalizations due to methylphenidate. Most cases concerned effects on the central or peripheral nervous system. Brain atrophy was evident in more than half of 24 adults treated with psychostimulants.[151] Peter Breggin, author of *Toxic Psychiatry* (Fontana), notes that long-term use of Ritalin causes irritability and hyperactivity – the very problems the drug is supposed to treat.[152] The latest side-effect is a possible causal link with liver cancer. In animal studies of mice given high doses of methylphenidate for two years, a signicant percentage developed hepto-blastomas, or liver cancer.[153] These are animal studies, which don't neces-sarily apply to humans. Nevertheless, the carcinogenic potential of methylphenidate has now been included as one of the official potential risks of the drug in material given to doctors.

Although many (if not all) children on Ritalin and its cousins are subdued in the classroom and at home, the research that has been done on methylphenidate shows that it doesn't really solve the problem. Parents asked to rate the drug's effectiveness on a special scaled rating system concluded that it doesn't really have any long-term effects on ADHD behaviour.[154] The Institute of Mental Health has concluded that the research shows no evidence of a short-term, positive effect on learning and no long-term effect on 'any domain of child functioning'.[155]

CHEMOTHERAPY

If antibiotics and steroids are the Sherman tanks of medical chemical warfare, chemotherapy for cancer is its nuclear warhead. No other illness is subject to the sophisticated combinations of chemicals that have been developed for cancer treatment.

Chemotherapy was first proposed as a treatment for cancer directly after the Second World War, when research on mustard gas demonstrated that it has the ability to kill living cells, particularly those which rapidly divide, such as those in the intestinal tract, bone marrow and lymph system. Doctors soon came up with the idea that they could use mustard gas to poison cancer, which constitutes the most rapidly dividing cells of all. In fact, many of the drugs we use today are close cousins of mustard gas – one reason we find them so toxic.[156]

In the early 1970s, medicine discovered that certain rare cancers would respond to chemotherapy and result in a person living longer. These include combinations of drugs for Hodgkin's disease, certain non-Hodgkin lymphomas, some germ cell tumours, testicular cancer and certain cancers in children, such as Wilm's tumour, acute lymphocytic leukaemia and choriocarcinoma, in which foetal cells transform into cancer and threaten the mother's life.

However, more than three decades later it is safe to say that virtually no progress has been made since then-US President Richard Nixon declared the 'War on Cancer' in 1971. No cancer incurable then is curable today. Chemotherapy's modest successes are almost identical to what they were then.[157] Since then, all the billions of dollars of research we've thrown at cancer haven't influenced survival one little bit. *For most of today's common solid cancers, the ones that cause 90 per cent of the cancer deaths every year – most breast, lung, colon and rectal, skin, liver, pancreatic and bladder cancers – chemotherapy has never been proved to do any good at all.*[158]

Giving out chemotherapy after surgery as a 'just in case' measure to kill any 'secret' pockets of cells has appeared to improve the survival prospects of certain groups of patients with particular types of breast, colon, or lung cancer. Recurrence rates are supposed to be reduced by a third, and survival improved.[159]

However, this evidence is only empirical (that is, only based on observation, not scientific studies). It is very likely that it was other factors that helped the survival of these patients. In one of the few reviews of all studies comparing chemotherapy against another form of treatment, chemotherapy proved no better than tamoxifen alone in women over 50 with breast cancer.[160]

Chemotherapy has been shown to increase the survival of patients with ovarian and small-cell lung disease, intermediate- and high-grade non-Hodgkin's lymphoma, and localized cancer of the small intestines – although, again, this is not proven beyond a shadow of a doubt.[161] Sometimes these advantages are major, as with ovarian cancer, where it has been shown that it may extend the lives of patients for years. More often the effect is modest, as with lung-cancer patients, increasing survival by only a few months.[162]

The other problem is that cancer doctors define 'cure' and 'response' in different terms than you or I might. In the main, oncologists look only at 'response' – that is, shrinking the tumour – as a measure of success, without considering whether this increases survival or improves quality of life. Dr Ralph Moss, former employee of the prestigious Sloan-Kettering Institute, has made it his life's work to examine the scientific evidence of orthodox and alternative cancer treatment. He describes a textbook on medicine in which a top National Cancer Institute (NCI) scientist said that for most forms of cancer, many patients initially respond to chemotherapy. But in only three forms of cancer – ovarian, small-cell lung cancer and acute non-lymphocytic leukaemia – did any appreciable percentage survive without disease, and even then this percentage represented, at best, less than a sixth of the total group of patients. In all the other types of cancer, disease-free survival was rare.[163]

Major chemotherapy manufacturer Bristol Myers discloses that only 11 per cent of patients taking carboplatin, and 15 per cent of patients taking cisplatin, had a complete response to these drugs; remission lasted, on average, about a year, and both types of patients survived, on average, only two years. And this is for the two major drugs given primarily for ovarian cancer, which is one of the cancers which most responds to chemotherapy![164]

In the majority of studies, the most important question of all – *Does chemo help you to live any longer than you would have done if you hadn't had the treatment?* – is never even asked! In the rush to be seen to be doing something about cancer, the US Food and Drug Administration has now officially sanctioned that new drugs for cancer can be fast-tracked on the market so long as they show they shrink tumours. There is no need to show that they lengthen the survival of cancer patients.[165]

You'd never know any of this if you talked to the average oncologist. Most would talk of the great strides made in chemotherapy, the new drugs, the new protocols (that is, combinations of drugs). But the measure of how much this constitutes the treatment of desperation is the language used — 'rescue' therapies and 'salvage' operations — and also the types of treatments being resorted to. The latest are termed 'rescue', as in rescuing you from the brink of death. Doctors harvest bone marrow from the patient before launching into treatment, then administer high-dose chemotherapy in the hope that replanting the bone marrow will somehow 'rescue' the patient before he dies from the drugs. Other researchers are experimenting with growing immune-system cells in the test tube in a last-ditch attempt to restore blood formation in patients who have undergone murderously high doses of chemotherapy.

Recently, one doctor returned from an autopsy with the proud announcement that his patient, who'd had widespread, disseminated cancer, had died 'cancer-free'. What he did not mention was that it was the lung disease, induced by chemotherapy, that killed him.

In oncology, more is always considered better. After the success with Hodgkin's disease with a quartet of cancer-killing drugs and steroids, medicine has applied this protocol to many other types of cancer, even though there is no evidence that it does any good at all. For many forms of cancer, multiple use of drugs appears to be no more effective than single drugs, which carry many fewer side-effects. In one of the only studies of its type, reported at a meeting in Dallas of the American Study of Clinical Oncologists, a double-dose of chemotherapy given to breast cancer patients was found to be no more effective than the standard dose.[166] But even when medicine admits that drugs haven't a prayer of curing, chemotherapy is given as palliative cure (that is, to improve the time the patient has left). This argument, of course, ignores the terrible effects of chemotherapy, which can hardly be said to improve the quality of life.

One of the most-used chemotherapy drugs is cyclophosphamide, which comes from mustard gas. It can cause nausea, vomiting, hair loss and anorexia, and can damage the blood, heart and lungs. Another drug, cisplatin (Platinol), made of the heavy metal platinum, can damage nerves and kidneys and cause hearing loss and seizures. It can also cause deafness, irreversible loss of motor function, bone marrow suppression, anaemia and blindness.

Mechlorethamine, an analogue of mustard gas (the 'M' of MOPP treatment, the standard protocol for Hodgkin's disease), is so toxic that those administering the drug are advised to wear rubber gloves and avoid inhaling it. A most dreaded complication is mucositis (or inflammation of the mucous membranes, particularly of the gut and mouth), possibly leading to life-threatening infection.[167] Various types of chemotherapy can cause heart problems, destroy bile ducts, cause bone tissue death, restrict growth, cause infertility, lower white and red blood cell counts and lead to intestinal and lactose malabsorption.

If a patient is lucky enough to be one of the few for whom chemotherapy actually does treat the illness successfully, chances are high that it will cause a worse cancer to develop many years later. In one study, one third of women treated for Hodgkin's disease as children, for instance, ended up developing breast cancer by the time they were 40. This risk is at least three times greater than among the general population.[168] Adults who had chemo as children also have a risk of bone cancer. Thus far, some 13,000 children who'd survived cancer for three years have been identified as bone cancer victims.[169] By using chemotherapy to treat cancer, many survivors could be trading one type of cancer for a more deadly one later on.

VIAGRA

Although Viagra has become a virtual synonym for virility, new research shows that the drug may, in fact, *reduce* a man's fertility. New research from the Queen's University in Belfast suggests that the drug may sort out one problem only to cause a host of others – including infertility.

The drug works by blocking an enzyme called phosphodi-esterase-5 (PDE-5). This enzyme normally breaks down the messenger-molecules involved in the energy process of cells. The effect of this is to increase energy levels in the cells, thereby increasing blood flow to the penis while, at the same time, constricting the outflow of blood. Although this will undoubtedly aid potency, it also appears to speed up other sperm activity, including motility (sperm movement) and the timing of a particular chemical reaction that is vital in enabling sperm to penetrate and fertilize an egg.

Speeding Up Sperm

A process called the 'acrosome reaction' occurs when the head of the sperm releases digestive enzymes to break down the egg's protective outer layer, thus enabling the sperm to enter. Sperm that are spent of these enzymes are said to have 'fully reacted'. The Queen's University researchers, led by Dr Sheena Lewis, discovered that Viagra accelerates this entire process, causing the acrosome reaction to occur earlier in the sperm's journey. This means that, by the time the sperm reaches the egg, it has exhausted its supply of digestive enzymes.

The researchers obtained 45 samples of sperm and treated half of them with Viagra, using the equivalent concentration of what would be in the blood of a user taking a single 100-mg dose. Within 15 minutes and for the next several hours, the sperm started speeding up. After two hours, nearly 80 per cent of the Viagra-treated samples had fully reacted.

This latest study is particularly worrying because of the change in the type of men now comprising the vast population who use Viagra and other similar drugs. When first made available in 1998, Viagra was aimed at middle-aged men with erectile problems. However, of the 16 million men who have taken it, an increasing percentage are young men who use it simply to enhance their sexual activity. Furthermore, the Queen's team discovered that more than 45 per cent of men attending fertility clinics with their partners are using the drug to help produce sperm samples. These are men who may be using Viagra when trying to start a family.

Although these are test-tube studies, which may produce different results from those in the body, they do have parallels with research by Lewis' team on mice (although, of course, animal studies may not apply strictly to humans). Male mice that were given Viagra and allowed to mate with females produced 40 per cent fewer embryos than those given a placebo. The embryos that were produced were less likely than normal to survive.

Dr Lewis says she is concerned about the effects of such misfiring on human embryos, too. The acrosome reaction causes the channelling of charged calcium ions, which can affect the mechanisms of other cells – including those involved in the early development of an embryo.

The Queen's University team has now started another study of sperm from men taking Viagra. The preliminary evidence based on 17 men shows that the drug indeed has a pronounced effect in speeding-up sperm.

Besides messing up your fertility, 'Pfizer's riser' causes vision problems[170] and has been linked with heart attacks, although a final association has yet to be proven.[171]

Dr John Urquhart, professor of Biopharmaceutical Sciences at the University of California, San Francisco, discovered that a higher percentage of men die taking Viagra (some 49 men per million) than those using other drugs for potency problems.[172] It also reacts with nitrate heart medications (such as nitroglycerin), vasodilators or alpha-blockers, all of which can cause a sudden drop in blood pressure.

DRUGS TO TREAT THE SIDE-EFFECTS OF DRUGS

With so many drugs causing so much illness, an entire medical industry has grown up just to counteract the ill-effects of medical 'treatment'. There are now drugs to combat the nausea caused by chemotherapy, and drugs to counter the terrible side-effects of transplant drugs. Zantac, or ranitidine, is one of a family of drugs called histamine-2 receptor antagonists. They work by blocking the H2 nerve receptors in the stomach, which histamine ordinarily stimulates to produce gastric acid. By inhibiting this action, the H2-blockers reduce both the amount of gastric acid in the stomach and its pepsin content. They also block the effects of the hormone called gastrin, produced in the stomach to stimulate the production of stomach juices. The drug is relatively long-acting, suppressing gastric acid secretion for 12 hours at a stretch. In most cases, claim Glaxo Laboratories, 'healing occurs in four weeks' or, in those who don't initially respond, four weeks after that.

NSAID-caused ulcers have been a lifesaver for drugs such as Zantac. Recently it was discovered that most ulcers are caused by the *Helicobacter pylori* bug and can be cured with a one-time, largely antibiotic drug treatment. Because of ulcers, Zantac was the best-selling drug in the world. The *H. pylori* breakthrough may strike a major financial blow to ulcer-drug manufacturers such as Glaxo, who rely on a steady stream of users taking Zantac indefinitely as 'maintenance'. Consequently, the ulcer-drug makers have been searching around for new long-term uses for what are among the biggest money-spinners of all time.

Nowadays, Glaxo has advertised Zantac for NSAID users to take as preventive medicine for ulcers. (As for healing NSAID-induced ulcers that are already there, there is less convincing evidence. In one study, under a third of NSAID patients healed after four weeks; about half after eight weeks.)[173]

The problem with using H2-blockers as a just-in-case measure is that patients have to stay on them (as well as NSAIDs) long term and risk suffering one or more of a long list of potential side-effects: headaches (often severe), insomnia, vertigo, depression, hallucinations, blurred vision, irregular heartbeats, pancreatitis (inflammation of the pancreas), diarrhoea, nausea/vomiting, abdominal discomfort, hepatitis and other liver disorders – even death. Other problems include blood count changes (usually reversible); rare cases of agranulocytosis (a severe blood disorder) have been reported, as have occasional cases of impotence, hair loss and anaphylactic shock. Taking H2 antagonists may mask any warning symptoms that you've got cancer of the stomach and so delay your diagnosis. I wonder how long it will be before there is another drug developed to counteract the effects of the drug taken to counter the effects of the first drug.

A DRUG CHECKLIST

Before your doctor writes you a prescription for any drug, it's a good idea to check if another drug isn't causing your problem in the first place. According to the Health Research Group, the American lobbying organization founded by consumer advocate Ralph Nader, 15 categories of drugs can bring on depression: barbiturates, tranquillizers, beta-blockers, heart drugs (particularly those containing reserpine), including drugs used to treat cardiac arhythmias, ulcer drugs, high blood-pressure drugs, cortico-steroids, antiparkinsonian drugs, amphetamines, painkillers, arthritis drugs, anticonvulsants, antibiotics, and drugs used to treat slipped discs or alcoholism. If your feelings of depression have come on about the time you started on a new drug, look first to that drug as the cause.

Unfortunately, in too many cases the treatment for drug-induced depression is an anti-depressive, which can react with the original drug and cause further physical or mental problems. The only treatment for this kind of depression is to stop or gradually cut down on the original drug or, if absolutely necessary, to switch to a similar acting drug that will not cause depression.

As with medical tests, before you take *any* drug it is vital that you learn as much as you can about it – indeed, more than even your doctor knows. Every drug marketed in the UK has a data sheet, which is essentially a profile of the drug at a glance, listing when it should or shouldn't be taken and also its side-effects. All these data sheets are bound up in a publication entitled the *Compendium of Data Sheets*.[174]

You can also find out information about drugs from the journal *MIMS*, the drug bible of most doctors (although copies are expensive), or on the Internet.

Once you've read up on the drug being proposed for you (and if you have only the one surgery appointment, ask for the data sheet on the drug right then and there), put the following questions to your doctor:

- **Is drug therapy really necessary for this problem?** Many conditions, such as premenstrual tension or depression after a bereavement, can be treated by diet or the loving attention of friends and relatives. A new study finds that people suffering from major depression can be aided just as well by help in facing up to and solving their problems as by taking anti-depressants. Unless you can be persuaded that your condition will definitely worsen, why introduce a substance that could also introduce a whole new set of problems?

- **What will happen if I don't take the drug?**

- **What is this drug supposed to do for me? How will it do that? How are you going to monitor the use of the drug? Do your instructions differ from those on the data sheet?**

- **What sorts of drugs or substances (including non-prescription drugs, food, vitamins or alcohol) should I avoid when taking this drug?** Many vitamins react with drugs, but rather than stopping the vitamins, consider stopping the drug instead, which is bound to do you more harm.

- **With what other drugs does this drug dangerously react?**
  Although one drug used alone might carry a small risk, when
  combined with another drug that risk can be multiplied several times
  over, as can the strength of the toxicity.

- **What are the known side-effects of this drug, as reported by
  the manufacturer?** (Don't settle for vague assurances from your
  doctor; request that he read out from *MIMS*, if he can't give you a
  data sheet.)

- **What are the latest reports in the medical literature about this
  drug's side-effects?** Magazines such as *The Lancet* publish new
  studies all the time demonstrating that the risks of a certain drug are
  far higher than the manufacturer originally thought. If your doctor
  doesn't know, go to a science reference library. Most large science
  libraries will have the *American Physician's Desk Reference* or the
  Compendium of Data Sheets. The British Library's medical section holds
  both. Another possibility is to do a search on Pubmed, a computerized
  version of the *Cumulated Index Medicus*, a summary of most scientific
  studies performed on most treatments. Pubmed is available free on the
  internet (www.ncbi.nlm.nih.gov/PubMed/). Otherwise, visit a large
  medical bookshop. Many useful books about medications can also be
  found in general bookshops. Your best source for full information
  about a drug's side-effects is to own your own copy of the US
  Physician's Desk Reference, since the US authorities require more
  disclosure about drug side-effects than does the British government.
  Check with major medical bookshops, such as the British Medical
  Association bookshop in London, to see if they can order it for you.

- **May I discontinue any other drugs I am currently taking?** The
  American Health Research Group suggests that if you are taking
  other drugs, you have a 'Brown Bag Session' with your doctor – that
  is, you place all medication you're taking (including non-prescription
  drugs) in a brown bag and take it to your surgery visit so that you and
  your doctor can determine if any complicate the effects of the others.
  (It also makes sense to write out a list of all the drugs, including the

frequency with which, and times of day when, you take them – so that you don't mix up what you are taking.)

- **Under what conditions and how should I stop taking this drug if I notice certain side-effects? What sorts of tests are available to monitor my reactions to the drug?**

- **If I don't wish to take this drug, what other possible therapies are there for me to consider?** Here you might have to prod your doctor gently into enumerating the possibilities he's heard of, not just to offer his opinion. Many doctors will tell you they simply don't believe in non-drug therapies – when in fact, very few doctors know anything about them.

If all else fails, contact the American Food and Drug Association. Anyone around the world has right of access to information about drugs licensed by the FDA, courtesy of the American Freedom of Information Act.

The first port of call is to visit the FDA's website and consult the Center for Drug Evaluation and Research pages (www.fda.gov/cder.htm). The FDA's site offering all information about clinical trials, side-effects and the like is www.fda.gov/cder/drug/default.htm.

If you don't get all the information you need, you could also write a letter to the address below, asking for a Summary Basis of Approval (SBA) on the drug in question (make sure to find out the generic and, if possible, American brand name first, as drug names can differ on either side of the Atlantic). An SBA will include detailed summary of the data, including results of any clinical trials, which influenced the FDA's decision to approve the drug. Also ask for Adverse Drug Reactions (ADRs) – unverified reports of any side-effects reported – including new MedWatch reports (the database of drug reactions set up by the FDA). Finally, ask for any reviews or assessments of the ADRs, which will put these isolated reports of reactions in context. (Bear in mind that American drugs can be licensed in different doses than British ones, and for different conditions.) (In your letter you can ask for an estimate of how much your search will cost.)

The address to write to is:

Food and Drug Administration
Freedom of Information Office
5600 Fishers Lane
Rockville, MD 20857-0001

They must respond within 10 days, if only to say that your request is being investigated.

WONDER DRUGS

The problem with wonder drugs is that they breed in the public mind a sense that medicine can and always should work miracles, even with benign problems. What gets forgotten is the price we always pay by tampering with mother nature.

Many benign problems will clear up by themselves. When my eldest daughter was small and still nursing, I suffered from a couple of bouts of severe mastitis. I phoned my hospital and convinced my doctor, who usually treats the problem with antibiotics, that I wanted to wait 24 hours to see what happened. During that time (and on subsequent occasions) I bathed the affected breasts with heat. My daughter, as if sensing my problem, nursed more than usual on the affected breast. A day later I was back to normal.

Other than for emergencies, where orthodox medicine comes into its own with the most brilliant of modern technologies, there are invariably better and far less invasive ways to treat – and often cure – most medical conditions. And most of these unorthodox methods have as much, if not more, scientific evidence of success than what we consider the 'tried-and-tested' conventional route. For arthritis, asthma, eczema, hypertension, hyperactivity and migraine there is solid evidence that such cases have mostly to do with food allergies, environmental causes (such as pesticides or gas cooking) or nutritional deficiencies. Locating both can alleviate, if not cure, the condition.[175] Even mental illness such as depression has been shown to respond to nutritional medicine.[176] With epilepsy, much progress has been made at such orthodox medical centres as Johns Hopkins

248

Medical Center in Baltimore, Maryland, using a high-fat diet to control seizures. In one review of 58 cases, seizure control improved in two-thirds of patients.[177] Some researchers speculate that the high fat intake helps to repair the myelin sheath around the nerves.

Even for cancer, many alternative methods have scientific evidence of success – certainly more than either chemotherapy or radiation.[178]

9

Dental Medicine:
Safe until Proven Dangerous

What would you say if you heard that doctors had selected one of the most toxic substances known to man, hadn't bothered to do any safety testing before placing it permanently in your body, and continued to maintain steadfastly that there was no danger whatsoever that any of it was doing you any harm?

AMALGAM FILLINGS

The British Dental Association and American Dental Association continue to insist that 'when mercury is combined with the metals used in dental amalgam, its toxic properties are made harmless'. This is the same position adopted by the British Dental Association. However, this position has been based upon reverse logic: that amalgam fillings are safe because the evidence does not prove irrefutably otherwise.

Although we refer to our fillings as 'silver' or mercury, amalgam is actually made up of about 52 per cent mercury, with the remainder copper, tin, silver and zinc. At the end of the 19th century, amalgam, which literally means 'mixed with mercury', was discovered as a cheap compound to replace gold, which was too expensive, and lead, which was considered too dangerous, as a dental filling. It was introduced in Britain in 1819 and in the US in the late 1820s. The National Association of Dental Surgeons (ADS), the US dental association of the time, held a debate as to whether dentists should use mercury amalgam fillings. The Association came out against mercury, and said it should be eliminated. But because amalgam was so much cheaper than other materials of the times, it became the filling of choice, particularly among dentists whose patients were poor, and in fact was promoted as a political issue – the filling everybody could afford. Most dentists chose to ignore the warnings about and known toxicity of mercury, arguing that those who favoured gold did so solely for pecuniary reasons and were denying medical help to patients on lower incomes. By 1840, the ADS had disbanded, undermined because of what hotted up to a raging battle over the amalgam issue.[1]

Nearly 60 years later, a new dental association, the American Dental Association (ADA) was established, which endorsed mercury amalgam as safe – a position the current ADA has maintained ever since. Dr Murray J. Vimy, clinical associate professor of the Department of Medicine at the University of Calgary in Canada, who has spent more than 20 years studying the effects of amalgam, makes the point that amalgam slipped through the cracks of safety regulation because it has been around so long. Drugs or substances such as this, which prefigured regulatory agencies like the US Food and Drug Administration, are said to be 'grandfathered' into practice if they were used before safety testing began. 'If the information we have about the effect of amalgam fillings were presented before the Food and Drug Administration today, they would not pass it for use because it hasn't even passed the required animal tests, let alone the human ones' says Dr Vimy – referring to the animal trials required by the FDA today.[2]

In 1993, the US Public Health Service issued a report evaluating the safety of dental amalgam. The report allowed that small amounts of mercury vapour are released from your fillings and can be absorbed into the body, and that these could cause small responses in that rare group of allergic individuals. Nevertheless, it concluded that 'there is scant evidence that the health of the vast majority of people with amalgam is compromised, nor that removing amalgam fillings has a beneficial effect on health'.[3] The US PHS reaffirmed its conclusions in 1995 and 1997.

In the UK, the British Dental Association conceded that 'about 3 per cent of the population are estimated to suffer from mercury sensitivity', although they resisted stating that mercury fillings may affect the public at large. The UK Department of Health has now also advised pregnant women not to have mercury amalgam fillings, following the lead of a number of leading amalgam manufacturers who issued data sheets warning that amalgam fillings should not be used in pregnant women, in children under six or in patients with kidney disease.[4] Nevertheless, this approach still lags behind those of other countries.

The American Food and Drug Administration's position continues to be that there is no valid data to demonstrate clinical harm to patients, nor that removing a patient's amalgam fillings will prevent any adverse health effects or reverse the course of existing diseases, although it and other agencies have began to study the issue.[5]

It's a position that is proving at variance with the doctrine of several other countries. In Germany the Federal Health Agency (Bundesgesundheitsamt, or BGA) decided in early 1992 that amalgam fillings should be used only for molars. The BGA also announced that amalgam containing gamma-2, a compound of tin and mercury, should be banned because of its inherent instability and the risk of mercury being released while a tooth is being filled. The German government has been cagey, denying there is scientific evidence that amalgam can cause long-term disease other than for people who are allergic or have electro-chemical reactions. Nevertheless, they also say that amalgam shouldn't be used for women of child-bearing age, patients with kidney failure, or toddlers.[6] The Germany Federal Registry of Dentists has sent a letter to the Minister of Health, requesting that he rule that no dentist in Germany be allowed to use dental amalgam.[7] The Swedes took the first step in an outright ban of amalgam fillings, adopted in 1997; Austria banned them in 2000. Health Canada proposed that alternatives be used in children and at one point that amalgam be avoided in those with impaired kidney function or allergies or in pregnant women, and the New Zealand Ministry of Health is currently reviewing its policy on amalgam fillings.[8] And some German companies such as Degussa, one of the world's largest manufacturers of dental amalgam, have stopped the production of amalgam – even though it once represented half their turnover – and have moved into the manufacture of composite fillings (the plastic alternative to amalgam). In a British television report on amalgam, Dr Matthias Kuhner, a senior manager at Degussa, admitted that one consideration for their move was potential lawsuits.[9]

The Canadian and American Dental Associations claim that dental amalgam exposure is minuscule compared with dietary exposure – that people get most of their mercury, in effect, from tuna fish. However, when the World Health Organization assembled some of the world's authorities on mercury poisoning, they concluded, after reviewing the scientific literature, that the public's highest daily exposure to mercury comes from dental amalgam fillings. They determined that human daily retained intake is from 3 to 17 mcg/day from dental fillings, compared with about 2.6 mcg/day from fish and seafood, and other food, air and water.[10] The committee also concluded that, regarding mercury vapour, a 'specific no-observed-effect level (NOEL) cannot be established' – which means that no level of exposure to mercury vapour, however slight, has been found to be completely harmless. Dr Lars Freiberg, chief adviser to the World Health Organization on mercury safety, and perhaps the world's leading authority on mercury poisoning, has said: 'There is no safe level of mercury.'[11]

A TIME-RELEASED POISON

Without a doubt, mercury is extraordinarily toxic to humans. The well-respected Toxicity Center at the University of Tennessee, which rates poisons for their lethal toxicity to humans, scores mercury at 1600 – plutonium, the most deadly, scores 1900. This rating places mercury among the most toxic substances known to man.

Dentists themselves show overwhelming evidence of mercury poisoning; autopsy reports of a group of dentists showed higher concentrations of the metal in their pituitary glands and double the number of brain tumours than among the ordinary population.[12] Female dentists and personnel are at least three times more likely to suffer sterility, stillbirth and miscarriage,[13] and all dental employees have a higher concentration of mercury in the central nervous system, kidneys and endocrine system.[14] More worrying, amalgam appears to cause subtle brain damage in dentists exposed regularly to amalgam fillings. Several years ago in Singapore, the neurological functions of a group of dentists were assessed and found to be less efficient than those of a similar group who hadn't been exposed regularly to amalgam, although the dentists did just as well as the control group on intelligence tests. The higher their exposure to mercury, the worse their performance on the neurological tests.[15] Dr Diana Echeverria, a neuro-toxicologist at the University of Washington, also tested American dentists to see whether they showed any evidence of mercury poisoning. Her study found subtle losses of manual dexterity and concentration – both evidence of central nervous system disorders.[16]

Further proof of the highly toxic nature of mercury comes in the form of the meticulous recommendations by the American Council on Dental Materials and Devices concerning its storage and use. This organization recommends that dentists use tightly sealed containers, avoid any contact with the mercury, and perform annual mercury level tests on all dental personnel.

The party line of both the British and American Dental Associations is that the mercury in amalgam fillings becomes inert, or 'locked in', when mixed with the other metals and placed in the mouth.[17] But numerous researchers have proved that mercury vapours are continuously released from the fillings, particularly when you chew or eat hot or acidic foods. The University of Calgary in Canada, which has been at the forefront of amalgam research, found that chewing increases the 'intra-oral' (within the air of the mouth) mercury content six-fold if you have amalgam fillings, making it 54 times higher than the intra-oral mercury content of patients without amalgam fillings. The greater the number of fillings, the more mercury vapour was released;[18] eight biting surface amalgams release about 10 mcg of mercury a day, says Vimy. At a conference in King's College, Cambridge, Professor R. Soremark of the Department of Prosthetic Dentistry of the Karolingska Institute of Sweden announced: 'The absorption rate is close to 90 per cent, 74 per cent of which is retained by the lungs. In 10 minutes, 30 per cent of the mercury absorbed in the lungs is transferred to the blood.'[19] Mercury can 'corrode' in the mouth, which is to say, rust, as metallic ions and vapour form on the amalgam surface – once it comes into contact with heat, saliva and such elements as fluoride or large gold fillings. Although most of these products get excreted, about 10 per cent accumulate in the various organs and tissues of the body. Furthermore, the five metals contained in amalgam can combine to produce some 16 different corrosion products, all floating around in the body to unknown effect. Professor J. V. Masi of Western New England College in Springfield, Massachusetts, who has studied this issue in detail, has written that all metals used as restorative dental materials are capable of corroding.[20]

A BODY OF EVIDENCE

Although much of the evidence about mercury used to have an element of speculation about it, there is growing proof that this released mercury settles in tissues in the body. Until recently, although we knew that mercury was released by chewing, we didn't know where it ended up. In December 1989, Dr Murray J. Vimy, clinical associate professor of the Department of Medicine, along with numerous other medical researchers from the Departments of Radiology, Medicine and Medical Physiology at the University of Calgary in Canada, published a study in which radioactive amalgam fillings were placed into the teeth of adult sheep. (Using radioactive amalgam effectively 'labelled' the mercury so it could be easily traced. It also eliminated the need for a control, as mercury present in food, air or water wouldn't be so labelled. Sheep were chosen because their physiological responses were thought to be most like those of humans.)

Within 29 days, substantial quantities of mercury appeared in the lungs, gastrointestinal tract and jaw tissue of the sheep. Once the mercury was absorbed, said the study, 'high concentrations of dental amalgam rapidly localized in the liver and kidneys'.[21] Over the course of the 29 days, the mercury vapour measurements taken from the mouths of the sheep closely approximated those taken from people in previous studies. The brain, the heart and several endocrine glands also contained substantial quantities of mercury, visible on a whole body scan. The study concluded:

Our laboratory findings in this investigation are at variance with the anec-dotal opinion of the medical profession, which claims that amalgam tooth fillings are safe. Experimental evidence in support of amalgam safety is at best tenuous ... From our results we conclude that dental amalgams can be a major source of chronic [mercury] exposure.[22]

In a number of successive studies where amalgam fillings were placed in animals, Dr Vimy found that kidney function (determined by the rate of insulin clearance) was drastically reduced – by as much as 50 per cent within one month. The mercury also increased potassium and sodium levels in the urine, and reduced levels of albumin, a water-soluble protein found in blood excreted in the urine. Altered sodium and potassium ratios quickly lead to symptoms such as muscle weakness, fatigue and heart irregularities. When sodium levels in the blood are low, the kidneys are prompted to release an enzyme called rennin, which causes increased blood-pressure. Dr Vimy and his colleagues have spent nearly two decades examining the effects of amalgam fillings on sheep, monkeys and, more recently, humans. Although 12,000 papers have been published to date on the dangers of amalgam, it is only because of the interest of respected medical departments like that at the University of Calgary, and their devastating findings, that the issue began to hot up, particularly in North America.

The evidence that Dr Vimy and others have published demonstrates that mercury from amalgam fillings migrates to tissues in the body, causing harm – a type of 'timed-released poisoning', as Vimy has called it.

The extent of the harm is still under study. 'The evidence shows there is some risk, we're not sure of the extent of the risk, but it certainly is prudent to study and consider it,' Vimy says.[23]

In Dr Vimy's initial experiments on sheep, the radioactive mercury landed in the stomachs, liver, left and right kidneys, in the oral cavity, the lungs and the gastrointestinal (GI) tract, the brain, the heart and the endocrine glands. 'The denser the tissue, the larger the volume of mercury which collected there,' Vimy said.[24]

Sheep were originally chosen for the University of Calgary's study because they are especially ruminant – that is, they chew all day. Dr Vimy's team felt that, if the mercury didn't go into the tissues and organs of sheep, it wouldn't go into the tissues or organs of any other living creature. 'Sheep,' they summed up, 'were a worst-case scenario.'[25]

Although sheep have a physiological response similar to that of humans, Dr Vimy and his colleagues were ridiculed for using sheep because they have a higher frequency of chewing than humans and more than one stomach, and so more bacteria for digestion. (The medical press tended to disparage the findings with such headlines as: 'Sheep Baaad Amalgam Recipients').

So Dr Vimy's group decided to repeat its experiment, this time using monkeys. They chose monkeys because their rate of chewing is more similar to that of humans, as are their teeth, their diet, feeding frequency, chewing pattern and organ physiology. They found the same pattern of mercury deposits in these monkeys – in the oral, lung and GI tract – as they had seen in the sheep.[26]

Vimy's animal studies were vindicated by the work of Professor H. Vasken Aposhian, head of the Molecular and Cellular Biology Department of the University of Arizona in Tucson. Aposhian and his team counted the number of amalgam fillings of volunteers, from which they were given an amalgam score. The study participants were then given a salt of 2,3-dimer-captopropane-1-sulfonic acid (DMPS), a chelating agent which binds to mercury and removes it from the body through the urine. An analysis of the results showed that the more amalgam in the teeth, the higher the amalgam in the body as excreted with the DMPS. Aposhian's team was also able to show that two-thirds of the mercury excreted in the urine of those study participants with dental amalgams came from their fillings.[27]

Dr Vimy and his researchers then conducted another sheep experiment to find out the effect of mercury's migration round the body, primarily on organs such as the kidneys. After placing regular (rather than radioactive) fillings into the mouths of several sheep, Vimy's group measured the flow rate of inulin, a starch, through the sheep's kidneys. This is a standard index of kidney function, since inulin is neither secreted or absorbed. 'Thirty days after the placement of amalgam fillings, kidney function and its filtration capacity was reduced by 50 per cent,' Dr Vimy said. A control group of sheep given white plastic fillings showed no change in kidney function.

The research team found a rapid rise (by 300 per cent) of sodium in the urea, even though the sodium diets of the animals were restricted. This indicated that substantial amounts of sodium were being lost. They also found a rapid decline in albumin excretion – by 68 per cent.[28] This showed that the reabsorption of urea was impaired and that kidney blood flow was reduced. Noted Vimy: 'That's like walking around with one kidney.'[29]

POSSIBLE DISEASES FROM MERCURY AMALGAMS

There is no conclusive proof that amalgam fillings produce certain diseases, particularly since whether mercury will be toxic to any given person has a lot to do with genetic predisposition, length of time in the body, other environmental factors and so forth. However, a number of new studies and clinical observations show a possible relationship between amalgam and a number of diseases.

Mercury and the Immune System

Mercury from amalgam fillings appears to lower T-lymphocyte cells, one of the most important components of our immune system.

The immune system contains T-lymphocyte cells and B-cells. Very generally speaking, of the numerous kinds of T-cells the most important are the T-4 lymphocytes, called the 'helper' cells, whose job it is to identify foreign bodies and cancer cells for the B-cells to engulf and destroy. Without these helper cells, the B-cells cannot do their job. Hence, in the case of AIDS, although B-cells are available to attack the offending viruses, there aren't enough T-cells around to label them the enemy.

The T-8 lymphocytes ('suppressor cells'), on the other hand, keep the B-cells from attacking normal body tissues. Any lowering of the total T-cell population or disturbance in the delicate T-4:T-8 ratio can lead to autoimmune diseases such as multiple sclerosis, lupus erythematosus (a chronic inflammatory disease), inflammatory bowel disease, and the like.

David Eggleston, a Californian dentist who has studied the effects of mercury exposure, measured the T-lymphocytes of three patients before and after removing their amalgam fillings. In all three cases their percentage of T-lymphocytes went up substantially (from 47 per cent to 73 per cent in one case, an increase of 55.3 per cent). Eggleston then reinserted amalgam in the dental cavities of two of the patients and measured the percentage of T-cells. In both cases, the percentage of T-lymphocytes decreased again (in the above-mentioned patient, to 55 per cent — a 24.7 per cent decrease). Finally, when Eggleston removed the new amalgam and put in a non-amalgam filling, the T-cells were up again in all patients — 72 per cent in the case mentioned above, an increase of 30 per cent.[30]

At a 1990 conference, Eggleston announced 30 such trials with an average improvement in T-cells of 30 per cent. Colorado dentist Hal Huggins, author of *It's All in Your Head* (Avery), who has himself studied the toxic effect of amalgam fillings on patients, claims that number is conservative. 'At the University of Colorado, I've measured T-cell rises of 100 per cent to 300 per cent after fillings were removed,' he says.[31] These findings could mean that amalgam may have a role in causing or exacerbating allergies, autoimmune diseases and even leukaemia. In fact, white blood cell level abnormalities such as those found in leukaemia have been shown to normalize when the patient's fillings are removed properly.[32]

The most recent study of a group of patients with central nervous system disorders showed evidence of mercury poisoning in 88 per cent of the patients and an immune system response to mercury in nearly two-thirds.[33]

ME and Multiple Sclerosis

There may also be a relationship between mercury poisoning from amalgam fillings and ME (myalgic encephalomyelitis), and also multiple sclerosis (MS) and other sclerosing diseases, such as ALS, the wasting disease which afflicts cosmologist Dr Stephen Hawking. In one study, conducted in Sweden, the mercury levels in MS patients were on average 7.5 times higher than in the control group. In many cases, treatment with antioxidation therapy (that is, vitamins A, D and E, selenium and/or removal of amalgam fillings) helped patients to improve – sometimes completely.[34] In another study, when mercury-sensitive patients had their fillings removed, most showed an immediate significant improvement.[35]

The UK's Dr Patrick Kingsley, noted for his work with MS and cancer patients, and Hal Huggins of the US, both of whom have treated hundreds of MS victims, almost always find evidence of mercury toxicity. Furthermore, many patients sensitive to amalgam report classic symptoms of MS: numbness and tingling in the extremities, facial twitching, tremors or shaking of hands and feet. In 1984, a Swedish patient with numerous neurological problems was diagnosed with ALS, thought to be invariably fatal. The dentist, who recognized many symptoms similar to those of mercury poisoning, suggested that the patient have her copious amalgam fillings replaced, particularly as she could date her neurological problems from the placement of the fillings. Six weeks after the fillings were replaced, the patient was able to walk up stairs without experiencing back pain. Four months later she returned to the same University Hospital at Umea, Sweden which had diagnosed her illness, for a week-long follow-up investigation. The following notation was placed in her medical records: 'The neurological status is completely without comment. Hence the patient does not show any motor neuron disease of type ALS. She has been informed that she is in neurological respect fully healthy.' The hospital concluded that the problem had been to do with mercury in the spinal cord. Nine years on, this woman is still in good health.[36]

Frequently, mercury poisoning also causes unexplained chronic fatigue. Hal Huggins says that over 90 per cent of his 2,000 patients have ME-like symptoms of fatigue which improve when their fillings are removed. Biologically, says Huggins, this is easily explained. Mercury interferes with the oxygen-carrying capability of red blood cells; in most of his patients, who are given an 'oxyhaemoglobin' test, the oxygen-transport ability of the red blood cells is about half what it should be. This explains why they are chronically tired even though they have normal haemoglobin levels.

Amalgam in Pregnancy

Mercury fillings in pregnant women may also affect the growing foetus. In another University of Calgary study, Vimy and his colleagues placed radioactive-tagged amalgam fillings in the 12 molar teeth of five pregnant sheep on their 112th day of pregnancy. As early as three days after the fillings were placed, mercury was evident in the blood of the foetuses and amniotic fluid; 16 days later it was evident in foetal pituitary glands, liver, kidney, as well as part of the placenta. By 33 days later (around the time of birth), most of the babies had higher levels of mercury than the mothers did. And during breastfeeding the mothers had eight times as much mercury in their milk as in their blood.[37]

More recently, a study on humans showed that mercury from a mother's fillings can cross the placenta and pollute the brain of her unborn child. Professor Gustav Drasch (a forensic toxicologist) and his colleagues at the Institut fur Rechtsmedicine in Munich examined the brains, liver and kidneys of dead babies and of foetuses aborted for medical reasons. They found that the level of mercury in the babies was significantly correlated with the number of amalgam fillings in their mothers. The babies were even found to accumulate mercury in their kidneys from the amalgams to the same degree that adults do from their own fillings. As most of these children obviously were not breastfed, or if so were fed for only a short period, the researchers concluded that the mercury must have crossed the placenta.[38]

Fertility

There's also evidence that amalgam fillings may affect fertility. A group of German women with hormonal irregularities were studied to see whether they had excessive levels of any environmental agents such as mercury, pesticides or industrial chemicals in their bodies. By far the most common problem was mercury contamination, levels of which again significantly matched the number of the woman's fillings and the amount of mercury released while chewing.[39] Mercury can also affect the fertility of men: A study of occupational workers exposed to mercury at work found that their fertility was significantly reduced.[40]

Hair Loss

Mercury fillings may even affect hair loss. In one study, nearly half of women with unexplained hair loss had evidence of elevated mercury in their bodies; in two-thirds the condition disappeared once they'd had their fillings removed.[41]

Allergies Caused by Mercury

Although there is no hard scientific evidence that mercury in some way contributes to allergies, there are copious case studies among dentists whose patients suffering from food or environmental ailments improved in some way once their fillings were removed.

Tara, a Swedish patient, had suffered with allergic problems – including eczema – from birth. At five she had developed severe asthma and had to take daily medication. During the whole of her adolescence she was often hospitalized. She also suffered from severe headaches and double vision. At three, Tara had had her first amalgam filling; she was ultimately to have seven fillings in total over 11 surfaces. Researchers, on examining her history, realized that her asthma had come on following the placement of two deep fillings. They also realized that her mother had received a large amalgam filling during her pregnancy.

Tara and her mother consented to have all their amalgam fillings removed. Six weeks after the procedure was completed, Tara's eczema began to disappear and she no longer required asthma medication. Seven months later, both conditions completely cleared up, and stayed clear over the eight years her progress was followed.[42]

The closest we have to a scientific study is a consolidated report of six separate studies of patients who had their amalgam fillings replaced. Eighty-nine per cent of the nearly 1,600 participants reported cure or improvement of 31 types of conditions. In the studies compiled from data from four countries, 83 per cent reported improvement in general gastrointestinal problems and 76 per cent in urinary tract problems; 87 per cent cured or improved their migraines, and 75 per cent of those with multiple sclerosis reported that they were better or cured.

If this data were extrapolated to all Americans with amalgam fillings, 17.4 million would have conditions like allergies improve or disappear simply by having their mercury dental fillings exchanged for non-mercury ones.[43]

Even though there are many success stories, Hal Huggins cautions that, unlike his MS patients, 85 per cent of whom improve, only 60 per cent of his 'environmentally ill' patients get better, suggesting that mercury is only one of many contributory factors.[44]

Upset in the Gut

What has been studied scientifically is mercury's ability to upset gut bacteria and create a resistance to antibiotics. The University of Calgary team combined forces with Dr Anne O. Summers and her colleagues at the Department of Microbiology at the University of Georgia in Athens, who are expert in matters concerning the gut. Calgary sent their raw statistics on the six monkeys to Summers and her colleagues to analyse in terms of the effect of mercury on intestinal flora.

The University of Georgia researchers found increased mercury-resistant bacteria in the gums and intestines of the monkeys, once they'd had amalgam fillings placed. In earlier work, Dr Summers had shown that when there is a high mercury resistance in gut bacteria, there is also a high level of resistance to antibiotics. In her study, the mercury-resistant bacterial strains such as streptococci were also resistant to ampicillin, tetracycline, streptomycin, kanamycin and chloramphenicol.[45]

To simplify greatly, the presence of mercury creates a change in the chemical make-up of the 1.15kg (2½lb) of 'friendly' bacteria living in the intestine, making it resistant to antibiotics. This means that the bacteria, which are essential for the smooth operation of the immune system, are, in effect, 'otherwise engaged' and no longer able to keep fungi such as candida albicans (which causes thrush) in check. The altered bacteria also enhance the reabsorption of mercury vapour as it migrates from the teeth. This sets up a basic dysfunction in the gut, upsetting protein metabolism and gut flora, and leading to a situation whereby food particles go undigested. Dr Vimy believes that amalgam fillings could be responsible for candida and the proliferation of allergies suddenly developing in people in their middle years, as well as for the general problem of resistance to antibiotics and superbugs present in the population at large.

Alzheimer's Disease and Mercury

Although Vimy showed only that mercury from fillings travels to the brains of sheep, we now have evidence that it settles in the brains of humans, too. American dentist and researcher David Eggleston spent months in the local county morgue examining the accumulation of mercury in the brain tissue of 83 accident victims with amalgam fillings, and discovered that the number of amalgam fillings correlated with the level of mercury in the brain.[46] Patrick Störtebecker of the Störtebecker Foundation for Research in Stockholm has described studies demonstrating that mercury poisoning reaches the brain directly from the nasal cavity.[47]

When considering the possibility that Alzheimer's disease could be an environmental illness, the finger of blame has always been pointed at aluminium. But increasing evidence shows that it is mercury, rather than aluminium, that is found in greatest concentration in the brains of Alzheimer's disease victims. W. R. Markesbery and his medical research team in the departments of Chemistry, Pathology and Neurology at the University of Kentucky and also the Sanders-Brown Center on Aging in

Lexington, Kentucky, have been investigating Alzheimer's disease and its association with mercury for several years. In one study they examined the brains of 10 autopsied Alzheimer's patients for concentrations of trace elements. The trace element found in the highest concentration was consistently mercury; the study also noted diminished zinc and selenium levels in the subjects examined.[48] In the view of the researchers, a high level of mercury in the brain of Alzheimer's patients is the most important of the imbalances they observed. But they also consider the lower zinc levels significant, since zinc and selenium are known to protect against heavy-metal toxicity.

Minute doses of mercury in the brain produce identical changes to those seen in Alzheimer's.[49] Tubulin is a protein needed for the healthy formation of neurofibrils, or connective nerve tissue. Alzheimer's patients have impaired tubulin, which causes what is known as a 'neurofibril tangle', where messages in the brain don't connect properly. Professor of Medical Biochemistry Boyd Haley and the other colleagues at the University of Kentucky fed rats aluminium but observed no change in tubulin levels, whereas mercury-fed rats displayed a diminished tubulin level similar to that of typical Alzheimer's patients.

Vimy and his team at the University of Calgary Medical School also used rats to show that mercury markedly inhibits tubulin levels. In fact, concentrations of mercury in the brains of these rats were similar to those recorded in monkeys 28 days after placement of dental amalgam fillings.[50]

Jim, now 80, had a mouth full of 15 large amalgam fillings, some covering virtually the entire tooth. Periodically his dentist of 35 years had replaced old silver fillings with new ones. Five years ago, his wife, Martha, noticed that Jim's motor skills began deteriorating. By last summer his walking had become quite poor; when he fell over at a lunch party she was astonished to realize that he didn't remember how to get up and refused to co-operate with friends attempting to assist him. Later that summer, Martha also noticed that a 'fog' seemed to have descended over Jim. He couldn't walk or climb stairs without assistance. During a holiday in Austria he seemed to have forgotten how to swim – formerly a favourite activity. 'Mentally, he just wasn't with it at all,' she says.

In September, Martha took Jim to a geriatrician who diagnosed Alzheimer's disease and predicted that Jim would need to be placed in a nursing home in three months' time. The shock of this diagnosis jolted Jim into listening to his wife, who'd been trying to get him tested for amalgam poisoning for years. Positive test results showing high amalgam levels persuaded Jim to have the fillings out.

Jim had the fillings removed in two sessions at the dentist. On his way there, Jim needed to hang on to Martha to climb the several flights of stairs to the surgery; after the final session, he walked down the stairs unaided. Soon after the fillings were removed, his GP agreed with Martha that Jim had 'woken up'. Five months later, once he'd undergone a detoxifying programme to get the amalgam out of his system, Jim now goes out again by himself. He is once again able to prepare his and Martha's tax returns and to write letters. Although his walking can be poor, it is getting better, and, most important, Jim now recognizes when he isn't walking properly and corrects himself.

Some among the anti-amalgam lobby consider that aluminium may well be a red herring in the quest to find the cause of Alzheimer's. Nevertheless, it is difficult to dismiss mounting evidence of some role for aluminium in the development of the disease.[51] It could be, as some suggest, that a brain depleted of zinc and overwhelmed by mercury is susceptible to the depositing of aluminium, but that aluminium itself doesn't cause the problem. Or it could be that both aluminium and mercury contribute. Although aluminium is ever present – in our water, commercially prepared orange juice, food, cosmetics, drugs, deodorants, cooking utensils and flip-top cans – the amounts of aluminium we are exposed to from these sources is nothing like the concentrated dose of mercury we receive when it is placed in our mouths and inhaled with every chew.

When not manifesting itself as full-blown dementia, amalgam poisoning causes 'brain fog'. This happened to Pam of Northamptonshire, who never made the connection until she visited a practitioner who suspected mercury leakage from her teeth and confirmed it with two tests.

My symptoms included chronic short-term memory problems (such as walking into a room and forgetting what for, forgetting people's names, losing the thread of my thought mid-sentence), slurred speech, blurred vision, a fuzzy head, swollen tongue and throat, a metallic taste in my mouth, asthma, IBS, pain in arms and legs (for 17 years), tingling and numbness all over, leg weakness (such that I had to give up driving), food allergies, chronic fatigue and collapsing after using an escalator. I couldn't enter a shop because clothing and carpets made me feel ill.

For the last few years of my illness, my symptoms were made worse after I had a nickel-backed crown put in. Not only did I have to give up work, but I also couldn't wear any jewellery, especially earrings, which would make my ears itch. It took me three years of special detoxification to remove all the metal from my brain and body.

Now that she's had the fillings removed, Pam can drive safely and again wear earrings.

Mercury and the Heart

New evidence has implicated mercury in the epidemic of congestive heart failure and other heart disease. Researchers at the Catholic University in Rome examined trace-element concentrations of mercury in biopsies from the left ventricle of patients with idiopathic dilated cardiomyopathy (IDCM) and those without heart disease. Those with IDCM showed hugely elevated concentrations of mercury in the heart tissue – 22,000 times higher than normal. As none of the patients was exposed to mercury through their occupations, researchers at the University of Calgary concluded that dental amalgams were the most likely source of the mercury.[52]

Major research from Finland also shows a clear link between mercury and heart disease. Although many men of eastern Finland are hardy fish-eaters, they have an extraordinarily high mortality rate from cardiovascular disease. Researchers ultimately isolated the local fish, which is high in mercury, as the cause; high levels of mercury doubled the risk of having a heart attack and trebled the risk of dying from heart disease. (This did not apply to those men who ate fatty, ocean-caught fish such as salmon, herring and tuna, which are high in omega-3 fatty acids.)

Mercury is thought to cause heart disease by promoting the creation of free radicals and inactivating the antioxidants glutathione and selenium, eventually causing an increased level of lipid peroxidation, a precursor of heart disease. A number of studies have shown a correlation between the number of amalgam tooth fillings in a patient's mouth and his subsequent risk of heart attack.[53]

Other studies show that mercury acts by contracting the smooth muscle of the blood vessels, which ultimately raises blood-pressure, affecting the heart's ability to contract and the electrical conductivity which regulates heartbeat.[54]

According to research from the former Soviet Union, mercury produces functional changes in cardiac activity and in heart muscle, and accumulates in heart muscle and valves largely because mercury profoundly affects hormones from the pituitary gland. Mercury has also been shown to increase the tendency of the blood to clot – a risk factor for heart attacks and strokes.[55] Studies comparing patients with and without amalgam fillings show that those with the mercury fillings have far higher blood-pressure, lower heart rate, a greater tendency to chest pains, abnormal heart beat, anaemia and fatigue than those without.[56]

Problems with other Metal Alloys

Aside from causing electrical problems, metal alloys (nickel, beryllium, chromium and molybdenum) may also affect the basic function of human cells. Researchers from Alabama exposed cells from human gums to solutions of alloys for short periods, and discovered that the cells slowed their energy-production and decreased their intake of oxygen. The effect was felt in the mitrocondria of cells, where ATP (energy) is produced. Abnormalities in this process are involved in many diseases, and a slowing of energy-production is considered the first stage in the eventual development of cancer.[57]

Mercury and Mental Illness

Mercury fillings have even been implicated in some cases of bipolar disorder. In one small study, patients who'd had their fillings replaced suffered significantly less anxiety, depression, paranoia, hostility and obsessive-compulsive behaviour, and indeed some were able to discontinue taking medication.[58]

Mercury Lawsuits

Even if the dental associations in Britain and the US have not alerted the public about the dangers of amalgam, companies that manufacture amalgam (and which could be most open to liability claims) had to take the warning signs seriously. California passed a law (Proposition 65) prohibiting Californians from being unwittingly exposed to chemicals known to cause cancer or birth defects. Any work environment containing such potentially harmful materials must carry a warning.

The US Environmental Law Foundation decided to test this by taking Jeneric, one of the biggest manufacturers of dental amalgam, to court on this issue. The court ruled in favour of the ELF, and Jeneric became the first such company to issue health warnings on its product, in the form of an alert to dentists, dental staff and patients in California about the potential dangers of birth defects from exposure to mercury.

Jeneric has added warnings to all amalgam containers shipped to California and agreed to supply dental surgeries with a warning sign to be displayed prominently in their waiting areas: 'This office uses amalgam filling materials which contain and expose you to mercury, a chemical known to the State of California to cause birth defects and other reproductive harm. Please consult your dentist for more information.' It also agreed to stop selling mercury fillings to dentists who fail to put up the warning notice.

After the Jeneric ruling, 10 other dental amalgam manufacturers banded together and challenged it. A US Federal court judge decision overturned the earlier one, on the grounds that the regulatory authority for amalgam was not Proposition 65, but the US Food and Drug Administration, which of course has ruled that mercury fillings are safe. In the summer of 1996, the lower court ruling was overturned upon appeal by the ELF. The appeal court ruled that the lower court had erred in granting the reversal; since Proposition 65 is a law passed by California voters, FDA regulation does not preclude the Proposition's mandate of a warning to patients. This means that California dentists must now disclose to their patients that fillings contain mercury. A bill introduced at the time of writing would ban amalgam fillings in California altogether.

Removing Your Fillings

Not everyone should get their fillings removed. If you do suspect that your fillings are making you ill, it might be wise to get proof of it, by undergoing a series of tests demonstrating mercury sensitivity. At Chelsea and Westminster Hospital, Drs Don Henderson and Michele Monteil of the Department of Immunology have developed a simple blood test to determine if your fillings are making you ill.

The test, called a Metal Specific Memory T Cell Test (MSMT), determines your immune system's 'memory' of dental and other metals. When your body is exposed to a foreign invader (say, a virus), your body mounts a defence and kills the infection. The next time you get exposed to the same virus, your body can attack it more quickly and powerfully, because of its immunological memory – the antibodies it has developed. These immune-system responses can actually be measured.

As for metal, although all people will demonstrate immunological memory of a variety of metals, including mercury, only those who have a serious reaction – for instance, those who get a rash from nickel – will show a strong memory response. A test like this to measure industry exposure to heavy metals has been available for years. Drs Henderson and Monteil have demonstrated that the strength of immune-system response to mercury and other dental metals can also be graded.[59] You should also be assessed for potential mercury toxicity on the basis of a comprehensive clinical medical and dental history. This includes all fillings, crowns, implants and dentures – any body-piercing and even amalgam tattoos.

Another possible means of checking the effect of the metal in your mouth is through a provocation urine test. This uses 2,3 dimercaptosuccinic acid (DMSA), which chelates, or chemically 'grabs' the mercury in your system, excreted in your urine. A urine sample is taken before and after taking DMSA; the result gives an indication of the total burden of mercury in your body. Other tests which will give you a crude indication of a heavy mercury body-burden are a hair mineral analysis and a sweat test for dental metals. (All three tests are available at Biolab in London: 020 7636 5959.)

In addition, each individual filling should be tested for electrical potential with a *millivoltmeter*, since each filling is a potential battery. This sort of test will show the amount of mercury vapour released from each filling. Some clinical ecologists will perform this function.

According to Huggins and the late UK dentist Jack Levenson, who led the fight against mercury in the UK, the most important aspect of removing fillings is removing them in the right sequence — that is, taking out the most negatively-charged ones first.

Many of the patients rushing to have their amalgam fillings replaced are getting more ill because no protocol is being observed to protect them from the onslaught of mercury vapours released. This happened to John, a scientist in Birmingham, who almost died after having his fillings carelessly removed.

Sophie from Gloucestershire got ill when her dentist removed all seven of her amalgam fillings without following any protective protocol:

I started to feel really ill and got progressively worse until I found myself in hospital with agonizing stomach pains. I was given morphine and thought I was dying. My legs were numb and tingly, I had muscle spasms and tremors and lost over a stone-and-a-half. After a month and various procedures (laparoscopy, endoscopy, colonoscopy, a barium meal, scans and blood tests), I was discharged as a 'medical mystery'.

Once home, I spent two months in pain — unable to sleep or move and barely getting better. In desperation I visited a homoeopath, who suspected mercury poisoning after a two-hour consultation. Tests confirmed this and I was referred to a London-based toxicologist, who started me on a course of detox. I am now beginning to lead a normal life, although I know that my body is still not totally rid of the poisonous substance.

It's a good idea to start your own supplement-and-detox programme two months before your amalgams are removed. This should include antioxidants to help bind and excrete mercury, a good multivitamin supplement, extra vitamin C and selenium (50 – 200 micrograms).

Make sure you are also eating a fresh, organic wholefood diet. Dr Levenson counselled that you should avoid foods that are salty, sour or eaten at a high temperature, or snacks between meals, since all of these increase mercury vapour.

It's also a good idea to take charcoal half an hour prior to treatment. This will help to pick up any mercury vapour that has been swallowed.

Before you have your fillings out, seek out a dentist who is experienced in removing amalgam fillings and interview him. Ensure that he is used to

271

removing fillings in sequence, depending on ammeter or voltmeter measurements.

Then once you've had your fillings replaced, you'll need to carry out an extensive detox programme for a number of months, using detox measures such as saunas and steam, lymphatic drainage and, if necessary, a chelator such as DMSA to flush mercury out of your system. Supplements such as MSM and N-acetylcysteine, charcoal tablets and Chlorella algae also may also be useful in helping to flush mercury out of your body. Many dentists report success with homoeopathic amalgam. As mercury can disturb the usual gut bacteria, probiotics may help, depending on symptoms. Finally, you need to be patient. As Sophie says, it is a long process.

Potential health problems with alternatives to amalgam certainly exist, but are fortunately much rarer in most people. Nevertheless, it's doubtful that any holistic dentist would describe any dental material as being completely without potential risk.

We do know that composites can make teeth sensitive when first placed. But some patients experience continued sensitivity when their filling is 'leaking' – that is, a gap exists between the tooth and its filling. With composite fillings, which are all based on resin-based materials, moisture like saliva, blood or gum fluids can adversely affect its ability to bond properly.

When liquid composites are placed in the mouth, these plastic substances must be 'cured' or polymerized, which hardens and sets the plastic through the use of a curing light. When the material is cured, the filling can shrink between 2 and 5 per cent. If the bond is inadequate, the composite will shrink and have a marginal gap between filling and tooth, which will never improve. According to Dr Stephen Dunne, Senior Lecturer and Consultant of the Department of Conservative Dentistry at Kings Dental Institute in London, 60 per cent of curing lights in general practice in the UK are operating below manufacturer's specifications.

Composites have always been expected to last only half as long as amalgam fillings. However, Carl Leinfelder of the University of South Carolina, who performs materials-testing on humans, says that the 'ideal' restorative materials least resistant to wear (even over fillings made of gold, classically considered the hardest substance) are certain makes of resin-based polymers placed in by a careful layering process.

Dentists using this method tend to etch the cavity, sealing it with a resin-bond layer. Next, they place in a soft, self-hardening substance of glass ionomer; over that goes more resin bond, then a macrofill material of high polymerization, which needs to be cured with the dentist's light. Another layer of bond follows and then a microfill substance after that, of high strength and low wear.

The most common type of composites today are composed of glass or porcelain particles in an acrylic base. If you are contemplating having resin-based fillings, choose a dentist who uses a rubber dam and meticulous isolating procedures prior to placing the filling, as well as a reliable curing light. Most of all, he should have plenty of experience and lots of contented patients. You can test your reaction to composite (white) fillings by sucking a sample of the material for two hours, and then doing so again two days later. Monitor any reactions and report them to your dentist. If you react to that specific composite, another one can be found for you.

With your children's teeth, the best course of all is prevention. Breastfeed if you can, avoid giving them sugary drinks or too many sweets, provide them with a wholefood diet including plenty of fruits and vegetables, and make sure they brush their teeth regularly and eat fruit after meals. As long ago as 1911, a survey in New Zealand of 1,500 schoolchildren found that if they ate alkaline, saliva-producing food after a meal, this food would neutralize the acidity of bacteria. This reduced the incidence of tooth decay enormously. One of the best alkaline saliva-producers is fruit.

PART V

SURGERY

10

Standard Operating Procedure

Of all areas in medicine, surgery is probably the least scientific. Most decisions about operations have more to do with the personal taste of individual doctors, the arbitrary consensus of professional bodies or just the fashion of the moment than with hard fact. For obvious ethical reasons, operations are almost never tested by controlled experiment, but are instead developed on an ad hoc basis and then taught to others – including trainees – more or less on the job. This means that many surgeons get enthused by new techniques before they know what they're doing or even whether the procedure is going to do any good at all.

Besides not knowing when to put down the knife, surgeons of all persuasions underestimate the simple risks involved in every type of surgery, no matter how 'routine'. A University of Oxford survey of some 225,000 operations in six nearby health districts found that one in 10 emergency prostatectomies and more than one in five emergency hip replacements ended in death a year after the surgery. Although emergency procedures had far higher fatality rates, a number of elective procedures also carried high risks. For instance, people electing to have cataracts or their prostate removed had a one in 20 chance of dying up to a year after their operation due to complications during surgery.[1]

A high proportion of deaths occur because routine procedures aren't followed properly. According to the third Report of the National Confidential Enquiry into Perioperative Deaths – information supplied voluntarily by over a thousand surgeons around Britain about postoperative deaths of patients in the month after an operation – many patients are needlessly dying after routine surgery. The Enquiry found that deaths from deep vein thrombosis and blood clots in the lungs were commonplace, simply because drugs that would have counteracted the problem weren't administered. Many deaths were due to preoperative preparations or even the surgery itself being undertaken too hastily, or to too much fluid being given the patient during surgery, causing heart attacks. *A considerable number of deaths were caused by the surgeon's lack of familiarity with the operation.*[2]

Many treatments are faddish, adopted in a flurry of enthusiasm and soon discarded in favour of the next new possibility when evidence proves the original procedures don't work. Just consider the history of treatment for back pain. Earlier in this century, sacroiliac joint disease was believed the culprit in many cases of back pain, leading to fusions (the joining of one vertebra to another) of the sacroiliac joints.

This was followed by such treatments as the removal of the coccyx, injections for slipped discs, lengthy bed rest, traction and even nerve stimulation – all, in their turn, discarded.

The latest fad to be discredited is steroid injections in the facet joints (the cartilage covering of the bony junction between two vertebrae). Recent evidence finally revealed that injecting steroids is no better than injecting salt water.[3]

Harvard Medical School once performed one of the few studies to see whether surgeons get it right when they recommend surgery. The Harvard researchers looked at the track record of over a hundred doctors in diagnosing one of the most common procedures – removal of non-malignant moles. In all, the correct diagnosis was made in less than half the cases. Dermatologists – who should be able to do this with their eyes closed – only got the diagnosis right two-thirds of the time, while other types of doctors were only half as good as that. Like the diagnosis, the appropriate procedure was carried out only half of the time.

Getting it wrong is nothing new with surgeons. In the US, some six million unnecessary operations and invasive tests get performed annually. In the US alone, 20,000 normal appendixes are mistakenly removed every year, up to a third of all operations.[4]

In fact, with the vast bulk of surgery patients often go under the knife unnecessarily. Most children with glue ear undergo operations needlessly,[5] as do women undergoing a D and C (dilatation and curettage – scraping of the lining of the womb) after complete miscarriage,[6] hysterectomy,[7] and even patients undergoing coronary bypass surgery. Bypass surgery might relieve symptoms in some patients, but there is no proof anywhere that this surgery actually prolongs life.[8] In one study involving researchers from 14 major heart hospitals around the world, up to one-third of all bypass operations were found to be unnecessary and actually to hasten the death of the patient. One-third of the patients, considered low-risk cases, might have lived longer if they had received drugs therapy rather than surgery.[9]

BYPASS SURGERY

Heart bypass – or coronary artery bypass graft (CABG) – is a radical procedure that has become the most frequently performed of all surgical operations, with around 500,000 carried out every year in the US alone. Around 10 per cent of all heart patients will undergo a cardiac bypass, especially if they have one or more coronary arteries that are either blocked or severely narrowed.

Coronary bypass operations are also one of the most unnecessary operations. Heart surgeons have known this since the 1970s, when several major studies revealed that bypass surgery did not improve survival except among patients with severe coronary disease, particularly to the left ventricle. Although earlier studies showed that it relieved severe angina,[10] the US National Institutes of Health has estimated that 90 per cent of American patients who undergo bypass surgery receive no benefits. A review of 37 studies of bypass surgery concluded that the heart function of the patients improves in only one-third to a half of all cases.[11] The rest had basically the same heart function they had before their operations.

During the operation, the surgeon removes veins from the patient's leg, forearm or chest, and grafts these onto a healthy portion of one of the main coronary arteries, thus bypassing the portion that is blocked. The traditional, or 'on-pump' method, is carried out while the heart is stopped and the patient and his blood supply attached to a pump, which oxygenates it and pumps it back into the patient. However, more than a quarter of all patients suffer a heart contraction after their bypass surgery,[12] and some 6 per cent suffer stroke, with some dying from it and others deteriorating mentally.[13] In fact, nearly a quarter of all bypass patients suffer deterioration of mental agility[14] because of the high risk that a blood clot will get dislodged and travel to the brain. CABG patients (as they're usually referred to) also suffer difficulties breathing, depression and other heart and circulatory problems, such as hypertension (high blood-pressure) and abnormal heart rhythms.

Consequently, surgeons have been experimenting with an 'off-pump' technique, also known as 'beating-heart bypass surgery', where the heart is kept going and stabilized through the use of special equipment – a procedure that surgeons maintain is far safer.

Nevertheless, this new procedure appears to have the same potential for causing permanent brain damage[15] and six times the risk of the grafts not taking and closing up.[16]

But even if a patient manages to get wheeled out of the surgery alive, he still faces substantial risks. More than 3 per cent of triple-bypass patients die in the first year after surgery, as do nearly 3 per cent of double-bypass patients, a figure that rises sharply with age.[17]

Most astonishing of all, bypass is far more dangerous and far less effective than conservative management with drugs. Some three times as many people die after this supposedly tried-and-tested surgery as those who eschew the knife and elect to sort out their triple-artery blockage with drugs.[18]

Indeed, perhaps the best medicine is to do nothing at all. New evidence shows that when left to its own devices, a heart with blockages of the main vessels somehow has the exquisite intelligence to know that it isn't getting enough oxygen and will embark on its own cure. In three-quarters of cases, the heart will engineer the growth of new blood vessels to form its own, natural bypass of the obstructed arteries. These 'collateral' blood vessels keep blood flowing to the heart when the main vessels are closed. Within three to six months, those patients who do absolutely nothing at all will experience a relief of chest pain.

Nevertheless, as if tacitly understanding that their work is done, the collateral vessels vanish in a patient given bypass surgery. If a bypass doesn't take, these patients are in more danger than they were if their temporary 'detour' vessels had remained intact. This suggests that the heart has its own self-healing mechanism, which is interrupted when doctors rush in too quickly after a patient has suffered an acute heart attack. In two studies of such patients, far more died if they were operated on, compared with those managed conservatively through drugs.[19] Similarly, in the US Veterans' Administration VANQWISH study, three times as many bypass patients died as those managed through 'watchful waiting'. Three years later, nearly a quarter fewer patients had died through conservative management than bypass.[20]

BACK PAIN

Treatment for back pain also aptly demonstrates how knife-happy many surgeons are without much in the way of evidence that operations will do any good. In most cases, medicine has shown a shocking ineptitude in diagnosing and treating back problems, often tending to make the problem worse.

Professor Gordon Waddell, orthopaedic surgeon at Glasgow's Western Infirmary, scathingly summed up this appalling track record: '... dramatic surgical successes, unfortunately, apply to only some 1 per cent of patients with low back disorders. Our failure is in the remaining 99 per cent of patients with simple backache, for whom, despite new investigations and all our treatments, the problem has become progressively worse.'[21]

For back patients who undergo surgery, 15 to 20 per cent will fall into the category of 'the failed back' – the official name given to people with chronic, considerable back pain that doctors can't fix. Some 200,000 to 400,000 patients go under the knife in the US every year. That translates into 30,000–80,000 Americans every year who will emerge from back surgery in considerably more pain than before they went to their doctor.

Many causes of disastrous residual pain are caused by inappropriate surgery for back pain. The most popular operations include: laminectomy, in which a disc and nearby bone are removed, to give the nerve branching off the central spinal cord more space to move without getting trapped or compressed by the spine; discetomy, where a disc is removed; and fusion, in which one vertebrae is surgically joined to another, in order to minimize what has usually been diagnosed as too much movement between the vertebrae. After fusion, this segment of the spine will be unable to move at all.

According to six studies of back operations, removing discs only relieves back pain in about half of all patients.[22] But of over a hundred cases of failed spinal surgery, primarily disc removal, surgery wasn't indicated for two thirds of them.[23] Three out of four studies comparing operations with to those without lumbar (lower back) spinal fusion surgery found no advantage for fusion; complications, including chronic pain, were common.[24]

Another study of 'failed back surgery syndrome' showed that in more than half of all such cases, the diagnosis missed or the surgery itself caused a condition called 'lateral spinal stenosis', or narrowing of a portion of the spine, causing compression of the spinal cord or an abnormally tight fit.[25]

Even more fundamental are the sheer number of bad diagnoses. Of those patients referred to him at Gordon Waddell's clinic in Glasgow, '60 per cent believe or have been told that they have a disc prolapse, although only 11 per cent show any evidence of nerve root involvement,' he says.[26]

Finally, postsurgical scarring ('epidural fibrosis') can itself cause failed surgery and chronic pain. US back specialist Henry La Rocca of Tulane University in Louisiana also found substantial evidence that surgeons cause nerve-root injury as the nerve is being separated from a herniated disc, causing scarring and therefore long-term pain and pressure on the nerve. 'Damage to the dura or the cauda equina [membranes covering the spinal cord] from poor surgical technique yielding possibly catastrophic results completes the list,' he writes.[27]

This is precisely what happened to Sarah of Woking. Her back problems developed after a hysterectomy, so she consented to surgery on her spine. The delicate layers of the spinal cord (meninges) became inflamed, and then thickened. This thickened membrane now presses constantly on her spine, incapacitating her with unbearable pain.

Gordon Waddell and others conclude that if there is a specific problem correctly identified – such as a spinal deformity or fracture or disc herniation – then surgery can help, but not for simple relief of unspecified back pain.[28]

In many cases, back pain may not be related to the back at all, but can be caused by an ulcer,[29] poor abdominal muscle tone,[30] pancreatitis[31] or even heart disease.[32] Indeed, the best results are achieved when doctors treat the back holistically, as part of the rest of the body, and advocate osteopathy, chiropactic manipulation, back exercises and mobility.[33]

SURGERY FOR BREAST CANCER

There is no doubt that the incidence of breast cancer is appallingly high. But the true number of cases of dangerous breast cancer may be vastly inflated by the 'tools' of modern medicine.

Perhaps the greatest scandal of breast cancer surgery is that up to half of all cases of so-called breast cancer are not cancer at all, but a harmless 'something' that has gone slightly awry but which, in the long term, is likely to sort itself out. Doctors believe that ductal carcinoma in situ (DCIS) is an early herald of breast cancer, much as they imagine that abnormal smear tests are an early warning sign of cervical cancer. But DCIS may well turn out to be a harmless aberration which, like abnormal smear tests, in the majority of cases does not progress to cancer. Indeed, women with DCIS might never become aware of it if medicine didn't insist on a blunderbuss means of screening for cancer. Insisting on surgery for DCIS is as barbaric as performing a hysterectomy on a woman with a dodgy Pap smear, a common practice a generation ago.

Ductal carcinoma in situ is a condition whereby the milk ducts are filled with little specks of calcium (referred to in medicalese as 'microcalcification'). Any abnormality is contained in the milk ducts of the breast and does not spread out to the fatty breast tissue or any other part of the body, such as the lymph nodes (hence the name 'in situ' or 'in place'). These microcalcifications are not large enough to be palpable, but are picked up only on mammograms. They are believed to be the precursors of cancer, but they are not in themselves cancerous – so even the name itself ('ductal carcinoma') is misleading. Nevertheless, DCIS is treated like any other invasive cancer and classified as a stage 0 cancer – that is, a cancer that hasn't spread anywhere.

DCIS is usually confirmed by either a fine-needle aspiration biopsy, which removes fluid and fragments of breast tissue, or a core-needle biopsy, which removes a larger chunk of breast tissue for examination under the microscope.

The American Cancer Society estimates that 41,000 new cases of DCIS are diagnosed every year, making up some 25 per cent of all diagnoses of breast cancer. The usual treatment is a lumpectomy or full mastectomy, followed by radiation.

Recently, a batch of Australian pathologists writing in to *The Lancet* noted that, in performing core biopsies for abnormalities picked up on mammograms, they routinely uncover cases of 'burnt-out' – that is, healed – ductal carcinoma in situ. These are cases of a calcified mass which was DCIS and which seems to have run its course.

The letter also indicated that this phenomenon – of a DCIS healing – was first described in the medical literature some 70 years ago.[34] The Australian pathologists repeatedly found a 'foci' of an abnormality at the centre of these microcalcifications, which had basically petered out. All that was left was a remnant of the old problem, which the body has effectively contained – an abnormal milk duct or a calcified mass surrounded by fibroid tissue.

The Australians were very wary of saying that this finding cannot always be counted on to be benign, and suggested continued follow-up. Nevertheless, UK breast cancer specialist Professor Michael Baum says that, in his experience, more than 80 per cent of all DCIS cases never progress to cancer.[35] Even when they do, mortality is extremely low and conventional treatment offers no survival advantage. According to a review of all breast cancer statistics by cancer expert Maryann Napoli of the Center for Medical Consumers in New York, 1 per cent of women with DCIS die of breast cancer – whether or not they are treated.[36]

Indeed, in many cases the surgery for cancer, including breast cancer or DCIS, may actually *precipitate* its spread. Dr Judah Folkman of Harvard University has carried out research showing that the creation of new blood vessels, a process known as *angiogenesis*, is responsible for the spread of cancer. Injury to skin and muscle, as occurs through surgery, and the consequent rush of blood and oxygen to the site, turns on this angiogenic 'switch'. Extra blood and blood vessels also offer the tumour cells a 'superhighway' to distant organs. Even biopsy can trigger angiogenesis.

'You take a latent cancer that would never hurt a woman,' says Baum, 'biopsy it, turn on the angiogenic switch, and it ceases to be latent – it becomes an aggressive disease.'

The implications of these findings are enormous. For many years doctors have admitted that they don't know whether DCIS spreads, and yet they perform mastectomies as a just-in-case measure. Now we have evidence that, in many instances, these could be little fires that the body is well equipped to stamp out by itself, without having to enlist the full support of the cut–and–burn fire brigade of modern medicine. These findings also suggest that many cases of so-called breast cancer are being mislabelled as such.

Finally, they also highlight how blunt an instrument mammography is as a form of detection. By indiscriminately detecting *all* abnormalities, including benign ones, mammograms are contributing to the problem of breast cancer, not the solution. Most cases of DCIS might resolve themselves with no one the wiser if they'd not shown up on a mammogram.

For the women with genuine breast cancer, doctors insist on surgery as the first port of call. Although many in medicine believe that cutting out the tumour reduces the cancer burden on the body, a number, including Dr Baum, a breast-cancer specialist for more than 30 years, believe that surgery is responsible for the vast spread of cancer,[37] particularly as surgery appears to increase the risk of relapse or death within three years of the procedure.[38] Even a tiny piercing of the flesh, as occurs through biopsies, is thought to bring on cancer in one in 15 women[39] and to spread cancer in a third of cases.[40]

Besides being unnecessary, a large number of surgical procedures still widely used are clearly obsolete. Despite a variety of surgical techniques, a host of back–up therapies and many confident headlines about breast-cancer breakthroughs, *the truth is that surgical treatment of breast cancer hasn't advanced one single step in the past century.* 'Over a period of 100 years,' says Dr Edward F. Scanlon of the Northwestern University Medical School in Illinois, who has studied breast-cancer incidence in depth, 'breast-cancer treatment has evolved from no treatment to radical treatment and back again to more conservative management, without having affected mortality.'[41]

Although governmental and most other official agencies recommend breast-conserving measures for breast cancer caught early, some surgeons persist in a full mastectomy, a mutilating operation developed in the 19th century and never really reviewed to see if it is still applicable to patients today – or indeed if it ever worked at all.

The standard procedure for breast cancer was developed by Dr William Halsted a century ago. (Dr Halsted is better known for advocating what was then a revolutionary notion: that surgeons should wear sterile gloves.) The operation he championed involves removing the breast, much of the skin, the chest wall and the lymph nodes.

Shortly after the Second World War, a study at three hospitals in Illinois showed little difference in five- and 10-year survival rates between radical mastectomies, simple mastectomies, or simple removal of the tumour. Then, some 25 years later, *The Lancet* reviewed 8,000 cases and again found no difference in survival rates among the patients who had received any of these procedures.[42] Nevertheless, the Halsted procedure maintained a tight grip on the mind of the average surgeon over the next two decades. In some areas it was then replaced by 'modified' radical surgery, which removed tissue and breast, but left the chest wall intact, or a simple mastectomy, which only removed the breast itself. But like its predecessor, the modified radical mastectomy was also put into place without any scientific studies proving its worth.

Like the earlier studies, evidence in the 1980s showed that mastectomy provided no benefit in terms of cancer recurrence or survival over breast-conserving surgery (BCS) such as simple lumpectomy (removal of the tumour itself) or quadrantectomy (removal of a portion of the breast). In the most famous study, headed by Dr Bernard Fisher and undertaken by the National Surgical Adjuvant Breast and Bowel Project in Pennsylvania, of nearly 2,000 women over nine years there was no difference in survival rates among those who had undergone lumpectomy, those who had had lumpectomy plus irradiation, and those who had had a total mastectomy.[43]

Several years later, the Chicago Institute discovered that the Pennsylvania trial – which had been the largest in the US on breast cancer – had been falsified. About 100 ineligible patients were included in the trial, which involved 5,000 patients in 485 academic and community hospitals. Once the fraud had been uncovered, two of the Pennsylvania teams pored over the research data again, excluding the ineligible patients, and nevertheless reached the same findings. After a second major US cancer study also headed by Dr Bernard Fisher was discredited, he resigned as research project chairman. In this second study, which tested the efficacy of tamoxifen to prevent breast cancer, Dr Fisher was accused of withholding data about the association of tamoxifen and the development of endometrial cancer. Informed consent forms, which women have to read and sign before agreeing to join the trials, apparently did not include the latest data showing that four women had died after taking tamoxifen.[44]

Luckily, more recent research from the National Cancer Institute (NCI) in Bethesda, Maryland, confirmed that lumpectomy and radiation are just as effective as radical mastectomy in controlling early-stage cancer. The NCI found that about three-quarters of patients given lumpectomy and radiation survived, which was comparable to the number of patients surviving after a radical mastectomy.[45] And in Italy, researchers found that a similar number of patients survived or had local recurrence of cancer, whether they were given radical mastectomy or a breast-conserving operation called a quadrantectomy (removal of only a quarter of the breast), plus radiation.[46]

Since 1990, the American National Institutes of Health has recommended that surgeons opt for breast conservation surgery over mastectomy for the majority of women with stage I or stage II breast cancer. By this they mean for tumours of less than 4 cm in diameter limited to the primary site (the single breast) without involvement of the chest muscle or overlying skin. In the past, doctors felt that cancer found in the axillary lymph nodes was evidence of spread, and grounds for radical mastectomy. With the NIH's announcement, whether or not lymph nodes are involved (so long as they are on the same side as the tumour) is now considered immaterial.

Despite all the publicity about the safety of lumpectomies, many doctors still think the more they cut out the better off a woman is, and refuse to offer breast-conserving surgery to many women with early breast cancer. A Seattle study examined cancer-registry information over five years. Fewer than a third of women were offered BCS, even though three-quarters of them clearly had early cancer. After 1985 (when publicity about BCS had died down somewhat) the practice of keeping breasts intact declined even further, and doctors returned to modified radical mastectomies even though there was no evidence to support their choice.[47]

Doctors also failed to offer radiation therapy to women with cancer who had already been through the menopause, and were more likely to sacrifice the breasts of older patients than younger ones, even for the same stage of breast cancer. In fact, the more affluent and well-educated the woman, the greater the chances of her breast being saved.[48] In many medical centres, the masectomy is still the operation of choice.

HERNIA REPAIR

In the field of other types of surgery, often no one can agree on the best technique to sort out a problem. Although a good hernia repair is as difficult as the most complex abdominal surgery, consultant surgeons leave this kind of surgery, which they consider routine and boring, to trainees to cut their professional teeth on. Juniors in England are allowed to go it alone after only six hernia repairs.[49] This is perhaps one reason for its dismal success rate. It is four times more dangerous to have a hernia operation than to go without one if you're over 65.[50] Up to 10 per cent of operations have to be repeated within five years.

Complications are also common. Up to 40 per cent of keyhole hernias and 33.4 per cent of open hernia repair cause problems.[51] These problems can include injuring the bowel, which occurs in 4 per cent of cases,[52] or producing persistent pain,[53] which occurs in 4 per cent of cases, or even causing pain or lack of feeling during sex.[54] There's also a question mark around the use of polypropylene mesh used for the repair.[55]

PROSTATE CANCER

In too many instances, surgeons rush in with the scalpel too early, when simple watchful waiting – that is, monitoring the situation to see if it gets worse – is called for. This is the case with prostate cancer. The commonest form of cancer (and surgery) for men over 40 concerns the prostate, the gland which lies just below the base of the bladder and produces some of the seminal fluid. Because it is so close to the bladder and urethra, problems in this area invariably cause problems with urination. Although the incidence of prostate cancer hasn't really gone up, the incidence of aggressive treatments such as radiation and surgery has – by a whopping 36 per cent.

Nine cancer registries throughout America, plus data compiled by the National Center for Health Statistics, together showed only a modest increase in prostate cancer incidence between 1983 and 1989 (due mainly to increased attempts at detecting early-stage disease). There was no increase in the types of cancer that spread and which can be fatal. Nevertheless, the rates of prostatectomy (surgical removal of the prostate gland) increased by nearly 35 per cent per year, and varied greatly from area to area.[56]

Nevertheless, all this aggressive cutting doesn't seem to make the slightest bit of difference to survival rates. Substantial evidence proves that conservative treatment of early prostate cancer – that is, maintaining a watchful wait-and-see attitude, and using other forms of therapy such as hormonal treatment rather than rushing into surgery – could be the best recourse, particularly in older men with a life expectancy of 10 years or less.[57] This is largely because prostate cancer can be, in the main, a slow-growing form of cancer. According to autopsy reports, a third of men in the European Community have prostate cancer, but only 1 per cent die of it.[58] Particularly in men over 70, patients are more likely to die with their prostate cancer than of it.[59]

There is plenty of evidence that most prostate cancer doesn't spread. In two studies during a decade of observations, tumours had only undergone local growth and hadn't spread to other organs in two-third of the patients. In these patients, hormonal treatment was usually successful.[60]

Among men over 70, radical prostatectomy not only isn't better than watchful waiting, but can also be downright harmful.[61] Thirty days after the operation, nearly 2 per cent of men over 75 die. Survival rates can be higher in groups for whom nothing is done (other than watchful waiting), compared with groups undergoing surgery.[62] Many patients who undergo surgery die from a number of major heart-related complications within a month after they've had their operation.[63]

Today one of the most common operations is the transurethal prostatectomy (known as TURPS), where an instrument inserted in the penis either cuts or burns away the prostate. This is one of the treatments of choice, not only for prostate cancer but also for enlarged prostate. Men are assured that this technique will maintain potency. However, the latest evidence shows that in 80 per cent of cases men are rendered impotent; a goodly number will also become incontinent and many suffer prolonged bleeding.[64] The reason for the sudden burgeoning of radical prostatectomies has to do with the introduction of the 'nerve-sparing' technique. In this operation, both the inner gland and the capsule of the prostate gland are removed. However, nearly 100 per cent of the nerves are spared, supposedly to maintain sexual potency.

For all the debilitating side-effects, prostate surgery won't even cure the problem. In a large percentage of cases after surgery, the cancer quickly returns. According to the US Mayo Clinic's own study, prostate cancer came back in some 8 per cent of patients after one year, and in 40 per cent after 10 years.[65] Besides not improving survival, having any sort of medical treatment, whether with drugs or surgery, negatively affects your quality of life. Prostate cancer patients given surgery or drugs have been found to be significantly worse off in terms of sexual, urinary and bowel function than those whose progress is simply monitored carefully. The incidence of complications with treatment are also much higher than generally thought.[66]

But the most important point is that radical surgery is indicated in only a very small number of cases: for those with a very early cancer (stage 1), confined to the gland itself and not the capsule containing it or any lymph nodes. It is also only effective if the margins around the gland are free from cancer.[67]

If you were in your seventies, and had early cancer, the decision would be easy: to elect for watchful waiting. However, if you are younger than that, much depends on which stage the cancer is at and whether you meet the criteria for surgery. For those with a substantially longer age-related survival rate than 10 years, the 'watchful waiting' approach supposedly is associated with a higher probability of living with cancer that spreads, or dying from prostate cancer.[68]

However, most evidence does show that conservative management can be a reasonable choice for men of all ages with stage I or II disease. It also admits that the benefit of aggressive treatment (as against conservative management) even for grade III cancer is 'less clear' and that new strategies for this stage of cancer are needed. Other research shows that even younger men – those who reach their sixties – with slow-growing prostate cancer are likely to live as long as men without tumours. In one University of Connecticut study, only 9 per cent of patients with low-grade cancer had died, even after 15 years. And only those with fast-growing – or higher-grade – tumours may die earlier, possibly losing between four and eight years off their life expectancy. Nevertheless, even those with higher-grade tumours may be better off without having radical surgery, as the years lost may not outweigh the significant problems associated with treatment.[69] This is as good as admitting that surgery for many patients may not be doing any good.

Aside from the fact that prostate surgery doesn't seem to improve survival, radical intervention and screening may simply bring to light many cancers which would otherwise remain dormant – and harmless – if left undetected.

There is also some worry in certain medical circles that radical surgery to treat prostate cancer (as with breast cancer) may only succeed in spreading the condition. Doctors have assumed that the poor survival rate had to do with the deadly ability of prostate cancer to spread. But it has now been discovered that surgeons are accidentally spreading cancer cells to other parts of the body while performing the surgery. In one study, among 14 monitored operations, prostate cancer cells were discovered in the blood of 12 patients afterwards. Only three had had such cell circulation before they'd been operated on.[70] Furthermore, as with breast cancer, piercing the skin through biopsy or surgery may contribute to the spread of cancer. Cases of prostate cancer have been shown to be spread by biopsy.[71]

HYSTERECTOMY

The hysterectomy is second only to caesarean section on the list of most common operations in the US, although Britain is fast catching up. If you are a woman in America, you've got a one in three chance of losing your womb by the time you're 60; in Britain, your chances are one in five.

But hysterectomy outranks all others when it comes to the most unnecessary of surgical procedures. Three-quarters of all hysterectomies are performed on women under 50 for highly dubious reasons. Indeed, a University of California committee of gynaecologists recently concluded that nearly three-quarters of all hysterectomies are inappropriate.[72] Although the only viable reasons for performing a hysterectomy are uterine or endometrial cancer or uncontrollable bleeding after childbirth, these account for only about 10 per cent of all procedures performed.[73]

The remaining 90 per cent of hysterectomies are carried out for a number of questionable purposes: fibroids, endometriosis, bladder prolapse, tipped wombs, heavy periods or unexplained period troubles, which are often given the fanciful gynaecological appellation 'pelvic congestion'. One measure of how little treatment rests on solid evidence or a strict criteria for recommending the operation is the enormous variation in the rates of hysterectomy between individual doctors or areas of the country, with the highest rates often among black or poor American women.[74]

Hysterectomy is often used to 'prevent' ovarian cancer in women who have had uterine cancer even though only 2 in every 1,000 women who've had a hysterectomy will go on to develop ovarian cancer,[75] and the disease itself is rare – there are only 2,000 cases in the UK per year. Besides just-in-case removal of ovaries, hysterectomy for other sorts of cancer prevention is equally unjustified. Fewer than 2 of every 1,000 fibroids, and fewer than 3 per cent of abnormal endometrial cells, will progress to cancer.[76] Since hysterectomy carries a mortality rate of 1 per every 1,000 procedures – a risk that increases with age – and serious complications occur 15 times more frequently than that, the risk of contracting cancer is far less than the risk of dying or being seriously injured from the operation. In fact, in abdominal hysterectomies, side-effects can occur in more than 40 per cent of operations.[77] One in six women suffer damage to internal organs, and half have some sort of major complication.[78]

These side-effects can include bowel problems,[79] urinary retention or incontinence,[80] and the risk of a fatal blood clot, particularly in women after the menopause,[81] which can occur in one in every 6,000 operations. One-third to nearly one-half of all women undergoing hysterectomy or removal of ovaries report a decrease in sexual response.[82] If a woman's ovaries are removed at the same time, she will experience severe menopausal symptoms.[83] Even if the ovaries are left in, hysterectomy may lead to early ovarian failure, bringing on the menopause far earlier than usual.[84] In many instances the surgery doesn't solve the problem; in nearly two-thirds of hysterectomies performed to correct endometriosis, the problem returns after surgery.

Other than the true indications for hysterectomy, virtually every other indication for hysterectomy can be treated with conservative surgery, medication, diet, nutritional supplementation, alternative medicine or, in the case of fibroids, waiting until you reach the menopause, when they will shrink.[85]

TRANSCERVICAL RESECTION OF THE WOMB

Surgeons are great enthusiasts of new procedures which haven't stood the test of time. In the 1990s, doctors were enthusing about a supposed gynaecological breakthrough, transcervical resection of the endometrium (TCRE), or removal of the lining of the womb, for women with abnormally heavy periods. This new procedure was meant to replace the more radical former treatment of choice: hysterectomy. Medical magazines proclaimed that 18,000 women a year could substitute out-patient TCRE surgery for hysterectomy. After one study – the source of all the fanfare – doctors noted that over 90 per cent of the patients enjoyed improved menstrual symptoms during the two and a half years of follow-up. There were a number of warning signals – out of 234 patients, up to 42 of the women stopped having periods, 16 needed repeat TCREs, two reported severe cyclical pain, 10 went on to have hysterectomies, and a majority were left with a severely shrunken uterus which had developed fibroids.[86]

Just two months later, journals that had been enthusing about the new breakthrough procedures were now issuing warnings following the deaths of five women who had undergone the procedure. In two other cases, a patient lost a leg and another suffered a hole in the aorta as a result of the procedure, even though she was in the care of very experienced surgeons. Uterine perforation is one of the main severe complications; endometrial resection can stimulate a particular nerve causing violent closing of the patient's thighs and thus causing the surgeon to 'miss' and perforate the womb.[87] One patient whose uterus was perforated nearly died, and since then she has suffered from chronic pelvic pain and diarrhoea. In one study, one in 20 of the women with resections went on to have hysterectomies.

Two years after the procedure, four healthy women who'd had the treatment for heavy periods went on to develop encephalopathy, or inflammation of the brain, and one died after suffering seizures. These conditions were caused by the 'irrigating solution', which is continuously infused into the uterus to wash away debris and tissue during the laser treatment. In the case of these four women, enough of the solution was apparently absorbed to cause encephalitis.[88]

For all the hoopla, the procedure has made no dent in the number of hysterectomies being performed. Oxford Regional Health Authority, which studied surgery rates in six local districts, discovered that endometrial ablation has simply created a new niche for surgeons. The number of hysterectomies performed has remained constant since before the procedure was introduced.[89] In fact, most women who have the lining of their womb removed by endometrial resection will end up having a full hysterectomy, anyway. About 87 per cent complain afterwards of continual vaginal bleeding and in some cases quite heavy loss of blood – one of the problems the technique is supposed to treat. Women who have the procedure are also more likely to suffer pain after surgery – in 11 per cent of cases, worse pain than before the operation, and about a fifth of women also experience worse premenstrual symptoms.[90]

BLOOD TRANSFUSIONS

Perhaps the biggest risk you face when you have an operation has nothing to do with the scalpel. The US Red Cross has even admitted that even in the most dire of emergencies, blood transfusions oftentimes only add to complications or increase a patient's chances of dying. Although the spectre of AIDS and HIV virus-contaminated blood has curtailed blood donation and transfusions, the latter are still routine in most surgical procedures and emergencies – in many cases without any medical justification whatsoever for their use, or any guidelines as to when they are necessary.

Like so many other practices in medicine, the guidelines doctors follow when deciding whether or not to give a transfusion have been adopted with very little in the way of scientific evidence. An estimated one-third to three-quarters of those given blood are transfused inappropriately to treat a diminished volume of blood or a low nutritional status (that is, anaemia). Anthony Britten of the American Red Cross Blood Services has admitted that there is 'gross over-use of blood products like albumin and plasma and also whole blood or red blood cells. Usage patterns vary so widely from place to place that it is clear that common standards do not exist for their use.'[91]

A US Office of Technology Assessment Task Force report estimated that as much as 20 to 25 per cent of red blood cells, 90 per cent of albumin and 95 per cent of fresh-frozen plasma transfused into patients are not needed. Indeed, a common 'transfusion trigger' is the measurement of haemoglobin (a compound in red blood cells transporting oxygen to the cells). Medicine uses the same 'trigger' level for men and women, even though women naturally have lower red blood cell counts than do men. 'Iron deficiency anaemia continues to be among the leading reasons for transfusions, even though it rarely warrants [them],' said the report.[92]

Many in medicine have begun to question some of the most established practices for administering blood before and during surgery. A survey of 1,000 American anaesthesiologists concluded that there were 'wide variations in transfusions practices' among anaesthesiologists, based on 'habit rather than scientific data'.[93] One such habit is the automatic administration of blood before operations in patients whose haemoglobin level is below 10 g/per 100 ml of blood. The practice apparently arose from a misreading by a haematologist of a study performed on dogs, which was accepted as gospel and preached to an entire generation of anaesthesiology students.[94]

Premature infants probably get more transfusions than any other body of patients in hospital (apart from haemophiliacs).[95] Transfusion is automatic if a baby is under 1,500 g (3lb), a practice that has little in the way of evidence.[96] Indeed, research shows that premature babies given fresh flozen plasma fare no better two years later in terms of disabilities or mortality than those not given the transfusions.[97] Blood components are also routinely irradiated, supposedly to reduce the risk of patients with immune-system problems rejecting the foreign blood. It has always been assumed that irradiation is harmless to red cells and has little effect on the function of the various components in the blood. But this irradiated blood may have too high a concentration of potassium, which could be especially hazardous to babies and pregnant mothers.

Besides giving blood for the wrong reasons, doctors often give out the wrong blood. In an informal questionnaire sent to 4,000 hospital haematology laboratories in Britain, one-third of the 245 labs that responded reported multiple incidents in which their patients received the wrong blood. In most cases, the patient was given the wrong blood while on the ward or in the operating theatre. Of some 111 such errors, six people died and 23 got ill.[98] And, since the question about handing out the wrong blood wasn't even asked on the questionnaire (but was volunteered by the labs), even the study had to admit that this was probably a gross underestimate of transfusion mistakes.

This questionnaire represented the first time that blood transfusions had ever been monitored in Britain, even though they have been practised for 50 years. However, this error rate corresponds with that of the US, which is supposed to have the tightest strictures on blood usage in the world.

After tallying the questionnaires, the study concluded that the wrong blood is given in one of every 6,000 red cell units given. In other research most errors have been found to arise when blood samples are inadequately documented or when information about which blood to be given to which patient is incorrect; two London teaching hospitals studied were shown to have inadequate information on the blood of a quarter of its patients.[99]

A Royal College of Physicians conference announced that transfusions have never been subjected to proper scientific study – that is, a random-ized, double-blind trial – to see if indeed there are any benefits. *Like much of modern medicine, what probably is a useful court of last resort has been introduced and adopted as a first-line standard practice on the a priori assumption of benefit without one shred of scientific proof.*

Evidence from Canada suggests that restricting blood transfusions is a matter of life and death. In the study, which compared liberal transfusion with more restrictive measures among patients, 24 per cent more patients died when blood transfusion was given more liberally than when it was restricted and transfusions given less than half as often or not at all.[100] As Paul Hébert, the trial's principal investigator, concluded: 'less transfusion is better than more transfusion.'[101]

Even blood components given in emergency situations, such as albu-min given to burn and shock victims to aid fluid retention, can be danger-ous. The Cochrane Injuries Group, based at the Institute of Child Health in London and part of the Cochrane Group for Evidence-based Medicine, studied 30 trials where patients were given albumin, and found that patients given albumin were more likely to die.[102] Even critically ill patients with low haemoglobin counts who receive transfusions are more likely to die than those who are not given blood.[103]

If you believe that giving and getting blood is warranted, the number of blood-borne diseases you can contract from other people might well change your mind. The arrival of AIDS has given blood transfusion the quality of Russian roulette. Because we really don't understand what causes AIDS or whether there needs to be another co-factor to convert HIV to AIDS, we also don't understand how long the HIV virus (if indeed it is the cause of AIDS) incubates before transforming into the full-blown disease.[104]

What we do know about is the considerable risk of contracting hepatitis from donated blood. Hepatitis from transfusions develops in an estimated 7 to 10 per cent of blood recipients from unpaid donors in the US.[105] This incidence multiplies three to four times among recipients of blood from paid donors and translates to up to 230,000 new cases of hepatitis in the US every year. The reason for the epidemic of cases is that there is, to date, no test reliable or sensitive enough to detect the agents that cause the disease. In fact, most cases of hepatitis C are due to blood transfusions or needle sharing among drug users. The Irish government has attempted to trace some 100,000 rhesus-negative mothers given blood transfusions in 1977 to see if they have developed hepatitis C, following an outbreak of hepatitis C among people who received transfusions in that year.[106] Italian researchers have even found that adults who had been given transfusions as premature infants are likely to contract adult hepatitis C, largely from infected blood.[107] New viruses which cause hepatitis have also been discovered in blood.[108]

Although the US Centers for Disease Control and Prevention claimed the Irish outbreak was the first of its kind, some among the medical community believe that anyone who received a blood transfusion before 1991 could be at risk of hepatitis C infection. Indeed, in Britain, some 3,000 haemophiliacs were recently found to have contracted hepatitis C. Doctors now wonder whether intravenous immunoglobulin, a protein given to stimulate the immune system, can actually trigger hepatitis C.

Since 1991, a screening test has been developed for the hepatitis C virus, showing that one in 2,000 blood donors supposedly is positive for hepatitis C antibodies.[109] However, even this screening test isn't necessarily going to protect you. A number of doctors once wrote to the *British Medical Journal* to complain about the inaccuracy of the test.[110] These doctors, from the virology departments of City Hospital in Edinburgh and John Radcliffe Hospital in Oxford, said that in the first eight months of screening for hepatitis C virus in the Oxford region, some 83,000 units of blood (from some 70,000 donors) were subjected to a second-generation enzyme-linked immunoassay (ELISA) test, the test most often used to detect hepatitis C.

In the sample, 358 donors showed up repeatedly as positive. When all those tested as positive were tested again by two other, more recently developed tests, the second-generation recombinant immunoblot assay (RIBA-2) or the Murex BCJ11 ELISA, the ELISA test was proved wrong more than three-quarters of the time.

Besides hepatitis, the risk of contracting human T-cell leukaemia (HTLV-1) from blood is ten times higher than the risk of contracting HIV.[111] This risk skyrockets when you consider that many blood recipients, including premature babies, are given the blood components from what can be, on average, as many as nine donors.

The medical literature is awash with studies about patients undergoing operations who have fared worse on foreign transfused blood than on autotransfusion (receiving their own stored or recovered blood). Blood transfusion has been linked with organ system failure, recurrence of cancer, a high risk of postoperative infection, and graft-versus-host disease – a condition affecting the joints, heart and blood cells in which the recipient rejects the transfused blood.

Besides the various diseases you can contract from someone else's blood, if you're a cancer patient a blood transfusion may depress your immune system, causing or in some way aiding a recurrence. In one study, the recurrence rate for patients with cancer of the larynx was 14 per cent among those who didn't receive blood transfusions, and more than four times as great among those who did. Of those with cancer of the oral cavity, pharynx and nose, the recurrence rate was 31 per cent without transfusions, more than double that with them.[112]

A poorer outcome was also experienced in patients receiving blood transfusions after surgery for lung cancer[113] as well as for those with colonic, rectal, cervical and prostate cancers.[114] There also seemed to be a higher incidence of recurrence if a patient received whole blood rather than simply red blood cells alone.

Having a transfusion during an operation also increases your chances of infection.[115]

In patients undergoing major abdominal surgery, blood transfusion has been the most significant contributor to organ system failure.[116]

Besides lowering your chances of surviving, you can suffer side-effects from blood that are every bit as severe as the worst reaction to a drug. Although the usual reactions include hives, fever or chills, some patients experience a severe reaction in the lungs, sometimes fatal, with some kinds of plasma, a risk that is higher than previously thought.[117] There are also substantial risks of general infection and life-threatening allergic reactions, as well as of contracting a sexually transmitted disease such as cytomegalovirus (CMV). Doctors are finally admitting that taking in someone else's blood may stress a person's immune system. It may well be, as one study concluded, that blood, like fingerprints, is uniquely – untransferably – individual: 'The unavoidable, biological (and now legally recognized) fact is that each person's blood contains a multiplicity of antibodies, antigens and infectious agents, many of which have yet to be identified by scientists and cannot presently be detected. "Pure blood" … is finally understood by courts to be imaginary.'[118]

JUST A MINUTE, SURGEON

Before you go in for surgery, it's important, in effect, to interview your surgeon, not least about his batting average. It is not automatically the case that surgery will make you feel better or that your surgeon is incapable of making a horrendous mistake. Ask your surgeon how many of these operations he's done and which procedure he follows. If he's just cutting his teeth himself and hasn't done more than 10 or 15, find a more experienced hand. It's also essential that you know exactly who is doing the operating. In many cases, particularly routine surgery, experienced surgeons supervise juniors, who get to practise routine procedures. Insist that the experienced surgeon does the job, or find one who will. And, most important, make sure you feel comfortable and confident with the surgeon; after all, you are going to be completely in his hands.

You can also help to make up your mind about risks and benefits by finding out about the complication rate for a procedure. Discuss the other treatment options with a variety of specialists. Ask about the scientific evidence supporting their claimed results. Carefully weigh up the risks of refusing surgery against the risks of the procedure itself on your future quality of life.

If you have any doubt concerning the surgeon's candour about treatment options or his ability to consider you an equal partner in any treatment decisions, reach for your hat, walk out the door and find yourself a surgeon who will.

As for transfusions, bear in mind that doctors have successfully transfused patients with their own blood, donated ahead of time, for all sorts of major surgery, including coronary bypasses, congenital heart surgery or cancer. Thirteen-year-old Lucy Buxton of England made the news in early 1994 for donating her own blood to have on hand before having her tonsils out. This technique can even be used during emergencies such as haemorrhage and trauma.

Doctors can also use haemodilution, a procedure that maintains the amount of fluid circulating around the body through artificial fluid-volume expanders. One study of some 10,000 surgery patients concluded that adult patients can undergo rapid loss of a third of the total volume of blood and not go into irreversible shock if haemodilution is adequate.[119] During emergencies, contaminated blood (which has been exposed to, say, intestinal contents) can be safely cleaned and recycled with a cell-washing system. Circulating blood volume can also be kept up with fluid replacements. Six thousand patients undergoing open-heart operations demonstrated that they had improved outcomes once blood transfusion was stopped and volume expanders substituted.[120]

11

Gee-whizz Technology:
The Video-games Wizard and
Blocked-drains Mechanic

Nearly 30 years since the first successful heart transplant, with the arrival of the computer chip and many highly specialized drugs, Western medicine is without parallel in offering miraculous solutions to what used to be considered the hopeless case. These days, medicine can give you a new heart or liver, install a new, artificial hip or knee, clear your arteries without the slightest incision and even make babies in women well past the menopause. The wheelchair-bound believe they are an operation away from walking; the infertile, a test tube away from a new baby. But like the rest of surgery (and most of these techniques are operations of a sort), every last one of these glamorous new technologies has been adopted incautiously, given the official seal of approval and employed on millions before the slightest shred of evidence exists that they work, especially over the long term, let alone whether they truly represent advances over any techniques they replace. It is only after millions of desperate patients rush to try the new miracle solutions that we begin to find out what the potential problems are.

The most insidious part of 'miracle-breakthrough' technology concerns the gushing public relations exercise surrounding it. The press often uncritically portray a new procedure as a miraculous breakthrough without reservation, before it has stood the test of time. The *Sunday Times* once proclaimed in banner headlines about foetal surgery: 'Unborn baby wanted by doctors for Miracle Op'. A week later, once the appropriate candidate had been found, the same newspaper published, with slightly less fanfare, the chilling results: 'Womb Operation Baby Dies in Mother's Arms'.[1]

There is no doubt that for many individuals with no alternatives, foetal surgery, joint replacement operations or organ transplants can prove life-saving. But in too many instances the idea of the 'miracle cure' captures the imagination of both doctor and patient and the new technique becomes the first (rather than the last) port of call for everyone, regardless of whether he is the right candidate. In the rush to embrace this new technique, and the doctor's eagerness to try his hand at the latest space-age gadgetry, the downside of the various techniques get played down, if not entirely ignored. We hear about the fact that heart, liver, pancreas, lung and intestinal transplants are now routine. We hear a good deal less about the fact that a third of these transplants get rejected, or about the Hobson's choice many patients face in choosing between the possibility that their body may reject the transplanted organ and the side-effects of powerful immunosuppressive drugs such as cyclosporine (which must be taken to prevent the body from rejecting a new organ as 'foreign'). Many patients who remain on cyclosporine keep the transplant, but at the expense of their own kidneys, which may develop chronic and progressive (and permanent) disease, and eventually fail, even after the immunosuppressive drugs are withdrawn.[2]

KEYHOLE SURGERY

For the past decade, the surgical fad *du jour* that has taken the operating theatre by storm is minimally invasive, or keyhole, surgery. This form of surgery has been hailed as one of the great medical innovations of the 20th century, and there's no doubt that the technology is impressive. Using the latest microtechnology, surgeons can perform major operations without the trauma (and cutting) of conventional open surgery. In theory, at least, the patient should be able to leave the hospital quickly – often, that same day – and enjoy a far less painful and far more speedy recovery, sometimes months sooner than he would after a conventional operation.

One of the fastest-growing techniques in the entire health field, keyhole surgery is already being used in one in five of all abdominal operations, and is likely to be used in 70 per cent of all operations by the end of this century. According to current levels, this translates to 2.1 million operations a year in the UK alone.

Video Games-Playing

Minimally invasive surgery (also known as MIS) involves making four or five minor incisions – between 5 and 7 cm (2 to 3 in) long – and feeding the laparoscope through one of them. A minute lens on its tip transmits pictures of the internal organs onto a video screen, which the surgeon views when operating.

The surgeon then threads his instruments down the other incisions, and commences the operation via the video screen. If a tumour or part of an organ has to be removed, it is compressed and squeezed through the incisions. Occasionally, a surgeon will also make use of light beams and lasers.

Although the laparoscope has been used for over 25 years by gynaecologists, only recently has the technology developed sufficiently to allow instruments to be fitted and used for investigative procedures (say, to check the state of a woman's ovaries), or to cut and perform ligatures (such as tying up arteries or cutting out tumours). The entire procedure can take up to seven times as long as conventional open surgery.

While keyhole techniques have been used most frequently to date for gall bladder surgery, hernias and a variety of abdominal operations, it is now being tried out on other types of surgery, even for cancer and the removal of organs, such as kidneys.

The biggest problem with this most sensational of surgical techniques is that most surgeons went at it with inadequate training. This was the tacit admission of a clinic in London where a woman died after receiving keyhole bowel exploratory surgery. Although the surgeon's name was cleared, the clinic where the operation was performed banned all keyhole surgery until independent experts confirmed that surgeons were qualified to perform the operations.

'It was merely the surgeons' enthusiasm for something new and the worry of being left behind if they did not master the technique that led to the explosion in popularity of this minimally invasive surgery,' Dr David

Lomax wrote in a letter to *The Lancet*,[3] commenting about the sudden explosion of this technique for any and all surgery, often inappropriately.

When first introduced, keyhole surgery was pounced upon by surgeons before they'd been adequately trained. Recognizing this, the British government set aside £4 million to train surgeons specifically in keyhole techniques, a training programme that came about as a result of a report by a working party headed by keyhole-surgery pioneer Professor Alfred Cushieri. The British government refused to publish the findings of this report – which led to speculation that the findings were particularly alarming.

'Adverse Incidents'

Some 158 reported 'adverse incidents' involved keyhole surgery between August 1990 and May 1992 in New York State alone. Twenty-four of these were life threatening or resulted in permanent disability, and more than two-thirds required further surgery to repair injuries.[4] In the first 26 kidney laparoscopic operations done at Washington University, nearly a third of patients suffered complications. Those with major complications had to be operated on again, this time with open surgery.

With laparoscopic cholecystectomy – the removal of the gall bladder by keyhole surgery – the number of complications and hospital readmissions has risen sharply with the increased use of keyhole surgery techniques. The number of bile duct injuries increased by 305 per cent in three years, now that keyhole surgery is used in 86 per cent of such gall bladder operations. Although the problem was always blamed on lack of skill, researchers now believe the dangers are inherent in the procedure itself, and that even after doctors become familiar with the procedures, the number of injuries don't go down.[5]

Serious complications arise in 15 out of every 1,000 laparoscopic procedures in gynaecological operations, where keyhole surgery is often used, according to figures from the American Association of Gynecologic Laparoscopists; three deaths among every 100,000 patients. As much as 5 per cent of patients who undergo keyhole hysterectomies suffer injury to their urinary tracts.[6]

With hiatus hernia repair, complications occur in as high as one-quarter of patients;[7] in one small study, one patient hemorrhaged so much blood that he required a special operation to control the bleeding. And even after the operation, nearly half of the patients still suffered from reflux disease.[8] With inguinal hernias, open surgery has fewer complications than keyhole surgery. Keyhole surgery is often used to correct carpal tunnel syndrome, but is almost never successful, leaving most patients with pain and sensitivity on the scar tissue.[9] The UK support group RSI Association urges anyone to think twice before accepting surgery. 'We are not aware of any surgery that has been completely successful. Ask the consultant for details of any patients whose surgery has been 100 per cent successful. He never can,' says association chairperson Wendy Lawrence, an RSI sufferer for more than 10 years.

Her view is supported by the medical trials. In one study, incisions for carpal tunnel-release (the standard procedure) on 47 patients resulted in pain and scar sensitivity.

Even the favourite of laparoscopic techniques, a gall bladder operation (known in medicalese as cholecystectomy), is not without a high error rate, considering the number of procedures now being performed. In a US survey of 77,604 of these operations, over half of the deaths due to the surgery were attributed to complications of the laparoscopic technique.[10] In Britain, the first damages of £22,500 were awarded to a woman who may need a liver transplant after a routine gall bladder operation went wrong when the surgeon accidentally cut her bile duct, which leaked and caused jaundice.

Most worrisome is new evidence showing that keyhole surgery may somehow trigger gall bladder cancer, or cause it to recur.[11] Lucy underwent a gall bladder operation by keyhole surgery:

> *Shortly afterward I experienced pain on walking. After various investigations I was diagnosed as having avascular necrosis of the head of the left thigh. [That means death of some of the cells in a tissue, not involving blood vessels but possibly caused by inadequate blood supply to the tissue, or injury.] The consultant who carried out the cholecystectomy stands by his opinion that there is no connection, even though he can offer no explanation as to why I should have contracted avascular necrosis – a condition usually associated with deep-sea divers, chronic alcoholics and people who fracture their hip.*

Lucy is now permanently disabled. Because the condition is so new, it has not been recognized by the Royal College of Surgeons as being caused by the operation. Nor is there any compensation scheme available to recompense patients who suffer this sort of injury.

Up until now, so long as a surgeon passed his general training he was allowed to have a go at this new technique, even if he hadn't a clue about how to do it. In many cases, surgeons were virtually experimenting with their patients, for fear of being seen to be old-fashioned.

Gynaecologists, in particular, as one surgeon put it, were particularly prone to rushing in too early as 'kamikaze surgeons', 'pushing the bounds of this surgery to the outer limits' or are clumsy at it – 'as maladroit as a beetle on its back'.[12]

Instead of this usual 'hands on' experience the surgeon has to have the skills of a video games player. Rather than being able to see the organ in front of him, he has to judge three dimensions via the screen, and then has to manipulate his instruments to do the work ordinarily done by his hands. It means that he is, in effect, operating without the sense of touch, and must get used to different way of viewing it – with a microtechnology that doesn't afford even the most experienced surgeon the normal full range of vision.[13]

A common complication is the puncturing of organs with the microscopic equipment. Three out of 10,000 complications in gynaecological surgery done in the US, and 0.05 per cent of laparoscopic cholecystectomies involve organ puncture. Of these, two patients died as a result of their injury. In a case in Australia which showed up the inadequacy of some of the microtechnology being used, a charge of negligence was filed because the surgeon in question did not fully appreciate that the field of vision provided through a laparoscope is limited.[14] Because the surgeon could not see what he was doing properly, a needle entered the patient's colon during the procedure (the surgeon was later found not to be negligent).

Another complication – usually among the elderly or those with a heart condition – involves the carbon dioxide used to inflate the abdomen, a standard procedure in order to give the laparoscope room to view organs properly. Once the carbon dioxide is introduced, some 17 per cent of patients report a sudden irregular heart beat, according to one British study. A third of patients in another study suffered a slowing heart rate.[15]

When first introduced in the US, some states did not allow surgeons to perform minimally invasive surgery unless they had been properly trained. In others, as in the UK, surgeons with little or no experience were able to carry out the procedure. The Society of American Gastrointestinal Endoscopic Surgeons suggested that surgeons should first carry out procedures on animals before being allowed to operate on people.

In early 1994, the senate of the Royal Surgical Colleges of Great Britain and Ireland introduced new quality assurance levels and a certificate of competence, which established surgeons now have to work for before they can practise keyhole surgery. Training, assessment and certification are mandatory, and those trainees not found up to scratch will not receive certification or be able to carry out the procedures.

Even open surgery for treating cancer carries a high risk of spreading diseased cells to healthy ones. But this risk multiplies with keyhole surgery, because the surgeon does not have full visibility or control, and also because cancerous organs and cells have to be squeezed through the small incisions, increasing the likelihood that the diseased cells will drop off and 'seed' themselves within healthy organs. This problem was highlighted once in Cardiff, where two women who underwent keyhole surgery for gall bladder cancer both went on to die from cancer. In both cases, as the surgeons pulled the malignant tissue through the small hole in the wall of the abdomen, cancer cells broke off and seeded themselves in the abdomen.

Longer and More Dangerous

Some of the risks associated with keyhole surgery might be worth it, if this technique definitely could be shown to offer real benefits to patients – such as a genuinely far speedier recovery rate than after conventional surgery. But the studies that have been done show that keyhole is not always best. One of the first major randomized studies comparing removal of the appendix with laparoscopic techniques and conventional open appendectomy showed there was no difference in postoperative pain and recovery rate among patients. This removes one of the primary rationales for performing laparoscopic procedures.

The study, by the Prince of Wales Hospital in Hong Kong, compared 70 patients who underwent open appendectomy with patients of similar ages undergoing keyhole surgery. Each study examined major complications in either group, although of the laparoscopic group had to convert to an open operation during their keyhole operation.

The Hong Kong research team found no difference between the groups in terms of severity of pain, need for painkilling drugs, timetable for reintroducing a normal diet, or hospital stay. After members of both groups attended follow-up examinations, similar percentages from both groups – 79 per cent of laparoscopic patients versus 74 per cent of open-surgery patients – had returned to work by three weeks after surgery.[16]

In the case of appendectomy, open surgery is no longer the major invasive technique it once was, but can now be performed by making a small, muscle-splitting incision. Hence the difference between keyhole and open surgery in this particular operation may be slight, compared to, say, gall bladder surgery.

Another study, setting laparoscopic hysterectomy against the standard vaginal procedure, concluded that keyhole surgery took nearly twice as long. A study team from the Royal Free Hospital in London found that the traditional method was not only much faster, but that recovery rates were similar for both groups.[17] A study done by the Indian Council of Medical Research revealed that the complication rate of keyhole sterilization surgery was seven times that of minilaparotomy (the usual open 'band-aid' approach).[18] Hernia operations are known to result in a high prevalence of internal scar tissue and salpingitis (inflammation of the fallopian tubes in women).[19] In one large study of some 900 patients comparing open and keyhole surgery for hernia repair, although the keyhole patients had less pain and could return to work earlier, they suffered serious complications – nerve damage, vascular and bladder injury – while those undergoing open surgery did not. This was the case despite the fact that the most senior surgeons were those performing the keyhole operations. This finding counters the usual argument that damage due to keyhole surgery is simply a matter of inexperience.[20]

Obviously what is needed is more research setting keyhole surgery against its conventional counterpart, to gauge the type of operations for which MIS is most appropriate. It may well become the procedure favoured for operations such as cholecystectomy, but may prove inappropriate for appendectomy and cancer.[21]

Surgeons eager to try their hand at the new technique also need to be reined in when the surgery isn't needed. A recent study found that gall bladder operations had increased by a fifth since the advent of keyhole surgery.[22]

JOINT-REPLACEMENT SURGERY

The joint-replacement surgical technique is another example of a faddish procedure embraced without proper testing. Joint replacement entails replacing the cartilage of hip or knee joints, worn away by osteoarthritis, with an artificial joint made of a mix of metal and polyethylene. Undoubtedly this procedure, which has transformed the lives of many older people, restoring the wheelchair-bound to normal activity, is justifiably regarded as miracle surgery. But largely because of the heady experience of making the lame walk, doctors are too quick to order up an operation without considering the consequences or any alternatives, particularly in young people. It's estimated that 10 per cent of people over 65 have a hip replacement, making it the most common form of surgery in the UK and the US.[23]

Old and New Technologies

Both knee replacement and hip replacement have a relatively good track record when performed with the older types of equipment. When artificial knee joints are cemented into place, an analysis of 130 studies shows that 89 per cent are successful and the knee remains functional for more than four years.[24]

During surgery, the surgeon removes the head of your femur (thighbone) and replaces it with a metal ball positioned on a long metal stem, which fits into the hollow middle of the thigh bone. He then replaces the worn socket of the hip with a plastic or metal cup with a plastic lining, which fits into the pelvic socket (acetabulum).

These days, surgeons will often use cementless balls in the thigh bone, relying instead on the porous metal to adhere to the bone, and manufacturers are experimenting with metal-on-metal components (a mix of cobalt–chromium and molybdenum alloys), to prevent the wear and tear experienced with plastic components, in the hope that these type will last longer and so can be used in younger patients.

The Royal Orthopaedic Hospital in Birmingham showed that the Charnley hip replacement – the original design which has been tested over time more than any other type of material – has a 91 per cent survival record after 10 years and 82 per cent survival over 20 years.[25]

Because even the most tried-and-tested design has a limited life-span (10 years in the case of knee replacements), medical technology firms have been trying since the 1980s to fix artificial joints biologically to bone via little metal beads or mesh. These products, called 'uncemented porous-coated' knee replacements, proved disastrous, resulting in a far greater need for 'revision' – that is, replacement of the joint replacement. This is a much more formidable operation, with far more bone loss and removal of tissue – and a far lower success rate. As Mike Wroblewski of the Wrightington Hospital in Wigan, which pioneered the operation over 30 years ago, puts it, 'First time is the best time. After that it's salvage.'[26]

In just one of the many studies demonstrating the high failure rate of knee replacement, of about 100 procedures roughly one-fifth failed due to problems with the lower leg component. After seven years, more than half the replacements were recommended for revision.[27] As for hip replacements, a Swedish study found that after 10 years, only about a quarter of the two new devices studied survived.[28]

If uncemented varieties of hip replacement have been found wanting, the other cemented versions don't fare much better. One study following a group of patients under 50 for 15 years found that a little less than a third needed revision because the parts had loosened and become infected.[29] In fact, in the last decade first-time failures requiring revision trebled, to 12 per cent.[30]

Complications

The operation has become ho-hum for most doctors, who boast success rates of 98 per cent; indeed, the age at which patients are recommended for a hip op is spiralling downward; in one recent study, the median age was 48.

That 98 per cent success rate refers to the number of patients who get wheeled out of the operation alive, with new hip intact. It doesn't account for all the casualties that occur subsequently, from death to permanent lameness or lifelong illness. Particularly if you are young, you should know about these side-effects *before* you agree to surgery. If it goes wrong you could die within a few months. Depending upon your age and state of health, you treble your risk of death. Three of every thousand people die within the first three months after hip replacement, most of heart attack or stroke.[31]

Among more than 11,000 cases of total hip replacement (THR) between 1976 and 1985, 11 out of every 1,000 THR patients died within three months of the operation, and 28 out of every 1,000 had to have emergency readmissions. This translates into one in every 91 patients dying and one in every 36 returning for an emergency readmission within a month of the operation. Most deaths had to do with heart attacks; most emergencies with strokes.[32]

As for knee replacements, a US analysis found an overall complication rate of 18 per cent, with the most common complications including infection, blockage in the lung (pulmonary embolism) or a blood clot in a vein.[33] Stroke from a blood clot in the lung remains the most common cause of death.[34]

Deep vein thrombosis remains a major risk after hip and knee surgery. The incidence of fatal venous thromboembolism after surgery – the risk of of a clot dislodging in a vein in the leg or lung, travelling and blocking the arteries to your lungs – will occur in about 1 in 32 patients, and fatal pulmonary embolism will occur in around 1 in 100 patients.[35]

George, a 75-year-old from Weymouth, tells this story:

I had two total knee replacements, which have become infected with staphylococcus as a result of mismanagement during a minor throat infection. After a long period of treatment with flucloxacillin tablets [antibiotics] I am told I shall have to continue with this for life.

His alternative to taking antibiotics for ever is to have the joints replaced yet again and to face potential failure, a prospect, at his age, he is loath to consider.

George's experience isn't as rare as it might be hoped. Associations have been made between oral infection and subsequent blood infection after total joint replacement operations, particularly if the patient has gum disease in his mouth. Nevertheless, few doctors take the precautions with hip-replacement patients that they do with heart-valve patients, who receive antibiotic treatment with dental surgery.[36]

New and Improved?

Most new 'designer hips' are put on the market without any sort of testing, as a stream of new, supposedly improved models with all manner of unproven claims are continually introduced and quietly withdrawn, a few hundred hapless patients later. In 1971 the only artificial hip was the Charnley design; 20 years later, 34 varieties had flooded the market.

'You can design a hip replacement in your garden shed today and be putting it in patients tomorrow,' says Chris Bulstrode, an orthopaedic surgeon at Oxford's John Radcliffe Hospital.[37] One particular problem is the prospect of wear debris chipping off and travelling to other parts of the body. These materials have been shown to break down and send parti-cles into the body, the long-term effect of which nobody knows. Emerging evidence shows that high levels of these microscopic metallic debris – all potential carcinogens – generated by constant contact between the artificial parts of the joint or by simple corrosion migrate to major organs of the body, causing constant infection or even autoimmune disease. The friction caused by the metal ball rubbing against the polyeth-ylene plastic lining causes flaking off of the small polyethylene or metal particles. The body's immune system reacts to the particles as foreign matter and attacks them. Since the particles typically settle near the implant, the immune system also attacks surrounding bone, a process known as osteolysis. As bone loss occurs, the hip implant can loosen and begin to function improperly. Osteolysis is considered the number-one reason for implant failure and the need for a repeat operation. In Britain, a group called the Bristol Wear Debris Analysis Team did a comparison study of patients who'd died with and without metal implants as used in joint replacement. The analysis team found high levels of debris in the liver, lymph glands, bone marrow and spleen of patients who'd had stainless steel and cobalt-chrome implants. But the highest number of particles migrated in people whose joint replacements were considered loose and worn. The main source of the debris was the matte coating of the joint. In one patient, the level of cobalt found in his bone marrow was *several thousand times* that considered normal.[38] Even particles of bone cement (which contains hard ceramic particles of barium sulphate or zirconia) chip off and travel.[39]

If you have osteolysis, you may have to have the hip cleaned out, and reset, which can leave one leg up to two to three inches shorter than the other.[40] In order to stabilize the hip so that it won't dislocate, many surgeons make one leg a bit long or short. To walk you will need to tilt your pelvis or build up a shoe. There's also the good possibility that your hip may dislocate, particularly in older patients with weak bones, possibly necessitating more surgery to reset or replace the hip.[41]

The Bristol researchers believe that an accumulation of metallic particles such as this is associated with chronic inflammation, lymph node disease, destruction of bone marrow, bone loss, and implant loosening. 'There is concern' they wrote guardedly, 'that metals used in prostheses may cause [cancer] since they are potentially carcinogenic in other situations.'[42] So far, at least two studies suggest an association between cancer of the lymph nodes or leukaemia and hip replacement.[43] This is quite worrying when you consider the increasing tendency to do joint replacements on young people, a situation given a fillip as celebrities such as Liza Minnelli have replacement surgery. And this shot-in-the-dark nature of joint replacement is likely to continue, since no one is keeping track of who develops cancer after replacement surgery. There is no adequate reporting system for implant-related tumours, despite appeals among researchers for an international register dating back to 1989.[44] Possibly because of the spectre of future litigation, several chemical companies have ceased selling polymers (used for coating the joints) to medical implant manufacturers.[45]

If you've exhausted all the tried-and-tested nutritional alternatives to prevent the progression of osteoarthritis and you must have a hip replacement, opt for the tried-and-tested models such as those produced by Charnley. In one study, two-thirds of Charnley prostheses were still operational after 25 years.[46]

For cementless varieties, the AML Total Hip Replacement (manufactured by DePuy/Johnson & Johnson) is the most widely used model in the world. Ceramic thigh-bone heads reduce wear, osteolysis and the need for revision. The lowest wear rate is metal-on-metal (alumina-on-alumina), although aluminium is a known poison to the body.[47]

ANGIOPLASTY: UNBLOCKING THE PLUMBING

In just a few short years, coronary balloon angioplasty – or percutaneous transluminal coronary angioplasty (PCTA), to give it its proper name – has grown to be the major method of treating heart problems, particularly angina. This has been largely in response to an epidemic: in 1989, 1 million people died of heart disease in the US, and 160,000 in the UK. Medicine has focused on it as a preventive measure because in the overwhelming majority of cases, the first heart attack is often the last. Of the 1.5 million people who suffer a heart attack in the US each year, only a quarter survive.

Coronary balloon angioplasty has been one of the most popular treatments for heart attack since 1978, and involves threading a tiny balloon through blocked arteries and expanding it to clear them – usually by pressing the atheromatous (fatty) plaques against the coronary artery wall.

When angioplasty first arrived on the scene, the wonder solution to arterial disease of the time was coronary bypass surgery. As angioplasty became more sophisticated it gained ground on heart surgery, representing as it did the cheaper, easier and less traumatic alternative. Before long it came to be regarded as a virtual cure-all for heart disease, offered to angina sufferers, those recovering from a heart attack, or even those with a high cholesterol count.

By 1990, 12 years after its first mention in the scientific literature, hundreds of thousands of people in the US and in Europe had been treated with the procedure, even though only a smattering of scientific prospective trials had thus far assessed its efficacy.[48] The extraordinary success rate of initial tests – some ranging above 90 per cent, with complications in fewer than 10 per cent of cases – tended to support the enthusiasts.

One of the most comprehensive early surveys seemingly vindicated the initial fanfare. Of 5,827 patients treated with angioplasty between January and June 1991 in the state of New York, 88 per cent were reported successful, although post-discharge complications were never studied.[49]

It wasn't until 1991 that *The Lancet* – the journal which first applauded the wonder treatment – began to voice concerns. A delegate from the journal attended an angioplasty course in 1991 and wrote that, based on his own observations, he tended to take a less favourable view of the outcome than the surgeon doing the procedure. 'In general the results of coronary angioplasty seemed inferior to those reported in journals.'[50]

Then, the American College of Cardiologists issued a statement: 'Observations raise the question of whether cardiology has focused too much on doing coronary angioplasty procedures rather than on addressing who needs it, what are the criteria, and what are the results. Is angioplasty being done for cardiologists or for patients?'

As the experience of nearly 20 years of use now demonstrates, angioplasty is not a miracle gee-whizz solution to all cardiac illness. First off, it is more effective for simple cases. A study in Boston, Massachusetts, discovered that angioplasty patients with two to three risk factors had a survival rate over five years of just 13 per cent.[51]

Stenosis (narrowing of the artery) has been found to recur within six months after angioplasty; the diameter of the blood vessels treated are only 16 per cent larger than before treatment, according to the American College of Cardiologists. In one Italian study, restenosis occurred in three-quarters of cases.[52]

Because of the need for continual retreatment and monitoring, the real costs of angioplasty may be much higher than those for medical therapy in cases of mild angina and single vessel disease. Hospital charges have doubled in the 10 years that angioplasty has been used, one study done in Maryland estimated.[53]

Angioplasty doesn't fare very well with patients who have triple-vessel disease – that is, where all the main arteries of the heart are clogged. An Italian study reported only a 52 per cent success rate in these cases. Angioplasty was also unsuccessful in more than two-thirds of cases of total blockage of the artery.[54]

Angioplasty also has a very poor success rate when used to treat blocked arteries in the lower part of the body. If those types of blockages aren't treated, the patient can end up having a leg amputated. Despite a 24-fold increase in the use of the treatment for lower-body blockages in one ten-year period in Maryland, the numbers of leg amputations remained constant, at 30 per 100,000.[55]

There is also strong evidence that many angioplasty operations may be unnecessary. A damning American study looked at patients who had been referred for angioplasty; the study concluded that, for half of them, the operation wasn't needed or could safely be deferred. And although coronary angioplasty was originally expected to replace bypass surgery, in fact the frequency of both techniques has grown exponentially, with an 'ever lowering threshold' for carrying out either procedure for even asymptomatic patients.[56]

In fact, new evidence shows that bypass surgery may be the more successful treatment for angina than angioplasty. In one study, nearly four times as many angioplasty patients needed repeat treatment or surgery as those who had had bypass surgery; angina was almost three times as common in angioplasty patients as in bypass patients within six months of the treatment.[57]

In other studies, the two procedures have shown that neither one makes a substantial difference in terms of saving lives, preventing heart attacks or increasing arterial blood flow after three years.[58] Actually both procedures have serious downsides: one scientific study found that those treated with angioplasty are more likely to need further intervention and drugs, whereas the bypass group were more likely to have an acute heart attack during the operation. And the latest research, which examined more than 1,000 patients from 26 heart centres around Europe, shows that the survival rate among patients in the first year after angioplasty is lower than among those who have major bypass surgery. Angioplasty patients also need to be on more medication than those given a bypass, and are more likely to need a repeat operation within the first year.[59]

ASSISTED CONCEPTION

Louise Brown — the world's first 'test-tube baby' — is 26 years old at this writing — and so is test-tube baby technology. In that time the media has largely painted a pretty picture of 'assisted conception', as it is known in medical circles, as a brilliant breakthrough for the infertile. As the percentage of infertile couples increases — the latest estimates are that one out of every seven couples of childbearing age has trouble conceiving — infertility drugs or techniques are becoming the first port of call for the childless.

Most doctors helping a couple investigate infertility are quick to rush into piecemeal investigations without a systematic overview to determine where the problem really lies. Mystifyingly, they also tend to look automatically to the woman as the source of the couple's infertility problem, even if the man is found to have a low sperm count.

There are three main ways that medical science plays at being stork:

- In vitro fertilization (IVF), or embryo transfer, is supposed to be used when a woman has blocked tubes, when the sperm cannot manage to get through the cervical mucus, or in other cases where for some reason sperm cannot unite with egg. This technique involves removing one or more eggs from the woman, fertilizing the eggs with her partner's sperm outside the body in a petrie (shallow) laboratory dish, and reinserting the embryos (fertilized egg) into the woman's uterus.

- Intracytoplasmic sperm injection (ISCI), where a single sperm is injected directly into the egg.

- GIFT (gamete intrafallopian transfer) is a means of giving nature a gentle nudge. Although eggs are removed from the woman, and sperm is taken from her partner, they are placed separately at the outer edges of the woman's Fallopian tubes. In this way, goes the theory, sperm of low motility won't have as far to go as they would if they had to travel the long and precarious journey through a woman's reproductive canal in order to make it to their target.

- Fertility drugs, now used for some 20 years, are supposed to be offered only to women who have trouble ovulating. Drugs such as clomiphene citrate (trade name Clomid or Serophene) work by blocking the production of oestrogen and fooling the brain into thinking the body is not ovulating. The brain then produces larger amounts of Follicle Stimulating Hormone (FSH), causing the ovaries to 'super-ovulate' – often producing two, three or more eggs.

Although Louise Brown resulted from the reimplantation of a single fertilized egg, test-tube pioneers Patrick Steptoe and Professor Bob Edwards then came up with the idea of improving what was ordinarily a low success rate. It stood to reason that a woman's chances of having a pregnancy 'take' would improve if they put back more than one egg. (It would also save the cost and trouble of going through multiple treatments.) They then began offering women fertility drugs to make them 'super-ovulate' and produce more than one egg at a go, which they would return all at once. Genetically-modified hormones are the latest in the increasing armentarium of fertility drugs. Drugs such as Pergonal, which are even more potent than Clomid, can make the ovaries produce anywhere from three to 30 eggs at a time.

In practice, many of these more potent drugs are employed as a matter of course at the first sign that a couple is having a problem, and even before the nature of the fertility problem is investigated. This is despite the fact that in the view of experienced IVF specialist Michael Ah-Moye, of Holly House Hospital, a noted infertility clinic, fertility drugs such as Clomid don't have a very good success rate other than with those clear-cut cases in which the problem is the fact that the woman isn't ovulating. Indeed, even the manufacturers of Serophene, one of these drugs, says that it is less effective after three goes and should not be used indefinitely.[60]

Women undergoing IVF are usually given three types of drugs: a GnRH (gonadotrophin-releasing hormone) agonist or antagonist to suppress the release of luteinizing hormone from the pituitary gland and to stave off ovulation until the follicles are mature; an FSH (follicle-stimulating hormone) product, to ramp up the ovaries into producing multiple follicles; and hCG (human chorionic gonadotrophin), to help mature the eggs in the follicles. In addition, when women undergo 'pituitary down-regulation' to postpone ovulation, they receive goserelin acetate and some-times yet more hormone drugs. Individual cases of ovarian hyperstimula-tion have occurred in women taking the two drugs in combination.[61] During such a cycle, a fertility specialist has basically seized control of a woman's entire fertility cycle, and so must keep careful watch over ovarian size and hormone levels to ensure that hormone levels don't rise too quickly.

Fertility drugs are also often given to men with low sperm counts, says Ah-Moye, even though most studies have shown these drugs do very little good.

Fertility drugs are known to have substantial side-effects – many of which will affect your pregnancy or baby if you do get pregnant while taking them. Doctors underplay the side-effects of the fertility drugs as limited to hot flushes or abdominal discomfort, but one of the manufac-turers, Swiss-based pharmaceutical firm Serono, warns that Serophene causes ovarian enlargement (in about 14 per cent of patients) and blurred vision (for reasons they don't understand). This has particular repercussions if you have endometriosis or ovarian cysts, as it will make the problem worse and possibly permanently affect your fertility. In addition, these problems cannot be detected immediately: 'maximum enlargement of the ovary … does not occur until several days after discontinuation of the drug.'

Besides ovarian enlargement, super-ovulation drugs such as Metrodin also cause Ovarian Hyperstimulation syndrome (OHSS), a serious medical problem causing a rapid accumulation of fluid in the abdominal cavity, the thorax and even the sac surrounding the heart, requiring immediate hospi-talization. This situation can worsen if the patient is also pregnant. 'With OHSS there is an increased risk of injury to the ovary,' says Serono in the US drugs bible, the *Physician's Desk Reference*. 'Pelvic examination may cause rupture of an ovarian cyst.' If this does occur, it may be necessary to remove the ovary surgically.

Seven years after more than two million women in the US alone had taken some sort of fertility drug, the first complete study to examine all the data was finally tallied. Its chilling findings were that fertility drugs such as clomiphene can double or even triple the risk of developing ovar-ian cancer if taken for longer than a year. The study, which looked at the records of nearly 4,000 infertile American women in Seattle, Washington between 1974 and 1985, discovered that 11 in the group reported an invasive or borderline malignant ovarian tumour, against an expected average of 4.4. Of these, nine were taking clomiphene, five of these for longer than a year.[62]

The American Collaborative Ovarian Cancer Group, of Stanford University in California, which analysed 12 studies, also concluded that infertile women taking fertility drugs face three times the risk of ovarian cancer as infertile women who haven't taken the drugs.[63] These findings have prompted the US Food and Drug Administration to now require that manufacturers of fertility drugs add the risk of ovarian cancer to the list of possible adverse reactions published about the drugs.

There's also a question mark about whether these drugs can trip off breast cancer, particularly following the death of Paul Merton's wife, who was undergoing IVF when she developed breast cancer. Hormone levels are sent sky-high – more than double the norm – for days at a time, and women's systems are cranked up to produce the number of eggs in a single month that she would normally produce in a year or two. With some women, who may undergo as many as 20 tries at an IVF baby, their bodies will churn out up to 500 eggs – as many as 20 years' worth of eggs in a few years.

One Australian study of nearly 30,000 women found that women undergoing IVF treatment had twice the incidence of breast cancer than usual a year after treatment.[64] If that isn't enough to make you think twice before taking one of these drugs, Serono also warns of pulmonary and vascular complications such as thrombosis in the veins or arteries which could result in a heart attack, stroke, or the loss of a limb. There's also the risk of an ectopic (tubal) pregnancy, which of course results in the removal of an ovary, thereby lowering your fertility even more.

The media has published lots of photos of boisterous triplets with cheery captions about how fertility drugs have increased the incidence of twins, triplets and quads, and that formerly childless couples are suddenly having to cope with a house-full of children. And there's no doubt that these drugs increase your chances of having anything from twins to quints. In clinical trials with Metrodin, Serono reported multiple births in 17 per cent of pregnancies; with Serophene, 10 per cent were twins, less than 1 per cent triplets or more. This percentage increases, depending upon the number of eggs replaced into the woman. In 1988 the overall multiple pregnancy rate was 24 per cent for IVF and 19.9 per cent for GIFT. The multiple pregnancy rate for GIFT increases to 31.2 per cent when five or more eggs are replaced.

The problem isn't so much coping with a house-full of children, however, as making sure any of them survive in the first place. According to a 10-year study by the UK Medical Research Council working party, multiple births of all kinds, whether natural or assisted, carry greater risks than singleton births. Of about 1,000 babies born as part of a multiple birth, 25 per cent were premature (compared with a usual rate in ordinary deliveries of 6 per cent in England and Wales) and nearly 33 per cent weighed less than 2.2kg/5½lb (compared with only 7 per cent of all deliveries born at that weight). More than 25 of the 1,000 IVF babies in the study died, at around birth (compared with the 9.8 per 1,000 national average).[65]

The working party claims that when allowances are made for the women's ages and multiple births, this death rate is similar to ordinary infant mortality rates, which isn't a very compensatory thought if they happened to be your babies. IVF babies are also five times more likely to be premature or born underweight.[66] If born alive, IVF babies also have a higher incidence of birth defects.

Fertility drugs can increase the chances of birth defects such as spina bifida by nearly six times (although other reports claim the risk is only doubled, still others that it is nonexistent).[67] One study found the risk was lower with clomiphene, which is only about three-quarters as risky as stronger fertility drugs. After examining all multiple births in Australia in the 1980s, one study concluded that triplet pregnancies produced a child with cerebral palsy eight times more often than twin pregnancies, and 47 times more often than singleton pregnancies. Some 86 per cent of the cases of cerebral palsy among the babies born in multiple births occurred in twins. Even when twins were of normal birthweight, they were still at a greater risk of developing cerebral palsy than singletons.[68] IVF babies also risk being born with anencephaly (a defect in the development of the brain and skull, which results in brain hemispheres that are small or missing altogether).

Other case reports suggest that IVF babies could carry a higher risk of developing cancer later in life. One Australian study found that IVF babies have a slightly higher risk than normal.[69]

Early reports of assisted conceptions found that 7 per cent were born with major congenital malformations, from heart malformations to club foot.[70] This compares with 2 per cent in the general population. Heart malformations were the greatest problem, accounting for almost 4 per cent of cases, compared with a ordinary rate of about between 0.4 and 0.5 per cent.

IVF babies have also been linked to rare genito-urinary birth defects, or cloacal-bladder exstrophy-epispadias[71] and genetic imprinting defects, such as Beckwith-Wiedemann Syndrome (BWS), which causes excessive growth of various tissues. IVF babies have six times the incidence of this syndrome than normal.[72]

ICSI is also suspected of causing imprinting problems, causing conditions similar to autism[73] and even brain defects. In one study, nearly one in six children had mild or significant delayed development – 17 times the norm.[74]

These days it is common practice to freeze embryos, or to delay placing embryos back into the body for up to five days. Even these delays are suspected of causing genetic defects.[75] A recent Spanish study found that the process of freezing distorts the structure of eggs during thawing, ultimately altering its number of chromosomes.[76]

A multiple pregnancy also introduces a Solomon-like decision for a mother – killing off one or more of the foetuses so that the other(s) may live. Because of the increased risk in multiple births, particularly for three or more embryos, some centres in the UK and on the continent quietly engage in what is euphemistically described as 'embryo reduction' or, even the more clinically neutral, 'reducing the products of conception'. What this amounts to is 'selective termination' of one or more of the healthy embryos through an injection of saline in order to decrease the risk of all of them dying.

This dilemma becomes more likely, the higher the number of eggs replaced inside the woman's body.

To try and pre-empt this problem, the Interim Licensing Authority recommends that only three eggs – and in extraordinary circumstances, such as advanced maternal age, four eggs may be replaced. But such figures only apply to licensed units. Unlicensed units may put back as many embryos as they wish.

There's also recent evidence that embryo reduction may harm those foetuses left behind. 'The obstetric outcome after pregnancy reduction in the first trimester is often complicated,' said the Interim Licensing report, which cited a case of triplet embryos 'reduced' by one. An ultrasound scan revealed that one of the remaining twins had developed an anencephaly-like malformation, after which he got the needle, too. The remaining baby was born healthy and normal at 39 weeks. The same occurred with a quadruplet pregnancy which was 'reduced' to twins – or, as the report put it, after 'a twin pregnancy was achieved as in the first case'. (Note the strict avoidance of emotive language.) One of these surviving twins was found to have an anencephaly-like malformation; he was then 'reduced', after which the only survivor was delivered premature at 32 weeks.[77] An Australian study also found that if one half of a set of twins dies in the uterus, the survivor is at higher risk of cerebral palsy.

Considering that GIFT and IVF still carry a low success rate (only about 20 per cent), are only indicated for about 20 per cent of infertile couples, and carry such high risks, anyone faced with a fertility problem should consider it the court of last resort. Furthermore, organizations such as Foresight: The Association for Preconceptual Care and the doctors they work with claim that a large number of 'unexplained' fertility problems and even blockages or low sperm counts, thought to be untreatable, can be resolved if a couple improve their nutritional status and resolve any allergies. Over 80 per cent of couples with previous histories of miscarriage or infertility go on to give birth to healthy babies, after following the Foresight diet and supplement programme.[78]

LITHOTRIPSY

Besides test tubes, doctors have been experimenting with waves of all sorts derived from light and sound. The latest surgical toy of the past decade is a high-tech invention with the unwieldy name of 'extracorporeal shock-wave lithotripsy' (ESWL), which has revolutionized the medical management of kidney stones. In ESWL, the lithotriptor creates shockwaves which, guided by x-rays, are aimed at the kidney stone, causing it to disintegrate. By use of sound, the lithotriptor is theoretically able to distinguish between the body's own tissues and those of the kidney stone.

Urologists all over the world rushed to embrace lithotripsy without subjecting it to proper clinical trials because it seemed, on the face of it, an improvement over surgery (the conventional method of handling stones). Plus, all the initial reports didn't show any short- or long-term damage to the kidney or its surrounding tissues. Lithotripsy is now recommended for three-quarters of all stone problems.

A number of the studies (which are only now being done) cast a few shadows over the initial rosy assumptions. It now seems evident that lithotripsy definitely causes damage to the kidney in a good percentage of cases. Most patients experience internal bleeding, ranging from a tiny haemorrhage to major bleeding requiring transfusion.

This bleeding also seems to change the dynamics of the blood in the kidney, causing kidney hypertension (abnormally high blood-pressure in the kidneys) in up to 8 per cent of patients.[79] Other studies show irreversible kidney failure,[80] a one-quarter reduction in the rate at which the kidney filters out impurities,[81] and a rise in blood-pressure[82] and heartbeat.[83] Rarely, it can even rupture the kidney.[84] The extent of damage appears to depend upon the intensity of shockwaves used, but in any case nearly a fifth of patients may sustain damage as a result of ESWL.[85]

A computed tomography (CT) scan performed two years after a group of French patients had undergone lithotripsy showed that 40 per cent had a recurrence of stones; 25 per cent had scarring.[86] Some patients followed over time suffered chronic changes to their kidney.[87] Apart from the risk of septic shock,[88] another worry concerns the bacteria within the stones, which is released when they are broken up and which can cause inflammation.[89]

Shock waves may also damage male sperm. In experiments on male rats, using ESWL, after five weeks the treated rat testes appeared to have atrophied and could no longer produce sperm. In human cells, sperm movement became frenetic and the percentage of abnormal sperm increased.[90] The procedure has also been known to cause haemorrhage in the scrotum.[91]

The problem with disintegrating kidney stones with shock waves is that it doesn't address the reasons why the body produced the stones in the first place. One major cause is prescription drugs: stones have now been linked to carbonic anhydrase inhibitors (acetazolamide or methazolamide), used to treat glaucoma;[92] to furosemide in infants, used for congenital heart failure;[93] to some anti-epileptic drugs;[94] to triameterene (used to combat hypertension);[95] to trisilicate-containing antacids (used for gastric discomfort and heartburn);[96] to ceftriaxone (which prevents the body from rejecting transplants);[97] and even to thiazide diuretics in patients with high blood-pressure.[98]

Numerous studies have made the connection between kidney stones and the use of sulphasalazine, particularly in AIDS patients given drugs such as Septrin over the long term as a 'just-in-case' measure against *pneumocystis carinii* pneumonia.[99] Laxative abuse can also bring on kidney stones.

STAR WARS IN THE SURGERY

The other bit of Star Wars-like gadgetry taking the medical world by storm is the laser, a light-sabre of a knife so precise that it can shave into a human hair without breaking the strand. Principally, it's being used for laser eye surgery and promises to cure mild myopia at a flash of light. Doctors are even experimenting with astronomical technology in order to diagnose and subsequently treat the smallest of aberrations.

The latest and most popular technique, called LASEX (laser subepithelial keratomileiusis), employs a beam of computer-controlled ultra-violet light directly into the cornea in order to reshape it, by shaving off little bits here and there. Other forms, like LASIK (laser in situ keratomileiusis), cut into the cornea with a standard surgical knife and use a laser only on the corneal bed.

Although more than a million Americans undergo the procedure every year, the popularity of LASIK has waned slightly amid new warnings about after-effects. Studies have discovered that one in five patients undergoing laser eye surgery required repeat surgery to fix problems left by the first procedure.[100]

The biggest worry appears to be a loss of contrast sensitivity (the ability to distinguish objects in low levels of light). The latest evidence from

Moorfield's Eye Hospital in London shows that more than half of patients undergoing LASIK surgery suffer loss of contrast sensitivity. At a special symposium, doctors admitted that, within a year, 56 per cent of patients undergoing LASIK develop permanent contrast sensitivity which cannot be corrected with either glasses or contact lenses.[101] Indeed, in Germany a study found that 75 per cent of patients had such poor contrast sensitivity after their operations that they failed basic night-vision tests for driving.[102]

You also risk permanently weakening your cornea, which occurs in more than a third of cases.[103] Other complications from surgery include a great risk of eye infections, damage to the macula or optic nerve, and astigmatism. The FDA has labelled laser surgery an 'option for risk-takers'.

Besides light waves, surgeons are experimenting with sound waves as a new way to carry out liposuction. The sound waves will liquefy fat cells – but the new techniques, like the old ones (where fat cells are drenched with water and then basically 'hoovered' out) are likely to carry the same risk of complications and even death from pulmonary thromboembolism or cardiac arrest.[104]

Even for the most tried-and-tested of gee-whizz techniques for aesthetic enhancements, there is no such thing in medicine as a sure thing.

PART VI

TAKING CONTROL

12

Taking Control

My maternal grandmother Stella, who emigrated to the US from Italy at the age of 15, had both her babies at home. This was not because she advocated home birth so much as because she had been taught to regard medical progress with a fair degree of suspicion. *'Don't go to hospital; they change your baby!'* her own mother had admonished her in broken English. My grandmother, being the good daughter she was, duly complied, for it would have been unthinkable not to: in all regards, in her native culture, mothers knew best.

As it turned out, not even home proved to be the safe haven Stella and her mother had anticipated. Stella's husband – my grandfather – agreed to go along with these 'female superstitions' only so long as a bona fide doctor was present at both deliveries. Many years later, on more than one occasion my grandmother would lament her second and final birth. 'The doctor – he *ruin* me!' she'd invariably exclaim. The force of her anger over the incident even a half-century later rendered the details too terrible for me ever to probe into, but I assumed that she was talking about a botched episiotomy.

During my childhood, the reason for my mother's birth at home was always recounted and held up to me with ridicule – an example of pig-ignorant hocus-pocus. *Imagine thinking that professionals like doctors could send you home with the wrong baby!* However, the more I reflect upon it over time, the more I realize the wisdom inherent in my great-grandmother's cautionary tale. Birth at home has since been proven to be safer than hospital births for low-risk deliveries,[1] and babies born in hospital have not only been mixed up but snatched on more than a few occasions. Furthermore, behind that terse pronouncement was a rather sophisticated philosophy about medicine in general: view any newfangled medical progress with the most profound suspicion; don't go anywhere near a hospital if you aren't really ill; trust that your own healthy body doesn't need much help; assume that doctors are capable of making the most basic and calamitous mistakes.

As it turned out, my grandmother's wariness about hospitals proved prescient on the single night of her life that she did spend any time in one. At the age of 90 she was rushed to the emergency room in the mistaken notion that she was having a heart attack, and kept overnight for 'observation'. Her problem turned out to be indigestion, but she was so utterly alarmed by the entire experience, was so moved to resist the parade of strangers poking at her and invading her privacy, that when we came to collect her the following morning we found her tied up in a straitjacket – the only means by which the hospital staff had managed to gain her compliance.

My Italian forebears correctly deduced what by now should be clear to you: that your doctor often doesn't know what he's doing – not because he isn't a good person with good intentions, but because the equipment inside his black bag doesn't work particularly well. In fact, most of the time, your body can manage things better than any doctor can.

Besides his decidedly inferior set of tools, there is something fundamentally wrong with a doctor's perception of the material he works with. As sophisticated as it is in many regards, medical science utterly lacks any understanding whatsoever of the extraordinary dynamics of the human body. With its emphasis on interrupting and often opposing your body's own processes, medicine never takes into account the exquisite mechanism of the organism it is trying to fix or the body's extraordinary potential to operate beyond the empirical. This includes the power of faith, hope and the will to live – what medicine now refers to as 'psychoneuroimmunology' – all long proven elements of so-called 'miracle' cures or spontaneous healing.[2] By reducing your body's own response to a stress – by lowering a fever, your body's best defence against outside agents – the doctor often ends up permanently weakening your body's ability to fight back.

Without a true appreciation of this wondrous ability, medicine is a blunt and clumsy instrument, a pointless meddler, a caveman being called upon to fix a mainframe computer, whose solution is to bash it with a club. And even this metaphor is crudely inexact, because even the most complex computer system cannot begin to approximate the body's mysterious ability to move from total disarray to order, in short, to heal itself.

Every medical solution appears clumsy and primitive beside some of the body's own highly sophisticated and shrewd mechanisms: the ability of a mother's breastmilk to create antibodies to fight her baby's infections. We also know that a component of breastmilk helps to complete brain growth, affecting areas such as visual acuity, for the entire first year of life.[3] Then there are the hormones in the brain that are produced whenever necessary to reduce anxiety. And new evidence shows that a woman's risk of developing high blood-pressure during pregnancy decreases the longer she's been with her partner.[4] This may mean there is something in her partner's sperm that keeps her and the pregnancy healthy. The most complex drug in the world cannot begin to match this subtlety.

Vitamin K

Medicine often operates on the premise that nature is imperfect. Figuring that all that's required is a little tweak here or there, it clumsily upsets an exquisite balance, thereby causing a load of new problems far worse than what it set out to resolve in the first place. This may be the case with vitamin K injections, which are meant to prevent children from dying from a rare haemorrhagic disease of the newborn. Recently, the Institute of Child Health in Bristol found that this practice could increase by 2½ times the risk of a child developing cancer.[5] Although the Bristol results haven't been replicated anywhere else, there is a private consensus that medicine doesn't really know what it is doing in this area.[6] When the practice first started in the 1950s, vitamin K3 was administered to babies – until it was discovered that K3 leads to high levels of blood bilirubin, damaging the brain and causing deafness, mental retardation and involuntary movement. It is also associated with haemolysis – where red blood cells are destroyed. Medicine then quickly changed to K1, which appears not to pose these risks.[7] Nevertheless, both the injected and oral varieties don't appear to last very long, and many babies with low vitamin-K stores appear to self-correct the problem.[8]

Another area where researchers have discovered that nature didn't make a big mistake after all is low iron stores during pregnancy. New evidence shows that this is not a sign of illness but of health, signifying good expansion in blood volume and resulting in bigger babies. All those iron pills and transfusions given to anaemic pregnant women all these years may have contributed to many premature births and small-for-dates babies.[9]

A Faulty Paradigm

Modern medicine doesn't work because the very paradigm on which it is based is faulty – that germs or genes alone are responsible for illness and that our bodies are akin to complicated machines. Medicine is largely based upon the 'germ theory', which holds that most illness depends entirely on the invasion of bacteria and viruses. According to this theory, disease is a random, stealthy entity that can strike down anyone at any moment, regardless of his nutritional, physical, emotional and environmental condition. This means that an undernourished child of the ghetto would have the same odds of dying from measles as a well-fed middle-class one.

This legacy from Louis Pasteur persists even though scientists are well aware that several pounds' worth of bacteria exist in a healthy body, providing either a positive service or there as the result, rather than as the cause of, disease. There is also growing evidence that the body's susceptibility to disease – its emotions, physical state and response to its environment – determines whether a patient succumbs to illness.

Blaming outside agents for every modern illness encourages a blinkered approach, which tends to justify the most basic solutions. When researchers discovered that babies in daycare were more likely to have earaches and respiratory diseases than those breastfeeding and at home with their mothers, they came up with a drug with eight species of bacterial extracts to prevent these recurrent respiratory infections among daycare children. The researchers centred on the notion that the bugs worked in isolation. They didn't consider such possible factors as lack of breastfeeding, the toddlers' lack of proximity to their mums, or the effects of placement in an institutional setting too early. Not surprisingly, vaccinating children against institutionalization didn't work.[10]

It's as well to keep in mind that what we think of as a long and distinguished tradition in medicine is only 50 years old. The flowering of drug therapy as we know it has mainly occurred in the wake of the big discoveries of the 1940s. Much as it gives the impression of being space-age, medical science, alone among the other scientific disciplines, is some four centuries out of date. In physics, for instance, the Cartesian view that everything works in predictable, reliable and hence measurable fashion, which still forms the basis of modern medicine, was long discarded in favour of relativity and, more recently, quantum theories, which hold that the universe and the way it works aren't quite as mechanical and bit-part as we used to think. Nevertheless, medical science still adheres to the notion of a static, clockwork universe, with human beings looked upon essentially as machines and the mind operating as a separate entity from the body.

Gene therapy is very much the new frontier in medicine. Scientists throughout the world working on the Human Genome Project claim to have cracked the three-billion letter code that constitutes our genetic makeup; by getting a handle on this genetic blueprint, medical researchers believe they will be able to conquer many diseases more easily.

In fact, the current vogue is to blame most illness on your genes – the idea being that one day doctors will be able to cut out your 'bad' DNA and paste in some better genetic instructions. Researchers are investigating interventions that would alter the DNA of your body in order to diagnose, prevent or treat genetic disorders.

One area where this has been tested out is Parkinson's disease using an unlikely solution: the herpes virus. Since the herpes virus lives in the body of victims forever, often quietly hibernating in nerve cells, scientists from King's College reasoned that if they could tinker with the genetic coding of the virus and get it to make dopamine, perhaps it could carry this genetic message to the brain cells of its host.

All they needed to do was to chop out a few chunks of the virus' 'bad' DNA, having to do with all the harmful bits like reproduction and infection, insert some new chunks with genetic instructions for making dopamine, and there you'd have it: Frankenstein's monster gets turned into the fairy prince in Snow White.

In practice, however, scientists have had to return to the drawing board since they discovered that the engineered virus is potentially fatal. Medicine's intention of 'editing' you and me to engineer all disease out of us has thus far proved elusive.

The biggest weakness with modern medical theory is that it assumes that we all get ill in the same way – that all illness stems from the same cause, all illnesses act alike, and there is only a single method of curing them. But as Dr Leon Eisenberg of the Department of Social Medicine, Harvard Medical School, argued in a lecture to doctors:

> *The premise is that as we go down the scale of magnitude from organisms to organs to tissues to cells to organelles to molecules, the understanding becomes ever deeper. The person whose body houses the collection of aberrant molecules is transformed into an incidental host, deserving of the physician's sympathy, of course, but essentially irrelevant. What 'really' matters is disease pathophysiology.*
>
> *How absurd! Between genotype and phenotype, a lifetime of individual experience has fashioned what began as an envelope of stochastic probabilities into a singular personal embodiment: the patient who faces us. In clinical practice, it is the particularities and the idiosyncrasies of the individual patient that challenge the physician. The same disease never presents in quite the same way in successive patients. Complaints vary; severity varies; response to treatment varies ... Medicine includes but cannot be reduced to molecular biology.*[11]

This theory that all illnesses (and therefore all patients) are alike also requires that every disease has a label. To hide their ignorance (and consequent fear), doctors need to turn what they don't understand into a 'syndrome', which makes it sound like something that they've managed to get under control. Not long ago, a phenomenon obviously due to bowel problems became 'tight-pants syndrome', infants being improperly fed by their parents were suffering from 'squash-drinking syndrome', and even itching whose source had not yet been identified became 'scratch-itch syndrome'. As for anything that doesn't fit a recognizable pattern, it is deemed 'all in the patient's mind'.

Food as Prevention

If much of the drugs-and-surgery interventionist approach to healing has proved useless or dangerous, except in emergencies, the most impressive and promising research at the moment concerns methods of providing the body with the appropriate tools to heal itself, particularly the role of food and nutrients in preventing or creating disease. Although they aren't publicized every day, studies showing the protective value of the vitamins and minerals (particularly vitamin A and beta-carotene, B_2 [riboflavin], B_3 [nicotinic acid], vitamin C, E and selenium) against cancer and a host of other illnesses now fill the medical literature. Antioxidants protect the body from damage caused by harmful molecules called free radicals, from oxygen. Besides respiration, the body's cells use oxygen to metabolize (and literally 'burn') food for its energy, and also for immune activity, to burn away germs and toxins. Free radicals are created from many sources – ultra-violet radiation, smoke pollution, heavy metals, or overheating of oils, such as in fast-food restaurants. They wreak havoc by destroying cell membranes, causing genetic damage, depressing immune function, hardening the arteries, disrupting hormone regulation, contributing to diabetes and other systemic disorders and, of course, causing the growth and spread of cancer.

But we're now learning that damage from free radicals can be prevented and even reversed if there are sufficient concentrations in the body of free-radical scavengers, the antioxidants.

One of the largest studies of cancer prevention, an investigation of 30,000 Chinese people in an area of historically high risk for a certain type of cancer, proved that certain antioxidants could protect people from developing cancer by as much as one-fifth. The same study found a 38 per cent reduction in mortality from stroke among people following the recommended diet.[12]

Antioxidants have been shown to prevent eye disease such as macular degeneration, heart disease and many of the diseases we associate with normal ageing.[13] For instance, people suffering from angina have been shown to have significantly lower levels of vitamins C, E and carotene than healthy individuals.

Besides the antioxidant vitamins, the vegetables containing them may have even more powerful protective effects. One study from Dartmouth Medical School in New Hampshire showed that vegetables are better than supplements in lowering the risks of developing cancer of the colon.[14] It may be that other factors we have yet to identify are at play in a diet high in vegetables and fruits.

We also have to examine the kinds of fats and oils we eat and to ensure that we are getting enough. Certain populations which consume great quantities of olive oil appear to have low levels of cancer. In Greece, where the average consumption of olive oil is 80 g a day, there is a very low rate of breast cancer. It is likely the components of olive oil have a protective effect.

Indeed, essential fatty acids in the right ratios have also demonstrated their importance in preventing everything from heart problems[15] to learning difficulties[16] and age-related macular degeneration.[17]

Many of what are now seen as healthy elements to a diet – large helpings of fruits and vegetables, unprocessed essential oils, meat and fish and unprocessed food – are present in the Mediterranean diet. Researchers have discovered that two populations with some of the lowest incidence of heart attacks are those on Crete and on Kohama Island in Japan. The people of these islands have high intakes of essential fatty acids, a fish-orientated diet, and a high intake of the natural antioxidants. In the Lyon Diet Heart Study, researchers found that a Mediterranean diet could protect you from a second heart attack if you'd suffered one already. Only eight of the 302 patients on the Mediterranean regime died from a second attack, against 20 in a similar-sized group on a traditional, low-fat diet. Levels of vitamins E and C were also found to be higher in the group on the Mediterranean diet.[18] The Mediterranean diet has also been shown to prevent stroke, as have the omega-3 essential fatty acids.[19] Clearly, this is where medicine should be directing more of its research efforts.

Despite this growing evidence, very little has filtered down to the rank and file. The average doctor still regards food and nutritional supplements with suspicion and doubt, or at best as an adjunct to the 'real' treatment – drugs and surgery. Although many now allow that pregnant women need folic acid, which has been proven to prevent spina bifida, so far few obstetricians have made the lateral mental leap that healthy living may prevent many other birth defects as well.

Government agencies even regard nutritional medicine as something virtually criminal. In May 1993, 15 US Food and Drug Administration agents with flak jackets, backed up by a batch of county policemen with guns at the ready, surrounded the clinic of noted nutritional therapist Dr Jonathan Wright in Kent, Washington. Instead of knocking, they kicked in the door commando-style and forcibly picked the locks of the three additional back- and side-door entrances so that armed police and agents could pour into the clinic from all sides. While pointing guns at some of Dr Wright's terrified staff, this SWAT team filled a lorry with nearly every important element of Dr Wright's practice.

Dr Wright's crime, it seems, was using injectable vitamins. A medical doctor with a Harvard degree, Wright now uses naturopathic methods. He imports pure vitamins from Germany because he can no longer get them in America; their US counterparts have preservatives that cause allergic reactions in his patients. In the eyes of the FDA, Dr Wright was guilty of smuggling.[20]

At this writing, a worldwide effort is afoot to make nutritional medicine illegal. The EU has passed the Foods Supplements Directive, which, if ratified in August 2005, will severely limit the levels and types of dietary supplements available throughout Europe, and in Australia many of the supplements are now illegal. Similar moves are in the offing in the United States and Canada.

Besides the role of vitamins and food as prevention, there is also growing evidence about the role of food in *creating* illness. A number of pioneers in medicine are discovering that allergies to food or modern-day chemicals are behind many of our chronic, so-called 'incurable' illnesses such as arthritis, eczema, asthma, hyperactivity, and even epilepsy and mental diseases such as schizophrenia. Copious research already exists in respected medical journals supporting the role of allergies or nutritional deficiencies in causing disease.[21] A respectable body of opinion among orthodox medicine, for instance, believes that gluten sensitivity may be one of the major causes of epilepsy. The largest study of this to date, performed in Italy, found that three-quarters of a group of epileptics passed the test for coeliac disease – a biopsy of the small bowel found the characteristic atrophy of the villi (the tiny hairs of the gut).[22]

Sharon, whose husband Gary prints our newsletter, is just one of many patients who've been helped by this approach. A young woman in her twenties, she was virtually crippled with rheumatoid arthritis and consigned to a lifetime of drugs. She'd also had no luck conceiving. When Gary mentioned her to us, we suggested that she see one of our panel members who has spent years investigating the role of allergies in illness, particularly migraine and arthritis. Sharon did go along to see him, and he isolated her problem as an allergy to potatoes, a common situation among arthritics. As soon as she eliminated potatoes from her diet, Sharon's arthritis disappeared. Several months after that, she became pregnant.

And of course 'hostile foods' aren't the only problem. We also need to look to some 25,000 chemicals – pesticides, plastics, by-products – now in common use in Britain alone, most of which humans have only been exposed to since the Second World War. Scientific evidence is mounting about the role of pesticides in virtually every illness.[23] Some scientists are pioneering important research into the more subtle effects of these chemicals on our bodies and their ability to cause many chronic, puzzling diseases such as arthritis.

One Swiss woman, called Irene, suffered from multiple joint pains and swelling that required cortisone treatments. Once she'd identified and eliminated certain foods from her diet, she improved somewhat but she was still left with residual pain – until she went to visit her mother in Zurich, where her pain and swelling disappeared completely. As soon as Irene returned home to Surrey, however, she was dismayed to find that many of her joint pains returned. When she sought out a doctor highly skilled in food and chemical sensitivity, he suspected that she might be reacting to household gas; her mother's flat in Zurich was all electric, while her home in Surrey had a gas cooker and gas central heating. Irene underwent a trial period of turning off her gas, and in a few days her joints were as good as they'd been in Switzerland. The gas central heating boiler was removed to an outhouse, and five years on Irene remains free of any arthritic symptoms.[24]

We are also only beginning to understand the precise role of exercise in preventing disease of all varieties. One report from the Harvard Alumni

Society, which was set up in the early 1960s to follow more than 17,000 graduates (of an average age of 46 when first recruited), reported that deaths from all causes were reduced by physical exercise. The amount of protection offered by vigorous exercise, as compared with not exercising, was the equivalent to the difference in the mortality rate between non-smokers and those who smoke 20 cigarettes a day.[25]

Many doctors have come to believe that the future of medicine depends upon a better understanding of how to boost the tools our bodies have for fighting disease. Michael Baum, one of Britain's foremost breast cancer specialists, bravely went on record in a letter to the *Times* to argue that the way forward in cancer was no longer high-dose chemotherapy and bone-marrow transplants, which, in his view, 'echoes the death throes of the conventional belief systems'. He continued:

Many of us believe that the future lies not in a blunderbuss attack attempting to eradicate all cancer cells present at the time of diagnosis, but a more sophisticated attempt to maintain a dynamic equilibrium controlling the disease by modulation of the body's natural defence systems.[26]

Medicine desperately needs to take a fresh, objective approach to many illnesses and discard any treatment that has no basis in fact. For several years, the buzzword in medicine has been 'evidence-based medicine' – which simply means looking up what has been proven in medical research before using it on patients.[27] The Cochrane Collaboration – named after epidemiologist Archie Cochrane, who spent most of his life pointing out the weakness of the evidence supporting much conventional medical evidence – has been set up to create and maintain a register of all random-ized controlled trials in biomedical research. But at the moment, this fresh approach – which might seem the obvious way forward to you and me – is only the subject of debate or thoughtful review in the medical literature. Whether the rank and file ever adopt it remains to be seen.

Suspicious of Alternatives

Doctors also need to suspend their preconceptions about other systems of medicine. Orthodox medicine has always taken a high-handed position against alternative medicine, denouncing it as experimental and unproven. Last year, the Royal College of Physicians and the Royal College of Pathologists criticized alternative treatments used to combat allergies as unscientific, warning that 'until the methods have been evaluated by reputable, randomized, double-blind, placebo-controlled trials they cannot be accepted into routine clinical practice.'[28] If alternative or complementary approaches are acknowledged at all, they are so only as 'integrated' adjuncts to the 'real' thing – as a feel-good practice akin to having a facial.

Actually, many so-called scientific treatments have far less proof than many medical systems such as homoeopathy or acupuncture that defy empirical logic. These treatments, along with herbalism and even arcane practices such as Romany medicine – have been proven by proper scientific trials to work for many ailments.[29] This doesn't take into account the evidence of clinical use over centuries, as compared with a paltry few years or decades of use in the case of most 'orthodox' drugs. Many alternative systems also have the superior advantage of diagnosing and treating people as individuals, creating remedies unique to the individual, and viewing the body, mind, emotions and environment as inextricable.

Not long ago, a doctor attempting to discredit alternative medicine proposed that he and a practitioner of acupuncture convene over a body on the operating table about to undergo surgery. Once the body in question was cut open, if it revealed the existence of meridians and physical evidence of the theories upon which Chinese medicine is based, the medical man would concede defeat and take the acupuncturist out to dinner. If, on the other hand, the work of the scalpel revealed a collection of organs such as a heart, liver and kidneys, concluded the doctor, with high-minded relish, then the acupuncturist should pick up the tab for the meal.

Actually, empirical evidence does prove the existence of meridians, but not in the strictly visual sense that this doctor required. Research has shown that many acupuncture points on the body demonstrate electrical resistance, which is dramatically decreased compared with points on the skin surrounding them (10 kilo-ohms at the centre of a point compared with 3 mega-ohms in the surrounding skin).[30] It's also been shown that slight stimulation of these points releases painkilling endorphins and the steroid cortisol, while more intense stimulation releases important mood-regulating neurotransmitters such as serotonin and norepinephrine. The same doesn't occur when the skin surrounding these points is stimulated.[31] We also know that acupuncture can dilate the circulatory system and increase blood flow to even distant organs in the body.[32]

Nine times out of 10 – with ordinary fever, colds and flu, common earache, or childhood illnesses – the body can sort itself out if you only wait before rushing to the doctor. In many instances of infection, chicken soup – so-called Jewish penicillin – is better for you than the real thing.

Of course, no matter how clever and self-healing your body is, there are times when it may need professional assistance. But if your doctor doesn't always know what he's doing, and you're never told what he's doing, where does this leave you? Because so little in orthodox medicine is really proven, taking control of your health requires that each of us view all medicines as both helpful and potentially dangerous, and do a good deal of detective work before consenting to treatment. It requires that we suspend our own preconceptions about how our bodies work and heal, and embrace other proven systems when they offer more help than we can get from a more conventional approach.

For some reason, the notion persists that there is something wrong with a patient knowing exactly what is being done to him. All of us hold doctors in such high regard that we view questioning them as something akin to treasonous disloyalty or extreme rudeness, a tactic that will undermine this special relationship. If anyone you knew were to avoid questioning a builder or plumber about to do work on his house because he thought it was rude, you would think him embarrassingly naïve. But the most assertive individual can turn into a blancmange when faced with asking for a simple clarification on a life-or-death procedure proposed by his doctor.

A Medical Consumer

No matter whether you are on the NHS or paying Harley Street prices, you have an absolute right to know everything you can about any medical treatments being proposed. Certainly you would never buy a car or a camcorder without painstakingly investigating the pros and cons. Why should something as vital as your health or that of your loved ones be any different? It's vital that you view yourself as a paying consumer and your doctor's advice as *services that you are purchasing*. Far from eroding trust, asking questions will cement the relationship between you and your doctor (if he's a good one, that is) to one of shared responsibility between two intelligent adults (rather than that of all-knowing adult and awe-struck child). Even though medicine, like most professions, protects its own through the use of convoluted language, all medical procedures can be explained in terms that you can understand. At one time, that fellow with all those complicated initials after his name was a lay person learning this gobbledygook from scratch.

This same vigilance applies to alternative medicine. Although in the main, tried-and-tested alternative medicine practised by experienced, qualified individuals can be more benign than orthodox medicine, it can also kill if in the wrong hands. Some years ago a short course of Chinese herbs screwed up my menstrual cycle for an entire year. When I had the herbs analysed by the Guy's Hospital Poison Control Unit, they discovered that they contained *11 different oestrogens – enough to rival HRT*. Another alternative heart treatment – beloved of Hollywood film stars – has been responsible for at least five deaths. In the wrong hands, acupuncture can bring on migraines and even stroke. Many alternative practitioners are given a licence to practise after a few weekend courses, even with highly potent substances such as Chinese herbs. Natural does not always equal better. It's vital that you grill your alternative therapist, as you would your GP, about his experience, track record and knowledge of your condition, and to exit immediately if you don't like his answers.

Although it is more difficult to obtain, scientific data does exist about many treatments in alternative medicine. Explore information about your treatment with your practitioner, or call the official registry or body regu-lating that therapy to see where they can direct you. Do an internet search or visit a medical library. Virtually nothing apart from a genuine medical emergency cannot wait a day or two while you do your homework.

There's also no reason why you have to take one set of answers as gospel. Get a second opinion (or a third or fourth) until you're confident and satisfied about the suggested treatment, but view all your healers as technicians and remain in control of all decisions.

Above all, refuse to accept a death sentence. These days it is fashionable for doctors to level with patients about whether or not they have a terminal illness. In fact, this would appear to be the will of the people: a US Harris Poll in 1982 found that 96 per cent of Americans said they would want to be told if they had cancer, and 85 per cent wanted a 'realistic estimate' of how long they would live if their type of cancer was one that usually led to death in less than a year.[33]

However, as many cases demonstrate, being straight with patients may only hasten their death. One British man in his mid-fifties was referred to the Department of Haematology at the Royal Gwent Hospital with a history of a highly benign form of leukaemia, for which he only occasionally required small doses of drugs such as steroids. He had never been told the true nature of his condition, and over the next couple of years remained well, with his blood profile stable. Although he was ordinarily quite punctilious about attending his outpatient clinics, one day he never showed up, and only later turned up on a surgical ward in a highly neglected state. It turned out that he'd looked over his GP's shoulder at his case notes and seen the word 'leukaemia'. From there he went rapidly downhill and in three weeks he was dead, even though his blood count was unchanged. None of his doctors or even the pathologists conducting his autopsy could find any biological cause for his rapid decline.[34]

This particular issue is especially close to home. Some years ago, my then 78-year-old mother-in-law, Edie, was diagnosed as having end-stage breast cancer. Privately her doctor told us, 'If I were you, I'd get her affairs in order.' When he'd examined her, he'd been shocked; her breast, he told me, looked like raw meat. In fact, so advanced was the cancer that it was too late to try chemotherapy or any other intervention. She had three months to live, at the very outside, we were told.

Her GP then wrote her a prescription for two drugs: tamoxifen, to slow the cancer, and metronidazole (Flagyl), to heal the open sores on her breast.

Two days later we heard from my father-in-law that Edie had nearly collapsed in town.

Her doctor then started Edie on morphine, since, he told us, she'd asked if she could have something for the pain. 'To be honest,' he added, 'I'd be looking into nursing home care as soon as possible.'

Two days later, Edie was unable to get out of her bathtub and was vomiting so violently that she couldn't eat.

One of the side-effects of metronidazole is a sudden drop in blood-pressure, particularly in the elderly, which could have accounted for Edie's loss of consciousness and falls. Tamoxifen can cause pain, and both Flagyl and morphine cause nausea.

In other words, every symptom she was displaying – besides the breast lumps themselves – appeared to be due mainly to the drugs – and also perhaps to the word 'terminal' on the various forms we were asked to fill in.

We told her to throw her drugs in the bin. Before long we'd managed to get the drugs out of her system, but not her GP's gloomy prognosis.

Fortunately, because of our work we knew of Dr Patrick Kingsley, a medical pioneer in Leicestershire who helped people with a variety of conditions. We didn't know how successful he would be with a case of terminal cancer, but were encouraged to hear that he had a local cancer group consisting of many other no-hopers who were apparently outliving the odds.

We contacted him and he examined Edie. I was in the room with them and he didn't flinch when he saw her breast. 'I think we can handle that,' he said with offhand confidence.

His regime consisted mainly of designing a modified healthy diet and vitamin supplement programme, tailored to the purse and tastes of someone reared on standard British fare, cutting out foods he'd found her to be allergic to and administering large doses of intravenous vitamin C twice a week. Several months later, Edie's GP, who'd delivered the death sentence on her in the first place, came to examine her. He was rendered utterly speechless. The cancer which had ravaged her breast, which he was so sure was beyond hope or treatment, *had completely disappeared*.

For seven years, little 7-stone Edie beat cancer, and we were never sure what exactly in her treatment was responsible. To a great degree, it may have had to do with my mother-in-law's optimism that Patrick would cure her, which in turn had something to do with his imperturbability during that first consultation, his refusal to be discouraged by cancer or to betray any doubt. Or perhaps it was the close rallying of her family round her and the courage of this ordinary pensioner in deciding (for we left it to her) to explore what must have appeared a bizarre and radical course. Some practitioners consider family support and personal commitment key elements in recovery from illness.

Although there is some scientific evidence for Patrick's treatment, I tend to believe that the success of his approach also had to do with the fact that my husband endorsed this treatment option. Edie's youngest son had told her it was going to work, and that was proof enough for her.

Edie did die in the end, after the first edition of this book was published, but it wasn't the cancer that got her. Her husband, 12 years her senior, began failing himself, and she decided at one point that she could no longer leave him on his own while she took the best part of a day travelling to Dr Kingsley's surgery for treatment. She stopped having treatments, and although the cancer reappeared in a limited form, she kept it at bay while tending to her husband. Then, several years later, when he died, she spent a few months staring at her hands. 'I just don't know what to do with myself now,' repeated Edie, who'd spent her life waiting on her partner. Within six months of his death, we buried her, too.

Edie was not the only one of Patrick's successes, however. He has treated hundreds of cancer and multiple sclerosis patients – many of medicine's 'no-hopers' – and been able to reverse the majority of them through his individualized dietary approach.

However, the most essential factor in our minds was Patrick's steadfast refusal to characterize the likely path of Edie's illness – to make a judgement call about 'how long' the illness would linger or how long she would live. Whatever the method, it had the single vital ingredient conspicuously left out of every potion dispensed by most doctors today: hope. Hope is the most important medicine there is. Everyone's confidence gave Edie hope, and hope is what gave her so many years of life.

Hope is what doctors used to provide before they presumed to have the knowledge to determine exactly how many months anybody's got left. Very few doctors have the humility to realize that no scientist, no matter how learned, can predict how a given patient will respond to the challenge of illness and healing, or say with certainty who will live and who will die.

Notes

CHAPTER 1

1. *British Medical Journal*, 1980; 280: 1–2.
2. *The Times*, 1 November 1994.
3. 'Cancer at a Crossroads', National Cancer Advisory Board, 1994; which notes that rates of cancer have increased 18 per cent since 1991 and the mortality rate grown by 7 per cent. See also *Journal of the American Medical Association*, 1990; 264 (24): 3178–83.
4. Dr Vernon Coleman, 'The Betrayal of Trust', *European Medical Journal*, 1994: 4.
5. Figures on the world's first study into hospital safety, carried out by the Australian Department of Health, June 1995.
6. *Journal of the American Medical Association*, 1995; 274 (1): 29–34.
7. *Journal of the American Medical Association*, 2000; 284 (1): 483–5.
8. http://news.independent.co.uk/low_res/story.jsp?story=471139& host=3&dir=505.
9. Edgar A. Suter, correspondence, *The Lancet*, 1993; 342: 112.
10. *New Scientist*, 17 September 1994: 23.
11. Robert S. Mendelsohn, MD, *Confessions of a Medical Heretic* (Chicago: Contemporary Books, 1979): xiii–xiv.
12. See I. Chalmer, M. Enkin and M. Keirse (eds), *Effective Care in Pregnancy and Childbirth* (Oxford: Oxford University Press, 1989).
13. *New England Journal of Medicine*, 1992; 326: 501–6; also 560–1. See also *Adverse Drug Reaction Bulletin*, June 1992 and *The Lancet*, 1993; 342: 818–19.

14. *The Lancet*, 1994; 344: 844–51.
15. *The Daily Telegraph*, 23 September 1994.
16. *Journal of the American Medical Association*, 1993; 269: 873–7, 878–82.
17. Interview with Norman Begg, December 1989.
18. *The Lancet*, 1993; 341: 343–5.
19. *The Lancet*, 1994; 344: 1601–6.
20. *The Lancet*, 1994; 344: 1585.

CHAPTER 2

1. Stephen Fulder, *How to Be a Healthy Patient* (London: Hodder and Stoughton, 1991): 26.
2. *The Lancet*, 1989; ii: 1190–1.
3. *The Lancet*, 1994; 344: 1339–43.
4. *The Lancet*, 1994; 344: 1309–11.
5. Mark Brown et al., correspondence, *British Medical Journal*, 1991; 303: 120–1.
6. *Behavioral Medicine*, Spring 1999; 25 (1): 13–22.
7. *Blood Pressure. Supplement*, 1997; 2: 91–6.
8. Ibid.
9. *British Medical Journal*, 1992; 305: 1062–6.
10. *Journal of Hypertension*, 1994; 12: 857–66.
11. *Annali Italiani di Medicina Interna*, Jan.–Mar. 2000; 15(1): 63–9.
12. *British Medical Journal*, 2001; 322: 531–36.
13. *Journal of Hypertension*, 1999; 17: 193–200.
14. *Clinical and Experimental Hypertension,* 1993; 15: 895–909.
15. *Blood Pressure Monitoring*, 1999; 4: 319–31.
16. *Blood Press Monitoring*, 2000; 5: 131–5.
17. Barnabus N. Panayiotou, correspondence, *Journal of the American Medical Association*, 1995; 274 (17): 1343.
18. M. J. Quinn, correspondence, *The Lancet*, 1991; 338: 130.
19. *The Lancet*, 1996; 347: 139–42.
20. *American Journal of Hypertension*, 2002: February 15 (2 Pt 2): 38S–42S.
21. *Archives of Pathology and Laboratory Medicine*, 1993; 117: 393–400.
22. *Health Devices*, 1990; 19: 343–71.

23. *Canadian Family Physician*, Feb. 1995; 41: 240–5.

24. *Archives of Internal Medicine*, 1995; 13; 155: 2146–7.

25. Robert Mendelsohn, *Confessions of a Medical Heretic* (Chicago: Contemporary Books, 1979): 2.

26. Dr Edward D. Folland, correspondence, *New England Journal of Medicine*, 1992; 327 (25): 1819; *New England Journal of Medicine*, 1992; 327: 458–62.

27. Mendelsohn, *Confessions*: 3.

28. Fulder, *Healthy Patient*: 26.

29. *The Lancet*, 1994; 344: 1190–2.

30. *Journal of Ultrasound in Medicine*, 2002; 21: 1347–56; discussion 1343–45.

31. *Echocardiography*, 2002 Aug; 19 (6): 495–500.

32. *Ultrasound in Medicine and Biology*, Mar. 2003; 29 (3): 473–81.

33. *Journal of the American Medical Association*, 1992; 268: 2537–40.

34. J. Isner, *Circulation*, 1981; 63 (5), as quoted in S. Fulder, *How to Survive Medical Treatment* (London: Century Hutchinson, 1987): 24, 27.

35. *Journal of the American Medical Association*, 14 April, and 28 April 1993.

36. *American Journal of Roentgenology*, Jun. 2001; 176 (6): 1385–8.

37. *Journal of Clinal Pharmacy and Therapeutics*, 2003; 28: 505–12.

38. *European Journal of Radiology*, May 1994; 18 (supplement 1): S115–9.

39. *The Lancet*, 2002; 359: 1037–8.

40. *The Lancet*, 2002; 359: 1643–7.

41. R. Wootton (ed.), *Radiation Protection of Patients* (Cambridge: Cambridge University Press, 1993): 16.

42. Ibid.

43. *The Lancet*, 2004; 363: 345–51.

44. *Journal of the American Medical Association*, 1991; 265 (10): 1290.

45. R. Wootton, op cit.

46. *Journal of the American Medical Association*, 1991; 265 (10): 1290.

47. *International Journal of Cancer*, 1990; 46: 362–5.

48. *British Journal of Cancer*, 1990; 62 (1): 152–68.

49. *New Scientist*, 1979; 82: 18, as reported in Fulder, *Medical Treatment*: 35.

50. Dr John Gofman, *Preventing Breast Cancer*, published by the Committee for Nuclear Responsibility, Inc., San Francisco, CA.
51. *New England Journal of Medicine*, 1993; 328 (2): 87–94.
52. *Journal of the American Medical Association*, 1994; 272 (15): 1160.
53. *Journal of Epidemiology and Community Health*, 1995; 49: 164–70.
54. Fulder, *Medical Treatment*: 29.
55. *British Medical Journal*, 1991; 303: 813–15.
56. *British Medical Journal*, 1991; 303: 811–12.
57. *British Medical Journal*, 1991; 303: 813–15.
58. FDA Consumer, January 1980, as cited in Fulder, *Medical Treatment*: 30.
59. Royal College of Radiologists and National Radiological Protection Board, 'Patient dose reduction in diagnostic radiology', (HMSO, 1990), as reported in *British Medical Journal*, 1991; 303: 812
60. *Journal of the American Medical Association*, 1991; 265 (10): 1290.
61. J. G. B. Russell, consultant radiologist, position paper, 'Reactions to the Recommendations from the Royal College of Radiologists': 1.
62. Russell, 'Reactions': 2.
63. *British Medical Journal*, 2001; 322: 400–5; *Journal of the American Medical Association*, 2000; 284: 2727–32, 2780–1.
64. *Journal of Neurology, Neurosurgery and Psychiatry*, 2000; 68: 416–22.
65. *The Lancet*, 1999; 353: 319–20.
66. *The Lancet*, 1989; ii: 1190–1.
67. *British Medical Journal*, 1991; 303: 809–12.
68. *Which?*, January, 1991: 41.
69. *British Medical Journal*, 1992; 304: 1411.
70. As reported in *The Independent*, 27 April 1990.
71. *British Medical Journal*, 1991; 303: 1497.
72. *Radiology*, 1977; 123: 523–7.
73. *New England Journal of Medicine*, 1994; 331 (21): 1449–50.
74. *The Lancet*, 2002; 359: 1037–8.
75. *Mount Sinai Journal of Medicine*, 1991; 58 (2): 183–7.
76. Charles V. Burton, 'Lumbo–Sacral Adhesive Arachnoiditis: the Modern New Guinea Syndrome'. Position paper: 9.
77. P. G. Bain and A. C. F. Colchester, correspondence, *The Lancet*, 1991; 338: 252–3.

78. K. Noda et al., correspondence, *The Lancet*, 1991; 337: 681.

79. *Mount Sinai Journal of Medicine*, 1991; 58 (2): 185–6.

80. Susan M. Ott, editorial, *British Medical Journal*, 1994; 308: 931–2.

81. Ibid.

82. David M. Reid et al., correspondence, *British Medical Journal*, 1994; 308: 1567.

83. 66th Annual Meeting of the American Academy of Orthopedic Surgeons, 1999.

84. *British Medical Journal*, 1996; 312: 296–7.

85. Angela Raffle and Cyrus Cooper, correspondence, *The Lancet*, 1990; 336: 242; Albert M. Van Hemert, correspondence, *The Lancet*, 1990; 336: 818.

86. *British Medical Journal*, 1996; 312: 1254–8.

87. Wootton, *Radiation Protection*: 2; also *The Lancet*, 1992; 340: 299.

88. *Radiology*, 2004; 232: 735–8

89. *American Journal of Roentgenology*, 2001; 176: 289–96.

90. *The Lancet*, 1976; i: 847–8. See also Joseph K. Lee (ed.), *Computed Body Tomography with MRI Correlation* (New York: Raven Press, 1989): 1117–18.

91. *British Medical Journal*, 1993; 306: 953–5.

92. *Lakartidningen*, March 11 1992.

93. *British Medical Journal*, 1994; 309: 986–9.

94. *New England Journal of Medicine*, 1994; 330: 25–30.

95. *American Journal of Public Health*, 1993; 83 (4): 588–90.

96. *RoFo. Fortschritte auf dem Gebiete der Rontgenstrahlen und der neuen bildgebenden Verfahren*, 1992; 156 (2): 189–92.

97. *British Medical Journal*, 1991; 303: 205.

98. *The Lancet*, 2002; 359: 1643–7.

99. *Radiology*, 1991; 178: 447–51.

100. Joseph Lee, *Computed Body*: 1119.

101. *New England Journal of Medicine*, 1993; 328 (12): 879–80.

102. *New England Journal of Medicine*, 1990; 323 (10): 621–6.

103. *Chicago Tribune*, 13 May 1984, as reported in *The People's Doctor*, 10 (11).

104. *Oral Surgery, Oral Medicine and Oral Pathology*, 1993; 76 (5): 655–60.

105. *Acta Oto-Laryngologica*, 1993; 113 (4): 483–8.

106. *British Medical Journal*, 1991; 303: 205.

107. Karl Dantendorfer et al., correspondence, *The Lancet*, 1991; 338: 761–2.

108. *IEEE Transactions on Biomedical Engineering*, 1993; 40 (12): 1324–7; *American Journal of Physical Medicine and Rehabilitation*, 1993; 72 (3): 166–7.

109. *American Journal of Roentgenology*, 1994; 162 (1): 189–94.

110. *American Journal of Roentgenology*, 1990; 154 (6): 1229–32.

111. *Journal of Magnetic Resonance Imaging*, 1992; 2 (6): 721–8.

112. *American Journal of Roentgenology*, 1990; 154 (6): 1229–32.

113. *The British Journal of Radiology*, 1984; 57: 1091–6.

114. Stephen Fulder, *Medical Treatment*: 24.

115. *The Lancet*, 1989; ii: 1190–1.

116. *British Medical Journal*, 1979; ii: 21–4.

117. *British Medical Journal*, 1994; 309: 983–6.

118. *Medical Hypotheses*, 1988; 25: 151–62.

119. *Nature*, 1985; 317: 395–403; *The Lancet*, 1989; ii: 1023–5.

120. *New England Journal of Medicine*, 1988; 318: 448–9.

121. Abstracts,VII International Conference on AIDS (Florence, Italy, 1991); 1: 326.

122. As reported in *The Sunday Times*, 22 May 1994.

123. *New England Journal of Medicine*, 1986; 314: 647.

124. *The Lancet*, 1986; i: 1090–2.

125. *AIDS*, 1988; 2: 405–6.

126. *Gut*, 1995; 36: 462–7.

127. *Gut*, 1995; 36: 462–7.

128. *Gut*, 1983; 24: 171–4; *Journal of Clinical Gastroenterology*, 1999; 28: 290.

129. *Endoscopy*, 1995; 27: 139–40.

130. *Journal of the American College of Surgeons*, 2001; 192: 478–91.

131. *Journal of the Society of Laparoendoscopic Surgeons*, 1999; 3: 331–4.

132. *Journal of the American College of Surgeons*, 2001; 192: 677–83.

133. *British Medical Journal*, Feb. 1998; 316: 562.

134. Charles Williams and Norman Frost, correspondence, *The Lancet*, 1994; 344: 1086–7.

135. *British Medical Journal*, 1993; 306: 953–5.

136. *Molecular Urology*, 2000; 4: 93–7.

137. *The Journal of Urology*, 1995; 153: 1543–8.

138. *What Doctors Don't Tell You*, 2004; 15 (1): 10–11.

139. *British Medical Journal* (Clinical Research Ed.), 1988; 288: 1254–6.

140. *American Journal of Roentgenology*, 1999; 173: 1303–13.

141. *Diseases of the Colon and Rectum*, 2003; 46: 454–8.

142. *Canadian Family Physician*, Feb. 1995; 41: 240–5.

143. *RoFo. Fortschritte auf dem Gebiete der Rontgenstrahlen und der neuen bildgebenden Verfahren*, Feb. 1992.

CHAPTER 3

1. Dr Christopher R. B. Merritt, editorial, *Radiology*, 1989; 173 (2): 304–6.

2. *Journal of the American Medical Association*, 1982; 247 (16): 2196.

3. *Acta Obstetricia et Gynecologica Scandinavica*, 1998; 77: 635–42.

4. *Acta Obstetricia et Gynecologica Scandinavica*, 1998; 77: 643–89.

5. *Mother and Baby*, May 1990: 20–2.

6. Ibid.

7. American College of Obstetricians and Gynecologists, Technical Bulletin No. 63, October 1981, as quoted in *Journal of Nurse-Midwifery*, 1984; 29 (4): 241–4.

8. Statement, Doris Haire, Chairman, Committee on Maternal and Child Health, National Women's Health Network, Diagnostic Ultrasound Education Workshop, April 26–28, 1990, Baltimore, MD.

9. *British Medical Journal*, 1993; 307: 13–17.

10. *New England Journal of Medicine*, 1993; 329 (12): 821–7.

11. Dr Richard Berkowitz, editorial, *New England Journal of Medicine*, 1993; 329 (12): 874–5.

12. *The Lancet*, 1992; 340: 1299–1303.

13. *The Lancet*, 1990; 336: 387–91.

14. *Journal of Epidemiology and Community Health*, 1990; 44: 196–201.

15. *American Journal of Obstetrics and Gynecology*, 1990; 162: 1603–10.

16. *British Medical Journal*, 1993; 307: 159–64.

17. *Epidemiology*, 2001; 12: 618.

18. *The Lancet*, 1993; 342: 887–91.
19. *Canadian Medical Association Journal*, 1993; 149 (10): 1435–40.
20. International Childbirth Education Association (ICEA) position paper: Diagnostic Ultrasound in Obstetrics, International Childbirth Education Association, March 1983.
21. Ibid.
22. *Obstetrics and Gynecology*, 1984; 63: 194–200.
23. *British Medical Journal*, 1975; 2: 62–4.
24. Presentation at the Annual Meeting of the Acoustical Society of America, Fort Lauderdale, FL, 2001.
25. *Journal of Nurse-Midwifery*, 1984; 29 (4): 241–6.
26. Robert Bases, correspondence, *British Journal of Obstetrics and Gynaecology*, 1988; 95: 730.
27. *Journal of the American Medical Association*, 1982; 247 (16): 2195–7.
28. Ibid.
29. ICEA position paper, op cit.
30. *British Journal of Obstetrics and Gynaecology*, 1982; 89: 694–700.
31. *Obstetrics and Gynecology*, 1983; 62: 7–10.
32. HHS Publication FDA 82-8190, July 1982, Bureau of Radiological Health, Food and Drug Administration, as cited in ICEA position paper, op cit.
33. *Obstetrics and Gynecology*, 1984; 64 (1): 101–7.
34. *The People's Doctor*, 11 (1): 7.
35. *British Medical Journal*, 1993; 307: 13–17.
36. *The Lancet*, 1998; 352: 1567–8, 1577–81.
37. *Acta Obstetricia et Gynecologica Scandinavica*, 1998; 177: 635–42.
38. *Acta Obstetricia et Gynecologica Scandinavica*, 1998; 77: 643–89.
39. *The Lancet*, 1998; 352: 1567–8, 1577–81.
40. *The Lancet*, 1990; 336: 387–91.
41. *Daily Mirror*, 3 June 1994.
42. *Journal of the American Medical Association*, 2001; 285: 1044–55.
43. *British Medical Journal*, 2001; 322: 1457–62.
44. *New England Journal of Medicine*, 1990; 322: 588–93.
45. *New England Journal of Medicine*, 1996; 334 (10): 613–18.
46. See *British Journal of Obstetrics and Gynaecology*, 1982; 89: 716–22; *British Journal of Obstetrics and Gynaecology*, 1982; 89: 427–33; *British*

Journal of Obstetrics and Gynaecology, 1983; 90: 1018–26 and *British Journal of Obstetrics and Gynaecology*, 1985; 92: 1156–9.

47. *What Doctors Don't Tell You*, 1990; 1 (6): 6.

48. Mr Chalmers recommends that readers consult the *Journal of Perinatal Medicine*, 1984; 12: 227–33 and P. Mohide and M. Keirse, 'Biophysical assessment of fetal wellbeing', in I. Chalmers et al., *Effective Care in Pregnancy and Childbirth* (Oxford: Oxford University Press, 1989).

49. Helen Klein Ross, *Mothering Magazine*, Summer 1990.

50. *British Medical Journal*, 1981; 282: 1416–18 as cited in Belinda Barnes and Suzanne Gail Bradley, *Planning for a Healthy Baby* (London: Vermilion, 1990): 164.

51. *American Family Physician*, 2002; 65: 915–20, 922.

52. *Obstetrics and Gynecology*, 1989; 74: 17–20.

53. *British Medical Journal*, January 13, 1996.

54. Roger Williams et al., correspondence, *The Lancet*, 1986; ii: 757, as cited in *The People's Doctor*, 11 (1): 3.

55. Ross, op cit.

56. Leaflet handed out by obstetric unit, St John's & St Elizabeth's Hospital, London, 1993.

57. *Prenat Diagn*, 1991; 11: 381–5.

58. *The Lancet*, 1991; 337: 1491–9.

59. Froas J. Los et al., correspondence, *The Lancet*, 1993; 342: 1559.

60. *The Lancet*, 1991; 337: 1491–9.

61. Karin Sundberg and Steen Smidt-Jensen, correspondence, *The Lancet*, 1991; 337: 1233–4.

62. M. J. Le Bris, correspondence, *The Lancet*, 1994; 344: 556.

63. *The Lancet*, 1991; 337: 762–3.

64. *The Lancet*, 1991; 337: 1091.

65. *The Lancet*, 1994; 343: 1069–71.

66. Ibid.

67. *The Lancet*, 1998; 351: 242–247.

68. *The Lancet*, 1994; 344: 435–9.

69. F. P. H. A. Vandenbussche et al., correspondence, *The Lancet*, 1994; 344: 1032.

70. *The Lancet*, 1994; 344: 1134–6.

71. Name supplied, Barking, Essex, *The Spectator*, 8 July 1995.

72. Robert Mendelsohn, *Male Practice: How Doctors Manipulate Women* (Chicago: Contemporary Books, 1981): 54.

73. *British Medical Journal*, 1994; 309: 158–62.

74. *Journal of Epidemiology and Community Health*, 1995; 49: 164–70.

75. *The Lancet*, 1990; 353: 7467–50.

76. Mortality and Morbidity Weekly Report, 1994; 43: 617–22.

77. Janet Carr, *Down's Syndrome* (Cambridge: Cambridge University Press, 1995).

78. Barnes and Bradley, op cit.

79. *What Doctors Don't Tell You*, 1997; 7 (12).

CHAPTER 4

1. *British Medical Journal*, 1992; 304: 463.

2. *The Lancet*, 1993; 341: 343.

3. Johannes Schmidt, correspondence, *The Lancet*, 1992; 339: 810.

4. *American Journal of Obstetrics and Gynecology*, 1941; 42: 193–205.

5. J. McCormick and P. Skrabanek, *Follies and Fallacies in Medicine* (Glasgow: The Tarragon Press, 1989): 103–4.

6. J. McCormick, 'Dogma Disputed', *The Lancet*, 1989; ii: 207–9.

7. *The Lancet*, 1990; 335: 97–9.

8. J. McCormick, op cit.

9. Vernon Coleman, *The Health Scandal: Your Health in Crisis* (London: Sidgwick & Jackson, 1988): 171.

10. *The Lancet*, 1993; 342: 91–6.

11. A. B. Miller, 'Evaluation of Screening for carcinoma of the cervix', *Modern Medicine Canada*, 1973; 28: 1067–9.

12. McCormick and Skrabanek, *Follies*: 104

13. Ibid.

14. Tom Bell, correspondence, *The Lancet*, 1990; 336: 1260–1.

15. *The Lancet*, 1995; 345: 1469–73.

16. Ibid.

17. *British Medical Journal*, 1986; 293: 659–63.

18. *Morbidity and Mortality Weekly Report*, 2000; 49: 1001–3.

19. McCormick, 'Dogma': 208.

20. *British Medical Journal*, 1988; 297: 18–21.
21. *The Lancet*, 1992; 339: 828.
22. *British Medical Journal*, 1993; 306: 1173.
23. *British Medical Journal*, 1986; 293: 659–63, as cited in *The Lancet*, 1990; 335: 97–9.
24. McCormick, op cit.
25. National Audit Office report, 'Cervical and Breast Screening in England', 1992.
26. *The Daily Telegraph*, 29 April 1993.
27. Coleman, *The Health Scandal*: 172.
28. Robert Mendelsohn, MD, *Male Practice: How Doctors Manipulate Women* (Chicago: Contemporary Books, 1981): 42–3.
29. National Audit Office report, op cit.
30. *The Lancet*, 1993; 342: 91–6.
31. *British Medical Journal*, 2003, 326: 733.
32. *What Doctors Don't Tell You*, 2004; 14 (11): 1–4.
33. *British Medical Journal*, 1995; 311: 1391–5.
34. M. Baum, correspondence, *The Lancet*, 1995; 346: 436; see also correspondence, *New England Journal of Medicine*, 1994; 331: 402–3.
35. *The Lancet*, 1993; 341: 1509–11.
36. Ibid.
37. *Journal of the American Medical Association*, 1994; 271 (2): 96.
38. J. A. Muir Gray et al., correspondence, *British Medical Journal*, 1991; 302: 1084.
39. Petr Skrabanek and James McCormick, correspondence, *British Medical Journal*, 1991; 302: 1401.
40. N. Wald et al., correspondence, *British Medical Journal*, 1991; 302: 845.
41. Skrabanek and McCormick, op cit.
42. *The Lancet*, 1995; 346: 29–32.
43. Ibid.
44. Ibid.
45. *The Lancet*, 2002, 359: 909–19; *The Lancet*, 2000; 356: 1087.
46. *British Medical Journal*, 2002; 324: 432.
47. *New England Journal of Medicine*, 1998; 338: 1089–96.
48. *Cancer*, 1997; 80: 720–4.
49. Johannes G. Schmidt, correspondence, *The Lancet*, 1992; 339: 810.

50. *Canadian Journal of Public Health*, 1993; 84: 14–16.

51. Michael Swift, correspondence, *The Lancet*, 1992; 340: 1538.

52. J. Mark Elwood, Brian Cox and Ann K. Richardson, correspondence, *The Lancet*, 1993; 341: 1531.

53. *British Medical Journal*, 1988; 297: 943–8.

54. Rob Boer et al., correspondence, *The Lancet*, 1994; 343: 979.

55. Schmidt, op cit.

56. *The Lancet*, 1992; 339: 810.

57. *Journal of the American Medical Association*, 1990; 263: 2341–3.

58. *Journal of the American Medical Association*, 1996; 275: 913–18. See also Cecily Quinn and Julian Ostrowski, correspondence, *The Lancet*, 1996; 347: 1259.

59. Personal interview with Dr James McCormick, 12 June 1996; see also *The Lancet*, 1994; 343: 969.

60. Mendelsohn, *Male Practice*: 110.

61. The Royal College of Radiologists, 'Making the best use of a Department of Clinical Radiology', London, 1993: 33–7.

62. *Glamour*, October 1992; see also *The Daily Telegraph*, 28 December 1991.

63. D. J. Watmough and K. M. Quan, correspondence, *The Lancet*, 1992; 340: 122.

64. E. J. Roebuck, correspondence, *The Lancet*, 1992; 340: 366.

65. J. P. van Netten et al., correspondence, *The Lancet*, 1994; 343: 978–9.

66. *Ultrasound in Medicine and Biology*, 1979; 5: 45–9.

67. J. Michael Dixon and T. G. John, correspondence, *The Lancet*, 1992; 339: 128.

68. J. Stevenson, correspondence, *British Medical Journal*, 1991; 303: 924.

69. Nicholas E. Day and Stephen W Duffy, correspondence, *The Lancet*, 1991; 338: 113–14.

70. *What Doctors Don't Tell You*, 1990; 1 (2): 4.

71. *British Medical Journal*, 1994; 308: 79.

72. D. Sienko et al., correspondence, *New England Journal of Medicine*, 1989; 320: 941.

73. *Journal of the American Medical Association*, 1993; 269 (20): 2616–17.

74. Graham Curtis Jenkins, correspondence, *British Medical Journal*, 1992; 305: 718.

75. *British Medical Journal*, 1994; 308.

76. Ibid.

77. Syed Bilgramia and Bernard Greenberg, commentary, *The Lancet*, 1994; 344: 700–1.

78. *Seminars in Urologic Oncology*, 1996; 14: 134–8.

79. *Journal of the American Medical Association*, 1995; 273: 289–94.

80. *New England Journal of Medicine*, 2003; 349: 335–42.

81. *Brazil Journal of Urology International*, 2000; 85: 1078–84.

82. *Urology*, 1996; 47: 511–16.

83. *The Lancet*, 1998; 351: 1563.

84. *British Medical Journal*, 1992; 304: 534.

85. Dr Joan Austoker, adviser to Britain's Chief Medical Officer, as quoted in *The Sunday Times*, 6 October 1991.

86. Daniel Kopans, correspondence, *The Lancet*, 1991; 338: 447.

87. *New England Journal of Medicine*, 1998; 338: 1089–96.

88. *Radiation Medicine*, 1994; 12 (5): 201–8.

89. *Anticancer Research*, 1994; 14 (5B): 2249–51.

90. *Geburtshilfe und Frauenheilkunde*, 1994; 54 (8): 432–6.

91. *Ultraschall in der Medizin*, 1994; 15 (1): 20–3.

92. *Journal of Clinical Pathology*, 1949; 2: 197–208, as cited in *The Lancet*, 1993; 341: 91.

CHAPTER 5

1. *The Lancet*, 1994; 344: 1182–6.

2. *British Medical Journal*, 1994; 309: 11–15.

3. *Circulation*, 1970; (Supplement 1): 1–211.

4. *Journal of the American Medical Association*, 1995; 274 (2): 131–6.

5. *The Lancet*, 1994; 344: 963–4.

6. *Atlantic*, Sept. 1989: 37–70.

7. *Journal of the American Medical Association*, 1995; 273 (24): 1926–32.

8. *Journal of the American Medical Association*, 1994; 272 (17): 1335–40.

9. *Atherosclerosis*, 1995; 117: 107–18; *Arteriosclerosis*, 1992; 12: 416–23.

10. *The Daily Telegraph*, 16 April 1993.

11. *Atherosclerosis Review*, 1983; 11: 157–246.

12. *The Lancet*, 1997; 350: 1119–23.

13. *The Lancet*, 1994; 344: 1383–9.

14. *Monitor Weekly*, 30 November 1994: 17.

15. *New England Journal of Medicine*, 1995; 333: 1301–7.

16. *Circulation*, 1995; 92: 2419–25; also *Journal of the American College of Cardiology*, 1995; 26: 1133–9.

17. Jan P Vandenbroucke, Rudi G. J. Westendorp, correspondence, *The Lancet*, 1996; 347: 1267–8.

18. Robert J. MacFadyen et al., correspondence, *The Lancet*, 1996; 347: 551–2.

19. R. Fey and N. Pearson, essay, *The Lancet*, 1996; 347: 1389–90.

20. William E. Stehbens, correspondence, *The Lancet*, 1995; 345: 264.

21. Vandenbroucke and Westendorp, op cit.

22. *Journal Watch*, 1995; 15 (24): 190, and 15 (23): 181–2.

23. Dr Nilesh J. Samani and David P. De Bono, correspondence, *New England Journal of Medicine*, 1996; 334 (20): 1333–4.

24. *New England Journal of Medicine*, 1996; 335: 1001–9.

25. *Journal of the American Medical Association* 1998; 278: 1615–22.

26. *New England Journal of Medicine*, 1998; 339: 1349–57.

27. *The Lancet*, 2002; 360: 7–33.

28. *The Lancet*, 2000; 355: 2185–8.

29. *New England Journal of Medicine*, 2000; 343: 317–26.

30. *Nature Med*, 2000; 6: 1004–10.

31. *Journal of the American Medical Association*, 2001; 285: 1850–5, 1888–9.

32. *Circulation*, 1992; 85: 1792–8.

33. *Journal Watch*, 1996; 16 (10): 83–4.

34. Donald R. Davis, Ph.D., correspondence, *New England Journal of Medicine*, 1996; 334 (20): 1334.

35. *Journal of the American Medical Association*, 1995; 274 (14): 1152–8.

36. Rodney Jackson and Robert Beaglehole, commentary, *The Lancet*, 1995; 346: 1440–1.

37. *British Medical Journal*, 1994; 308: 373–9.

38. *Annals of Pharmacotherapy*, 2002; 36: 288–95.

39. *Annals of Internal Medicine*, 2002; 137: 581–5.

40. *British Medical Journal*, 1997; 315: 31.

41. *Annals of Pharmacotherapy*, 2003; 37; 274–8.

42. *Neurology*, 2002; 14: 1333–7.

43. *Proceedings of the National Academy of Sciences of the United States of America*, 1985; 82: 901–4.

44. *Biofactors*, 1999; 9: 291–9.

45. Arzneim Forsch, 1999; 49: 324–9.

46. Drs George Davey Smith and Julia Pekkanen, debate, *British Medical Journal*, 1992; 304: 431–3.

47. *British Medical Journal*, 1995; 310: 1632–6.

48. *The Lancet*, 1993; 341: 75–9.

49. Bruno Bertozzi et al., correspondence, *British Medical Journal*, 1996; 312: 1298–9.

50. *The Lancet*, 1993; 341: 75–9.

51. *Psychological Medicine*, 1990; 20: 785–91.

52. Dr Melvyn Werbach, *Nutritional Influences on Mental Illness* (Tarzana, CA: Third Line Press, 1991): 145–9.

53. *Archives of Internal Medicine*, 1995; 155: 695–700.

54. M. R. Law and N. J. Wald, correspondence, *British Medical Journal*, 1995; 311: 807.

55. *American Journal of Clinical Nutrition*,1995; 62: 1–9. See also *What Doctors Don't Tell You*, 1995; 6 (6): 1–3.

56. *Journal of the American Medical Association*, 1996; 275: 55. See also *Journal Watch*, 1996; 16 (10): 83–4.

57. Newman and Hulley, correspondence, *Journal of the American Medical Association*, 1996; 275: 1481–2.

58. *New England Journal of Medicine*, 1996; 335: 1001–9.

59. *The Lancet*, 1990; 336: 129–33.

60. *Journal of the American Medical Association*, 1995; 274: 894–901.

61. *The Lancet*, 1992; 339: 563–9.

62. *New England Journal of Medicine*, 1996; 334 (20): 1298–1303.

63. *Circulation*, 1996; 93: 1346–53.

64. *The Lancet*, 1999; 353: 1045–8.

65. M. Montignac, *Eat Yourself Slim – and Stay Slim!* (UK, Montignac Publishing, 1999).

66. Drs Edward Siguel et al., correspondence, *Journal of the American Medical Association*, 1996; 275 (10): 759.

67. *The Lancet*, 1994; 343: 1268–71.

68. Ibid.

69. *Journal of Lipid Mediators*, 1992; 33: 399–410.

70. *British Journal of Preventive and Social Medicine*, 1975; 29: 82–90.

71. *The Lancet*, 1993; 341: 581–5.

72. *Townsend Letter for Doctors*, 1995; 139/40: 68–70.

73. *The Lancet*, 1995; 345: 273–8.

74. *Journal of Nutritional Medicine*, 1991; 2: 227–47.

75. *New England Journal of Medicine*, 1985; 312 (5): 283–9, as quoted in *Journal of Nutritional Medicine*, 1991; 2: 227–47.

76. *Journal of Nutritional Medicine*, 1991; 2: 227–47.

77. *American Journal of Epidemiology*, 1983; 117: 384–96.

78. L. Galland, *The Four Pillars of Healing* (New York: Random House, 1997): 103–5.

79. *American Journal of Epidemiology*, 1979; 109: 186–204; *American Journal of Epidemiology*, 1988; 128: 370–80.

CHAPTER 6

1. National Vaccine Information Center News, August 1994, as quoted in *Campaign Against Fraudulent Medical Research Newsletter*, Spring/Summer 1994; 2 (2): 10.

2. Correspondence, February 1994, between DOH and National Immunization Program, confirmed by interview with Mark Papania of the US National Immunization Program, October 1994.

3. *The Lancet*, 1995; 345: 567–9.

4. *Journal of Infectious Diseases*, 1999; 179: 1569–72.

5. Gordon Stewart, *World Medicine*, Sept. 1994: 17–20.

6. Personal interview with Dr J. Anthony Morris, December 1989.

7. *Journal of Pediatrics*, 1973; 82: 798–801.

8. *The Lancet*, 1995; 345: 963–5.

9. *Campaign Against Fraudulent Medical Research Newsletter*, 1995; 2 (3): 5–13, quoting statistics from the 'London Bills of Mortality 1760–1834' and 'Reports of the Registrar General 1838–96', as compiled in Alfred Wallace, *The Wonderful Century*, 1898.

10. *Bulletin of the World Health Organization*, 1975; 52: 209–22.

11. Derrick Baxby, correspondence, *British Medical Journal*, 1995; 310: 62.

12. Walene James, *Immunization: The Reality Behind the Myth* (South Hadley, MA: Bergin & Garvey, 1988): 26–7.

13. Neil Z. Miller, *Vaccines: Are They Really Safe and Effective?* (Santa Fe, NM: New Atlantean Press, 1992): 20.

14. James, *Immunization*: 27–8.

15. James, *Immunization*: 32.

16. *Health Freedom News*, Jan. 1983: 26, as quoted in James, *Immunization*: 28.

17. *The Herbalist New Health*, July 1981: 61, as quoted in James, *Immunization*: 28.

18. Richard Moskowitz, 'Immunization: The Other Side', *in Vaccinations: The Rest of the Story* (Santa Fe, NM: Mothering, 1992): 89.

19. *Science*, 1978; 200: 905, as quoted in Miller, *Vaccines*: 32.

20. Miller, *Vaccines*: 24, 33.

21. Michael Alderson, *International Mortality Statistics: Facts on File* (Washington, DC, 1981): 182–3, as quoted in Miller, *Vaccines:* 25.

22. Report from the Office of Population Censuses and Surveys, 1993, as reported in *The Independent*, 10 August 1993.

23. *Journal of the American Medical Association*, 1993; 269 (2): 227–31; also 269 (2): 264–6.

24. *The Lancet*, 1997; 349: 1197–1201.

25. Personal interview with Norman Begg, December 1989.

26. *Journal of the American Medical Association*, 1972; 220: 959–62.

27. *American Journal of Epidemiology*, 1980; iii (4): 415–24.

28. *The Lancet*, 1986; i: 1169–73; *British Medical Journal*, 1932; 2: 708–11, as reported in *Townsend Letter for Doctors*, Jan. 1996: 29. Also, *New England Journal of Medicine*, 1990; 323: 160–4.

29. *British Medical Journal*, 1998; 316: 561.

30. *World Medicine*, Sept. 1984: 20.

31. Ibid.

32. Moskowitz, *Vaccinations*: 92.

33. *Drugs*, 1998; 55: 347–66.

34. *Journal of Pediatrics*, 1974; 84: 474–8.

35. *The Lancet*, 1977; i: 234–7.

36. *World Medicine*, Sept. 1984: 20.

37. Gordon Stewart, correspondence, *British Medical Journal*, 1983; 287: 287–8.
38. *New England Journal of Medicine*, 1994; 331: 16–21.
39. Personal interview with Dr J. Anthony Morris, April 1992.
40. *World Medicine*, Sept. 1984: 19.
41. Dr J. Anthony Morris, testimony before the Subcommittee on Investigations and General Oversight, May 1982.
42. *Journal of the American Medical Association*, 1995; 274 (6): 446–7.
43. *CDR Weekly*, 21 June 2001; *Infection Control and Hospital Epidemiology*, 1999; 20: 120–3; *Can Communicable Disease Report*, 1995; 15: 45–8; *Communicable Diseases Intelligence*, 1997; 21: 145–8.
44. *Morbidity and Mortality Weekly Report*, 2002; 51: 73–6.
45. *Morbidity and Mortality Weekly Report*, 2002; 51: 73–6.
46. *New England Journal of Medicine*, 1995; 333: 1045–50.
47. *The Lancet*, 1996; 347: 209–10.
48. November 20–21, 1975, Minutes of the 15th meeting of the Panel of Review of Bacterial Vaccines and Toxoids with Standards and Potency (Bureau of Biologics and Food and Drug Administration), as quoted in Robert Mendelsohn, *But Doctor ... About that Shot* (Evanston, IL: The People's Doctor, Inc., 1988): 6.
49. *The Lancet*, 1995; 345: 963–5.
50. *Zhurnel Mikrobiologii, Epidemiologii i Immunobilogii*, 1994; 3: 57–61.
51. Mendelsohn, op cit.
52. Centers for Disease Control Mortality and Morbidity Weekly Report, June 6 1986, as reported in Mendelsohn, *But Doctor*. 81.
53. *Annals of Internal Medicine*, 1979; 90 (6): 978–80.
54. *New England Journal of Medicine*, 1987; 316: 771–4.
55. Centers for Disease Control Mortality and Morbidity Weekly Report, June 6, 1986, as reported in Mendelsohn, *But Doctor*. 81.
56. *New England Journal of Medicine*, 1989; 320 (2): 75–81.
57. *Pediatric Infectious Disease Journal*, 1994; 13: 34–8.
58. *Scandinavian Journal of Infectious Diseases*, 1996; 28: 235–8.
59. *Journal of Infectious Diseases*, 1994; 169: 77–82.
60. Dr Stanley Plotkin, professor of Pediatrics, University of Pennsylvania School of Medicine, as quoted in Mendelsohn, *But Doctor*. 12.

61. M. G. Cusi et al., correspondence, *The Lancet*, 1990; 336: 1071.

62. *Pediatric Infectious Disease Journal*, 1996; 15: 687–92.

63. *The Lancet*, 6 April 1996.

64. *Acta Paediatrica*, 1994; 83: 674–7.

65. Minnesota epidemiologist Michael Ostenholm, as reported in St. Paul Pioneer Press Despatch, quoted in Mendelsohn, *But Doctor*: 87.

66. *The Lancet*, 1991; 338: 274–7.

67. *British Medical Journal*, 2000; 321: 731–2.

68. *New England Journal of Medicine*, 1997; 337: 970–6.

69. *The Lancet*, 1994; 344: 630–1.

70. Ibid.

71. James, op cit.

72. S. O. Cameron et al., correspondence, *British Medical Journal*, 1992; 304: 52.

73. *British Medical Journal*, 1992; 302: 495–8.

74. *Medical Monitor*, 5 June 1992.

75. *The Lancet*, 1992; 339: 636–9.

76. *The Lancet*, 1995; 346: 1339–45.

77. Professor David Baum and Dr Susanna Graham-Jones, *Child Health: The Complete Guide* (Harmondsworth: Penguin: 1991): 89.

78. Dr Bob Chen and Dr John Glasser, 'Vaccine Safety Datalin, The National Immunisation Programs Large- Linked Database Study, Advisory Committee on Childhood Vaccines', presented on September 28, 1994.

79. *The Lancet*, 1995; 345: 567–9.

80. *New England Journal of Medicine*, 2001; 345: 656–61.

81. *Acta Paediatrica*, 1993; 82 (3): 267–70.

82. *Morbidity and Mortality Weekly Report*, January 24, 2003 (52), no. SS1: 1–10.

83. Harris L. Coulter and Barbara Loe Fisher, *A Shot in the Dark* (New York, NY: Avery Publishing Group, 1985): 8–9.

84. *World Medicine*, Sept. 1984: 17.

85. *The Lancet*, 1996; 347: 209–10.

86. Coulter and Fisher, *A Shot in the Dark*: 13–14.

87. Stratton et al., *Adverse Events*: 309–19.

88. Coulter and Fisher, *A Shot in the Dark*: 32.

89. Stratton et al., op cit.

90. Kathleen Stratton et al., 'DPT vaccine and chronic nervous system dysfunction: a new analysis', Division of Health Promotion and Disease Prevention, Institute of Medicine (Washington, DC: National Academy Press, 1994).

91. Gordon Stewart and John Wilson, correspondence, *British Medical Journal*, 1981; 282: 1968–9.

92. Gordon Stewart, correspondence, *British Medical Journal*, 1983; 287: 287–8.

93. House of Commons, Hansard, 3 December 1980; col. 262, as reported in Stewart and Wilson, correspondence, *British Medical Journal*, 1981; 282: 1968–9.

94. Mendelsohn, *But Doctor*: 19.

95. *Pediatric Infectious Disease Journal*, Jan. 1983, as reported in Mendelsohn, *But Doctor*: 42.

96. Ibid.

97. A. Kalokerinos, *Every Second Child* (New Canaan, CT: Keats, 1981), as cited in Coulter and Fisher, *A Shot in the Dark*: 131.

98. *Pediatrics*, 1981; 68: 650–60.

99. *British Medical Journal*, 1967; 4: 320–3.

100. DHSS, Whooping Cough: Reports from the Committee on the Safety of Medicines and the Joint Committee on Vaccination and Immunisation, HMSO, 1981.

101. Stratton et al., *Adverse Events*: 67–117.

102. *New England Journal of Medicine*, 1981; 305: 1307–13.

103. *Physicians' Desk Reference* (Montvale, NJ: Medical Economics Data Production Company, 1995): 1288.

104. Department of Health Press Release, 3 October 1988.

105. *Morbidity and Mortality Weekly Report*, January 24, 2003 (52), no. SS1: 1–10.

106. International Symposium on Immunization: Benefit Versus Risk Factors, Brussels, 1978. *Developments in Biological Standardization*, 432: 259–64 (S. Kurger, Basel, 1979).

107. *The Lancet*, 1989; ii: 1015–16.

108. *Annals of Internal Medicine*, 1979; 90 (6): 978–80.

109. *The Lancet*, 1995; 345: 1071–3; *The Lancet*, 1995; 345: 1062–3.

110. *The Lancet*, 1994; 343: 105; also Kohji Heda et al., correspondence, *The Lancet*, 1995; 346: 701–2.

111. Stratton et al., *Adverse Events*: 118–86.

112. *American Journal of Diseases of Children*, 1965; 109: 232–7.

113. *The Lancet*, 1985; i: 1–5.

114. W. Ehrengut, correspondence, *The Lancet*, 1989; ii: 751.

115. *Pediatric Infectious Disease Journal*, 1989; 8 (11): 751–5.

116. *Canada Diseases Weekly Report*, 1987; 13–35: 156–7, as reported in *The Lancet*, 1989; ii: 1015–16.

117. *Pediatric Infectious Disease Journal*, 1989; 8 (5): 302–8.

118. *Pediatric Infectious Disease Journal*, Mar. 1991.

119. *The Lancet*, 1993; 341: 979–82.

120. Ibid.

121. *The Lancet*, 1993; 341: 46.

122. *Physicians' Desk Reference*: 1575.

123. *The WDDTY Vaccination Handbook: A Guide to the Dangers of Childhood Immunization* (London: The Wallace Press, 1991): 7.

124. MacLean's, February 8 1982, as reported in Mendelsohn, *But Doctor*. 30.

125. *Morbidity and Mortality Weekly Report*, 2001; 50: 41–51.

126. The Washington Star, February 12, 1981.

127. *ASM News*, 1988; 54 (10): 560–2.

128. *Morbidity and Mortality Weekly Report*, January 24, 2003 (52), no 551: 1–10.

129. *British Medical Journal*, 1992; 305: 79–81.

130. T. Mertens and H. Eggers, correspondence, *The Lancet*, 1984; ii: 1390.

131. *American Journal of Clinical Nutrition*, 1977; 30: 592–8.

132. Yan Shen and Guohua Xia, correspondence, *The Lancet*, 1994; 344: 1026.

133. M. Uhari et al., correspondence, *The Lancet*, 1989; ii: 440–1.

134. A. D. Langmuir, 'The Safety and Efficiency of Vaccines for the Prevention of Poliomyelitis', paper presented for Committee to Study the Poliomyelitis Vaccine at the Institute of Medicine, National Academy of Sciences, March 14–15, 1977.

135. Interview with Dr J. Anthony Morris, April 1991.

136. *Journal of the American Medical Association*, 1997; 277: 873.

137. *Danish Medical Bulletin*, 1960; 7: 142–4.

138. *Clinical Toxicology*, 1971; 4: 185, as reported in Murphy.

139. *British Medical Journal*, 1979; ii: 12.

140. *American Journal of Public Health*, 1940; 30: 129, in Murphy.

141. *Contact Dermatitis*, 1989; 20: 173–6.

142. *Contact Dermatitis*, 1980; 6: 241–5.

143. *Toxicology and Applied Pharmacology*, 1983; 68: 218–28.

144. *Pediatrics*, 2001; 107: 1147–54.

145. Randall Neustaedter, *The Vaccine Guide: Making an Informed Choice* (Berkeley, CA: North Atlantic Books, 1996).

146. *Vaccine*, 1995; 13: 1366–74.

147. Murphy, *What Every Parent* …

148. *American Journal of Dermatopathology*, 1993; 15: 114–7.

149. *The Lancet*, 1988, i: 955–60.

150. *Pediatrics*, 1989, 84: 62–7; *International Archives of Allergy and Applied Immunology*, 1989; 89: 156.

151. *Biologicals*, 1994; 22: 53–63.

152. Murphy, op cit.

153. Randall Neufstader, *The Vaccine Guide.*

154. *The Lancet*, 1990; 336: 325–9.

155. Ibid.

156. *Gastroenterology*, 1992; 102: 538–43.

157. A. J. Zuckerman et al., correspondence, *The Lancet*, 1994; 343: 737–8.

158. *Pediatric Infectious Disease Journal*, 1992; 18: 6.

159. *The Lancet*, 1993; 341: 851–4.

160. See Harold S. Ginsberg, *The Adenoviruses* (New York, NY: Plenum Press).

161. *Transactions of the Royal Society of Tropical Medicine and Hygiene*, 1985; 79: 355–58 and 1989; 83: 545–9.

162. Mertens and Eggens, op cit.

163. *Transactions of the Royal Society of Tropical Medicine and Hygiene*, 1985; 79: 355–58 and 1989; 83: 545–9.

164. *New England Journal of Medicine*, 1995; 332 (8): 500–7.

165. *What Doctors Don't Tell You*, 1994; 5 (9): 12.

166. Ibid.

167. Michel Odent, *Journal of the American Medical Association*, 1994; 272 (8): 592–3.

168. *The Lancet*, 1998; 351: 637–41; *American Journal of Gastroenterology*, 2000; 95: 2285–95.

169. *The Lancet*, 1998; 352: 234–5; *Journal of Pediatrics*, 1999; 135: 559–63.

170. *Journal of Pathology*, 2000; 190 (Supplement): 1A–69A.

171. *Digestive Diseases and Sciences*, 2000; 45: 723–9.

172. *Gut*, 1995; 36: 564–9; *Journal of Clinical Pathology*, 1997; 50: 299–304.

173. *Journal of Clinical Pathology; Molecular Pathology*, 2002; 55: 84–90.

174. *Brain Dysfunction*, 1991; 3: 328; *Advances in Biochemical Psychopharmacology*, 1993; 28: 627–43.

175. *Acta Paediatrica*, 1996; 85: 1076–9.

176. *Gastroenterology*, 1999; 116: 796–803.

177. *The Lancet*, 2004; 363: 750.

178. *The Lancet*, 1998; 351: 1327–8; *The Lancet*, 1999; 353: 2026–9.

179. *Journal of American Physicians and Surgeons*, 2004; 9 (3): 70–5.

180. *New England Journal of Medicine*, 2002; 347: 1477–82.

181. *Journal of Pediatrics*, 1986; 108 (1): 671–6.

182. *Pediatric Infectious Disease Journal*, 1992; 11: 955–9, as reported in *Journal of the American Medical Association*, 1994; 271 (1): 13.

183. *The Lancet*, 1996; 347: 1792–6.

184. *American Journal of Diseases of Children*, 1992; 146: 182–6.

185. *The Lancet*, 1986; i: 1169–73.

186. *New England Journal of Medicine*, 1990; 323: 160–4.

187. *British Medical Journal*, 1987; 294: 294–6.

188. *What Doctors Don't Tell You*, 1996; 7 (2): 8.

189. *Przeglad Epidemiologiczny*, 1965; 19: 175–6.

190. *South Med Surg*, 1949; 111: 209–14.

191. *Pediatrics (Supplement)*, June 1986: 963.

192. *American Journal of Public Health*, 1990: 80.

193. See 'Alternatives' by Harald Gaier, *What Doctors Don't Tell You*, 1995; 5 (11): 9.

194. Gaier, *Thorsons Encyclopaedic Dictionary of Homeopathy*, (London: HarperCollins, 1991).

195. *British Medical Journal*, 1987; 294: 294–6.

CHAPTER 7

1. National Public Radio's 'All Things Considered' by Joe Neel as reported on www.npr.org/news/specials/hrt/
2. *Reviews in Cardiovascular Medicine*, 2003; 4 (2): 68–71.
3. *American Journal of Obstetrics and Gynecology*, 1989; 161: 1859–64
4. *Journal of the American Medical Association, 1991; 265 (15): 1985–90.*
5. *Obstetrics and Gynecology*, 1992; 79 (2): 286–94.
6. *New England Journal of Medicine*, 1989; 321: 293–7.
7. *New England Journal of Medicine*, 1995; 332 (24): 1589–93.
8. *Obstetrics and Gynecology*, 1993; 81 (2): 265–71; *Annals of Internal Medicine*, 1992; 177 (12): 1016–37.
9. *The Times*, 11 November 1994.
10. *Journal of the Royal Society of Medicine*, 1992; 85: 376–9.
11. Ibid.
12. Writing Group for the Women's Health Initiative Investigators, JAMA, 2002; 288: 321–33.
13. *Climacteric*, 2003; 6 (supplement 1): 11–36.
14. *The Lancet*, 2003; 362: 419–27.
15. *The Lancet*, 2004; 363: 453–55.
16. *New England Journal of Medicine*, 1993; 328 (15): 1069–75.
17. *British Medical Journal*, 1994; 308: 1268–9.
18. *New England Journal of Medicine*, 1993; 328 (15): 1115–17.
19. *Journal of the American Medical Association*, 1995; 273 (3): 199–208.
20. *The Lancet*, 1991; 337: 833–4.
21. *British Medical Journal*, 1994; 308: 1268–9.
22. F. M. Ward Posthuma et al., correspondence, *British Medical Journal*, 1994; 309: 191–2.
23. *Journal of the American Medical Association*, 1998; 280 (3): 605–13.
24. *Journal of the American Medical Association*, 1998; 280: 605–13.
25. *New England Journal of Medicine*, 2000; 343: 522–9
26. *Journal of the American Medical Association*, 2002; 288: 321–3.
27. *British Medical Journal*, 1995; 311: 1193–6.
28. *New England Journal of Medicine*, 1985; 313: 1038–43; and 1991; 325: 756–62.
29. *Journal of the American Medical Association*, 280: 605–13.

30. *The Lancet*, 1996; 348: 977–80.

31. *New England Journal of Medicine*, 2001; 345: 1243–9; *Annals of Internal Medicine*, 2000; 132: 689–96.

32. *Annals of Internal Medicine*, 2000; 133: 933–41; 999–1001; *The Lancet*, 1996; 348: 981–3.

33. *Annals of Internal Medicine*, 2000; 133: 933–41; 999–1001.

34. *Journal of the American Medical Association*, 1993; 269 (20): 2637–41.

35. *New England Journal of Medicine*, 1993; 329 (16): 1141–6.

36. *New England Journal of Medicine*, 1993; 329 (16): 1192–3.

37. *American Journal of Medicine*, 1988; 85: 847–50.

38. *Annals of Internal Medicine*, 1995; 122: 9–16.

39. Anne Szarewski et al., *British Medical Journal*, 1994; 308: 717.

40. See Kitty Little, *Bone Behaviour* (New York, NY: Academic Press, 1973); also Dr Ellen Grant, *Sexual Chemistry* (London: Cedar, 1994).

41. Dr John McLaren Howard, 'Current Research in Osteoporosis and Bone Mineral Measurement II', proceedings of the third Bath Conference on Osteoporosis Bone Mineral Measurement, Bath, 23–26 June 1992 (British Institute of Radiology, 1992).

42. *British Journal of Obstetrics and Gynaecology*, 1990; 97: 917–21.

43. *The Lancet*, 1992; 339: 290–1.

44. *The Lancet*, 1992; 339: 506.

45. *The Times*, 1 February 1992.

46. *British Medical Journal*, 1992; 305: 1403–8.

47. See Dr Ellen Grant, *The Bitter Pill* (London: Corgi Books, 1985) and *Sexual Chemistry*.

48. *British Medical Journal*, 1990; 300: 436–8.

49. *American Journal of Epidemiology*, May 1995.

50. *Clinical Therapeutics*, 1990; 12 (5): 447–55.

51. *Journal of the American Geriatrics Society*, 1992; 40 (8): 817–20.

52. *Australian and New Zealand Journal of Obstetrics and Gynaecology*, 1992; 32 (4): 384–5.

53. *Journal of Neurology*, 1993; 240 (3): 195–6.

54. *The Lancet*, 1979; i: 581–2.

55. *Obstetrics and Gynecology*, 1994; 83: 5–11.

56. *Journal of Women's Health and Gender-based Medicine*, 1999; 8: 637–460.

57. *British Journal of Obstetrics and Gynaecology*, 1990; 97: 1080–6.

58. *What Doctors Don't Tell You*, 2003; 14 (8): 5.

59. Gillian Walker (ed.), *ABPI Data Sheet Compendium, 1993–4* (London: Datapharm Publications Ltd, 1993). See also *What Doctors Don't Tell You*, 1995; 6 (8): 8–9 and 6 (11): 8–9.

60. *Townsend Letter for Doctors*, 1996; July: 125–7.

61. De Boever et al., 'Variation of Progesterone, 200 alpha-Dihydroprogesterone and Oestradiol Concentrations in Human Mammary tissue and Blood after Topical Administration of Progesterone', in P. Mauvais-Jarvis et al., *Percutaneous Absorption of Steroids* (New York, NY: Academic Press, 1980): 259–65.

62. *The Lancet*, 1999; 354: 1447–8.

63. *Maturitas*, January 30 2002; 41(1): 1–6.

64. *Menopause*, Jan.–Feb. 2003; 10(1): 13–8.

65. *Fertility and Sterility*, Apr. 1995; 63(4): 785–91.

66. *The Lancet*, 2004; 363: 453–5.

67. Klim McPherson et al., correspondence, *British Medical Journal*, 1995; 310: 598. See also Dr David Grimes, editorial, *Fertility and Sterility*, 1992; 57 (3): 492–3.

68. IARC Monographs on the Evaluation of Carcinogenic Risk of Chemicals to Humans, December 1979.

69. *British Medical Journal*, 2001; 322: 586–7.

70. *Archives of Pathology and Laboratory Medicine*, 1996; 120: 970–3. *Fertility and Sterility*, 1992; 57: 4992–3.

71. *Journal of Immunology*, 1988; 1491: 1–8.

72. *The Lancet*, 1998; 352: 905–6.

73. *British Medical Journal*, 1993; 303: 13–6.

74. Ibid.

75. *Obstetrics and Gynecology*, Aug. 1999; 94 (2): 225–8.

76. *American Journal of Clinical Nutrition*, 1991; 54: 1093–1100.

77. *Cancer Epidemiology, Biomarkers and Prevention*, 1996; 5: 785–94.

78. *Environmental Health Perspectives*, 1997; 105 (supplement 3): 633–6.

79. *American Journal of Clinical Nutrition*, 1998; 68 (supplement 6): 1431S–5S.

80. *Proceedings of the Society for Experimental Biology and Medicine*, 1995; 208: 44–50.

81. *Journal of the Department of Agriculture of Western Australia*, 1946; 23: 1–12.

82. *Archives of Toxicology*, 1999; 73: 50–4.

83. *Proceedings of the Society for Experimental Biology and Medicine*, 1998; 217: 369–78.

84. Ellen Grant, *Sexual Chemistry*: 144–5.

85. *Journal of Nutritional Medicine*, 1991; 2: 165–78.

86. *British Medical Journal*, 5 December 1992. See also *Journal of the American Medical Association*, 1994; 272 (24): 1909–14.

87. Ibid.

88. *Here's Health*, Mar. 1991: 13.

89. See Harald Gaier, 'Alternatives', *What Doctors Don't Tell You*, 1995; 6 (9): 9.

CHAPTER 8

1. John Mansfield and David Freed, 'Choking on Medicine', *What Doctors Don't Tell You*, 1993; 4 (6): 12.

2. Dr Sidney M. Wolfe and Rose Ellen Hope, *Worse Pills, Best Pills, II* (Washington, DC: Public Citizens' Health Research Group, 1993): 10.

3. *Journal of the American Medical Association*, 2000; 284 (1): 483–5.

4. *The Lancet*, 1994; 343: 871–81.

5. *Science*, 1994; 264: 1538–41, as reported in Minerva, *British Medical Journal*, 1994; 308: 1726.

6. *British Medical Journal*, 1994; 308: 283–4.

7. Ibid.

8. *Journal of the American Medical Association*, 1994; 271 (15): 1205–7; *The Lancet*, 1994; 343: 784; *British Medical Journal*, 1994; 308: 809–10.

9. Both examples taken from The Hon. John D. Dingell. Shattuck Lecture – Misconduct in Medical Research, *New England Journal of Medicine*, 1993; 328: 1610–15.

10. *Science*, 1994; 263: 317–8, as reported in Minerva, *British Medical Journal*, 1994; 308: 484.

11. *What Doctors Don't Tell You*, 1994; 5 (2): 3.

12. Charles Medawar, *The Wrong Kind of Medicine?* (Consumers' Association and Hodder & Stoughton, 1984): 79.
13. *Journal of Family Practice*, 2001; 50: 853–8.
14. Personal interview with Geoffrey Cannon, January 1991.
15. *The Lancet*, 1981; 2: 883–7; *Arch Otol*, 1974; 100: 226–32; *Clin Otol*, 1981; 6: 5–13, as reported in Harald Gaier, 'Alternatives', *What Doctors Don't Tell You*, 1994; 5 (12): 9.
16. T. T. K. Jung et al., in D. J. Lim et al. (eds), *Recent Advances in Otitis Media with Effusion* (Philadelphia: B. C. Decker, 1984), as reported in Harald Gaier, 'Alternatives', *What Doctors Don't Tell You*, 1994; 5 (12): 9.
17. *Journal of Family Practice*, 2001; 50: 853–8.
18. *Mims*, 1991; 18 (3): 32.
19. Personal interview with Professor Ian Phillips, January 1991.
20. See William Crook, *Solving the Puzzle of Your Hard-to-Raise Child* (New York, NY: Random House, 1981).
21. *Townsend Letter for Doctors*, October 1995: 9.
22. *British Medical Journal*, 1996; 313: 648
23. See Dr Lisa Landymore-Lim, *Poisonous Prescriptions* (Subiaco, Western Australia: PODD, 1994).
24. *Journal of Hospital Infections*, Feb. 1988.
25. *Journal of the American Medical Association*, 2003; 289: 885–8
26. *ABMJ*, 1996; 313: 897–91.
27. *Mortality and Morbidity Weekly Report*, 1995; 43: 952–3, as reported in *Journal of the American Medical Association*, 1995; 273 (6): 451.
28. *New England Journal of Medicine*, 1992; 326 (8): 501–6.
29. *Adverse Drug Reaction Bulletin*, June 1992.
30. *The Lancet*, 1995; 345: 2–3.
31. *Journal of Allergy and Clinical Immunology*, 1987; 80: 415–16, as reported in Mansfield and Freed, op cit.
32. *Adverse Drug Reaction Bulletin*, June 1992.
33. *The Lancet*, 1990; 336: 1391–6.
34. *British Medical Journal*, 1991; 303: 1426–31.
35. Gillian Walker (ed.), *ABPI Data Sheet Compendium, 1993–4* (London: Datapharm Publications Ltd, 1993): 45–6.
36. *The Lancet*, 1990; 336: 436–7.

37. *American Journal of Respiratory and Critical Care Medicine*, Mar. 1994.

38. *Annals of Internal Medicine*, 15, 1993; 963–8.

39. S. Teelucksingh, correspondence, *The Lancet*, 1991; 338: 60–1.

40. *Archives of Disease in Childhood*, 1982; 57: 204–7.

41. *Acta Paediatrica*, 1993; 82: 636–40.

42. *Science*, 1990; 250: 1196–8

43. V. D. Ramirez, commentary, *The Lancet*, 1996; 347: 630–1.

44. *European Respiratory Journal*, 1989 (supplement); 6: 566s–7s.

45. *British Medical Journal*, 1996; 312: 542–3.

46. J. K. H. Wales, correspondence, *The Lancet*, 1991; 338: 1535.

47. *The Lancet*, 1966; ii: 569–72.

48. *Clininical and Experimental Rheumatology*, 1991; 9 (supplement 6): 37–40.

49. J. K. H. Wales et al., correspondence, *The Lancet*, 1991; 338: 1535.

50. *Journal of Asthma*, 1986; 23 (6): 291–6.

51. Faruque Ghanchi, correspondence, *The Lancet*, 1993; 342: 1306–7.

52. *Pediatric Nephrology*, 1994; 8 (6): 667–70.

53. *Clinical Pharmacy*, 1993; 25 (2): 126–35.

54. *Arthroscopy*, 1985; 1 (1): 68–72.

55. *Journal of Rheumatology*, 1994; 21: 1207–13.

56. *British Journal of Dermatology*, 1993; 129: 431–6; *New England Journal of Medicine*, 1990; 322: 1093–7.

57. *Journal of Dermatology*, 1991; 18 (8): 454–64. *Skin Pharmacology*, 1992; 5 (2): 77–80.

58. *Dermatological Clinics*, 1992; 10 (3): 505–12; *Graefes Archive for Clinical Experimental Ophthalmology*, 1988; 226 (4): 337–40; C. J. McLean et al., correspondence, *The Lancet*, 1995; 345: 330.

59. *Zeitschrift fur Hautkrankheiten*, 1988; 63 (4): 302–8.

60. *Archives of Disease in Childhood*, 1982; 57: 204–7.

61. *Archives of Disease in Childhood*, 1987; 62 (9): 876–8; J. K. H. Wales, op cit.

62. *Journal of the American Medical Association*, 1980; 244: 813–14.

63. C. J. McLean et al., correspondence, *The Lancet*, 1995; 345: 330; *British Dermatology*, 1989; 120: 472–3; *Eye*, 1993; 7: 664–6; Dr Evan Benjamin Dreyer, correspondence, *New England Journal of Medicine*, 1993; 329: 1822.

64. R. H. Meyboom, correspondence, *Annals of Internal Medicine*, 1988; 109 (8): 683.

65. Hoffmann-LaRoche, Rituxan product monograph, 21 June 2000.

66. Drs Peter M. Brooks and Richard O. Day, *New England Journal of Medicine*, 1992; 327 (ii): 749–54; *The Lancet*, 1984; ii: 1171–4.

67. Drs Peter M. Brooks and Richard O. Day, *New England Journal of Medicine*, 1991; 324 (24): 1716–25.

68. *Physicians' Desk Reference* (Montvale, NJ: Medical Economics Data Production Company, 1995).

69. J. Hollingworth, correspondence, *British Medical Journal*, 1991; 302: 51; *British Journal of Rheumatology*, 1987; 26: 103–7.

70. *Journal of the American Medical Association*, 28 November 1990.

71. L. Theilmann et al., correspondence, *The Lancet*, 1990; 335: 1346.

72. *Journal of the American Medical Association*, September 14 1994.

73. Michael Gleeson et al., correspondence, *The Lancet*, 1994; 344: 1028.

74. *New England Journal of Medicine*, 1991; 325: 87–91.

75. *British Medical Journal*, 1999; 319: 1518.

76. *Tidsskr Nor Laegefor*, 2002; 122: 476–80.

77. *Journal of the American Medical Association*, 2001, 286: 954–9.

78. P. Sever, correspondence, *The Lancet*, 1994; 344: 1019–20.

79. *Archives of Internal Medicine*, 1993; 153: 154–83.

80. *Blood Pressure*, 1993; 2 (supplement): 5–9.

81. Wolfe and Hope, op cit.

82. Peter T. Sawick, correspondence, *British Medical Journal*, 1994; 308: 855.

83. *British Medical Journal*, 1993; 306: 609–11.

84. *Journal of Internal Medicine*, 1992; 232: 493–8, as reported in *Journal of the American Medical Association*, 1993; 269 (13): 1692.

85. *New England Journal of Medicine*, 1992; 327: 678–84.

86. *The Lancet*, 1993; 341: 967.

87. *British Medical Journal*, 1992; 304: 946–9.

88. *Journal of the American Medical Association*, 20 May 1992.

89. Larry Cahill et al., correspondence, *Nature*, 1994; 371: 702–4.

90. *American Heart Journal*, 1995; 130: 359–66; *Archives of Internal Medicine*, 1994; 154: 737–43; *Archives of Internal Medicine*, 1996; 156: 278–85.

91. *Scandinavian Journal of Primary Health Care*, Sept. 2003; 21 (3): 153–8; *Annals of Emergency Medicine*, Dec. 2001; 38(6): 666–71.

92. *Journal of Clinical Psychopharmacology*, Feb. 1982; 2 (1): 14–39.

93. *Pharmacotherapy*, 2001; 21: 940–53.

94. *Journal of Cardiovascular Pharmacology*, 1990; 16: 58–63.

95. *Journal of Cardiovascular Pharmacology*, 1990; 16: 58–63.

96. *New England Journal of Medicine*, 1989; 320: 709–18.

97. Ibid.

98. *The Lancet*, 1995; 346: 767–70 and 346: 586.

99. The Observer, December 1992.

100. *British Medical Journal*, 1994; 310: 177–8.

101. *Epilepsia*, 1988; 29: 590–600.

102. *British Medical Journal*, 1993; 307: 483.

103. *The Lancet*, 1991; 337: 406–9; Epilepsy Research, 1993; 14: 237–44.

104. *Neurology*, 1996; 46: 41–4.

105. *New England Journal of Medicine*, 1990; 323: 497–502.

106. Neurology, 1993; 43: 478–83.

107. *Journal of Neurology, Neurosurgery and Psychiatry*, 1995; 58: 44–50.

108. *The Lancet*, 1996; 347: 709–13.

109. *Townsend Letter for Doctors*, October 1995: 100.

110. *British Medical Journal*, 1995; 310: 215–8.

111. Harold Silverman, *The Pill Book: A Guide to Safe Drug Use* (New York, NY: Bantam Books, 1989): 278.

112. Ibid.

113. *Journal of Clinical Psychiatry*, 1995; 56: 3.

114. *Journal of Affective Disorders*, 1998; 51: 267–85.

115. *Australian Adverse Drug Reactions Bulletin*, Oct. 2003; 22 (5).

116. *Journal of Psychopharmacology*, 2003; 17: 121–6.

117. *New England Journal of Medicine*, 1991; 325: 316–21 and *Journal of the American Medical Association*, 1991; 265: 2831–5.

118. *The Lancet*, 1994; 344: 985–6.

119. S. Hood et al., correspondence, *The Lancet*, 1994; 344: 1500–1.

120. *New England Journal of Medicine*, 1993; 329: 1476–83.

121. *The Lancet*, 1993; 341: 1564–5.

122. *British Medical Journal*, 1993; 307: 1185.

123. *The Lancet*, 1993; 341: 861–2.

124. Theresa Curtin, et al., correspondence, *British Medical Journal*, 1992; 305: 713–4.

125. *New England Journal of Medicine*, 1993; 329: 1476–83.

126. *European Neurology*, 1991; 31: 306–13.

127. Carl Dahlof, correspondence, *The Lancet*, 1992; 340: 909.

128. *British Medical Journal*, 1994; 308: 113.

129. *The Lancet*, 1993; 341: 221–4.

130. *Neurology*, 2000; 54: 156–63.

131. *Neurology*, 2001; 56: 1243–4.

132. *The Lancet*, 1993; 341: 861–2.

133. *Neurology*, 2004; 62: 563–8.

134. *Headache*, Feb. 2003; 43 (2): 90–5.

135. *Headache*, Apr. 2001; Apr; 41 (4): 399–401.

136. *Neurologic Clinics*, Feb. 2001; 19 (1): 1–21.

137. *American Journal of Public Health*, 1999; 89: 1359–64.

138. *British Medical Journal*, 1996; 312: 657.

139. *Physicians' Desk Reference*, op cit: 897–8.

140. As cited in Peter Breggin, *Toxic Psychiatry* (London: HarperCollins, 1991): 384–5.

141. *Physicians' Desk Reference*, 1995: 897.

142. *Journal of Neuroscience*, 2001; 21: RC121.

143. *Canadian Journal of Psychiatry*, 1999; 44: 811–13.

144. *American Journal of Psychiatry*, 1979; 136: 226–8.

145. *Journal of the American Academy of Child and Adolescent Psychiatry*, 1987; 26 (1): 56–64.

146. *Pediatric Neurology*, 2001; 24: 99–102.

147. *Journal of Child Neurology*, 2000; 15: 265–7.

148. *Journal of the American Academy of Child and Adolescent Psychiatry*, 2000; 39: 517–24.

149. *Archives of Pediatrics and Adolescent Medicine*, 1994; 148: 859–61.

150. *L'Encephale*, 2000; 26: 45–7.

151. Breggin, *Toxic Psychiatry*: 382.

152. Breggin, *Toxic Psychiatry*: 380.

153. *Toxicology*, 1995; 103: 77–84.

154. *Research in Developmental Disabilities*, 1996; 17: 417–32.

155. *Journal of the American Academy of Child and Adolescent Psychiatry*,

1995; 34: 987–1000; Regier, A I Leshner, MH092-03, paper presented to the National Institute of Mental Health, Feb 1992. Dr Gerald B. Dermer, *The Immortal Cell* (Garden City Park, NY: Avery Publishing Group, 1994): 107.

156. See Ralph Moss, *Questioning Chemotherapy* (New York, NY: Equinox Press, 1995).

157. Ibid. See also Dr Urich Abel, *Der Spiegel*, 1990; 33: 174–6.

158. *New England Journal of Medicine*, 1992; 326 (8): 563.

159. *The Lancet*, 1996; 347: 1066–71.

160. *Current Opinion in Oncology*, 1995; 7 (5): 457–65.

161. Moss, *Questioning Chemotherapy*: 104.

162. See Moss, op cit.

163. *Physicians' Desk Reference*, 1995: 673.

164. *British Medical Journal*, 1996; 312: 886.

165. International Herald Tribune, 19 May, 1994.

166. *Current Opinion in Oncology*, 1995; 7 (4): 320–4.

167. *New England Journal of Medicine*, 1996; 334: 745–51.

168. *Journal of the National Cancer Institute*, 1996; 88: 270–8.

169. *The Lancet*, 1999; 353: 1442.

170. *Journal of the American Medical Association*, 2000; 283: 590–3.

171. *Journal of the American Medical Association*, 2000; 283: 590–3.

172. *New England Journal of Medicine*, 1989; 320: 69–75.

173. *Medicines Compendium 2002* (London: Datapharm Communication, 2002).

174. Although a comprehensive discussion of alternatives for various illnesses is outside the scope of this book, a number of publications (including my newsletter *What Doctors Don't Tell You*) cover such alternatives in detail. For arthritis, consult *The Arthritis Manual*, published by What Doctors Don't Tell You, 2003. For proof of what works in all natural therapies, consult *PROOF!*: a monthly newsletter by What Doctors Don't Tell You plc.

175. *What Doctors Don't Tell You*, 1995; 6 (6), and Dr Melvyn Werbach, *Healing Through Nutrition* (London: Thorsons, 1993), and his sourcebooks, *Nutritional Influences on Illness* and *Nutritional Influences on Mental Illness* (Tarzana, CA: Third Line Press, 1996 and 1991, respectively).

176. *Epilepsia*, 1992; 33 (6): 1132–6. See also *What Doctors Don't Tell You*, 1996; 6 (11): 12 and Werbach, op cit.

177. For discussion of the medical evidence of alternative cancer treatments, see Dr Ralph Moss, *Cancer Therapy: The Independent Consumer's Guide to Non-Toxic Treatment and Prevention* (New York, NY: Equinox Press, 1995), and Drs Ross Pelton and Lee Overholser, *Alternatives in Cancer Therapy* (New York, NY: Simon & Schuster, 1994). Also *The Cancer Files*, published by What Doctors Don't Tell You, 2004.

CHAPTER 9

1. For the history of amalgam, see Dr Hal Huggins, *It's All in Your Head: The Link Between Mercury Amalgams and Illness* (Garden City Park, NY: Avery Publishing Group, 1993): 59–61.

2. Dr Murray J. Vimy, symposium, 'Mercury from Dental Amalgam', British Dental Society, 14 April 1992.

3. *Journal of the American Medical Association*, 1993; 269: 2491.

4. *New Zealand Medical Journal*, 1998; 111: 326 (letters to the editor).

5. *Journal of the American Medical Association*, 1991; 265: 2934.

6. *The Lancet*, 1992; 339: 419.

7. *Bio-probe Newsletter*, 1994; 10 (3): 3.

8. *New Zealand Medical Journal*, 1998; 111: 326 (letters to the editor).

9. Panorama, 'Poison in the Mouth', transmitted 11 July 1994.

10. *Environmental Health Criteria 118: Inorganic Mercury* (World Health Organization, Geneva, 1991).

11. Panorama, op cit.

12. M. Nylander, correspondence, *The Lancet*, 1986; i: 442; also *British Journal of Industrial Medicine*, 1991; 48: 729–34.

13. *Polski Tygodnik Lekarski*, 1987; 42 (37): 1159–62; *International Archives of Occupational and Environmental Health*, 1987; 59: 551–7.

14. *Swedish Dental Journal*, 1989; 13: 235–43. *Advances in Dental Research*, 1992; 6: 110–13.

15. *British Journal of Industrial Medicine*, 1992; 49: 782–90.

16. Dr Diana Echeverria, as interviewed on Panorama's 'Poison in the Mouth', op cit.

17. *British Medical Journal*, 1991; 302: 488, and *British Medical Journal*, 1994; 309: 621–2.

18. *Journal of Dental Research*, 1985; 64 (8): 1072–5.

19. Professor P. Soremark, Department of Prosthetic Dentistry, Karolinska Institute, Sweden, 'Mercury Release in Dentistry – I', paper delivered 15–16 July 1985, 'Hazards in Dentistry: The Mercury Debate', Kings College, Cambridge.

20. Professor J.V. Masi, PhD, 'Corrosion of Restorative Materials: The Problem and the Promise'. Unpublished paper.

21. *FASEB Journal*, 1989; 3: 2641–6.

22. Ibid.

23. Dr Murray J. Vimy, symposium, op cit.

24. Ibid.

25. Ibid.

26. Ibid.

27. *FASEB Journal*, 1992; 6: 2472–6; *Clinical Toxicology*, 1992; 30 (4): 505–28.

28. *American Journal of Physiology*, 1990; 258: R938–45.

29. Vimy, symposium, op cit.

30. *The Journal of Prosthetic Dentistry*, 1984; 51: 617–23.

31. Hal Huggins, personal interview, April 1990.

32. Hal Huggins, *All in Your Head*: 126.

33. J. Levenson, Menace in the Mouth? What Doctors Don't Tell You Ltd, London, 2000.

34. *Journal of Epidemiology and Community Health*, 1978; 32: 155. *Swedish Journal of Biological Medicine*, Jan. 1989: 6–7.

35. *Neuroendocrinology Letters*, 2004; 25: 211–8.

36. *International Journal of Risk and Safety Medicine*, 1994; 4: 229–36, as reported in *Bio-Probe Newsletter*, 1994; 10 (3): 6.

37. *American Journal of Physiology*, 1990; 258: R939–45.

38. *European Journal of Pediatrics*, 1994; 153: 607–10.

39. *Zentralbatt fur Gynäkologie*, 1992; 14: 593–602.

40. *American Journal of Industrial Medicine*, 1985; 7: 171–86.

41. *Klinisches Labor*, 1992; 38: 469–76.

42. *International Journal of Risk and Safety Medicine*, 1994; 4: 229–36.

43. *Bio-Probe*, Mar. 1993.

44. Huggins, interview, op cit.

45. *Annual Review of Microbiology*, 1986; 40: 607–34; *Antimicrobial Agents and Chemotherapy*, 1993; 37 (4): 825–34.

46. *Journal of Prosthetic Dentistry*, 1987; 58: 704–7.

47. P. Störtebecker, correspondence, *The Lancet*, 1989; i: 1207.

48. *Brain Research*, 1990; 553: 125–31.

49. Duhr et al., FASEB 75th Annual Meeting, Atlanta, Georgia, April 21–25 1991, Abstract 493; *Journal of Neurochemistry*, 2000; 74: 231–6.

50. *Journal of Neurochemistry*, 1994; 62: 2049–52.

51. *The Lancet*, 1994; 343: 993–7; 343: 989. See also studies reported in *What Doctors Don't Tell You*, 1995; 5 (12): 1–3.

52. *Journal of the American College of Cardiology*, 1999; 33: 1578–83; *Journal of the American College of Cardiology*, 2000; 35: 819 (letter to the editor).

53. *Circulation*, 1995; 91, (3): 645–55.

54. *Proceedings of the Society for Experimental Biology and Medicine*, 1965; 120: 805–8; *Proceedings of the Society for Experimental Biology and Medicine*, 1967; 124: 485–90; *American Journal of Physiology*, 1970; 219: 755–61; *American Journal of Physiology*, 1971; 220: 808–11; *American Journal of Physiology*, 1975; 229: 8–12.

55. *Thrombosis Research*, 1983; 30: 579–85.

56. *Science of the Total Envirnoment*, 1990; 99: 23–35.

57. *Journal of Biomedical Materials Research*, 2000; 50: 598– 604.

58. *Journal of Orthomolecular Medicine*, First Quarter 1998; 13 (1): 31– 40.

59. London naturopath Harald Gaier has adapted a simple test developed by Max Dauderer, in Munich, which your dentist can use to see if you are 'leaking' excessive amounts of mercury. All you need is a stick of sugarless chewing gum, some zinc-free wads of cotton, two syringes and two sterile containers. Make sure before you start the test that you haven't chewed anything for at least two hours. Then, take one of the two small wads of cotton and place them in your mouth for a short while, so that they are soaked with your saliva. Don't chew the cotton.

   Take the plunger out of the syringe and insert the saliva-sodden cotton into it. Replace the plunger and squeeze the saliva out through the syringe into a sterile container marked 'Before'. Close it tightly.

Next, chew the stick of sugarless gum intensively (concentrating on those areas of your teeth covered with amalgam fillings). Discard the gum. Collect a second saliva sample the same way you did the first, with a second wad of cotton and the second syringe. Squeeze the saliva out into the second sterile container marked 'After'. Close it tightly.

Send both samples to a lab that can analyse each sample for its mercury content.

In Dr Gaier's experience, people with large amounts of amalgam have far higher mercury content in the 'After' sample. For instance, in 40 of his patients investigated for amalgam poisoning, the amount of mercury in their saliva went up by an average of 415 per cent after chewing the gum. Those patients with symptoms suggestive of mercury poisoning such as MS invariably had increased post-chewing mercury scores – often by as much as 1,800 per cent.

CHAPTER 10

1. *British Medical Journal*, 1994; 309: 361–5.
2. E. A. Campling et al., 'The Report of the National Confidential Enquiry into Perioperative Deaths', 1990 (National CEPOD, 1992). See also more recent editions of *CEPOD*.
3. *New England Journal of Medicine*, 1991; 325: 1002–7.
4. As cited in *Drugs and Therapeutic Bulletin*, 1980; 18: 7–8, as cited in Stephen Fulder, *How to Survive Medical Treatment* (London: Century Hutchinson, 1987): 90; *Digestive Surgery*, 2003; 20: 215–19.
5. *Effective Health Care*, Nov. 1992.
6. *GP*, 6 August 1993.
7. See studies mentioned in *The Lancet*, 1994; 344: 1652–3.
8. John G. F. Cleland, correspondence, *The Lancet*, 1994; 344: 1222–4.
9. *The Lancet*, 1994; 344: 563–70.
10. *New England Journal of Medicine*, 1992; 326: 10–16.
11. *Journal of the American College of Cardiology*, 1997; 30: 1451–60.
12. *Journal of the American Medical Association*, 1996; 276: 300–6.
13. *New England Journal of Medicine*, 1996; 335: 1857–63.

14. *Journal of the American Medical Association*, 2002; 287: 1405–12.
15. *Stroke*, 2000; 31: 707–13.
16. *New England Journal of Medicine*, 2004; 350: 21–8.
17. *Journal of the American College of Cardiology*, 1999; 33: 63–72; *Annals of Thoracic Surgery*, 1994; 58: 445–51.
18. Figures compiled by the Noninvasive Heart Center in San Diego, CA (www.heartprotect.com/mortality-stats.shtml.
19. *New England Journal of Medicine*, 1998; 338: 1785–92.
20. *New England Journal of Medicine*, 1998; 338: 1785–92.
21. Gordon Waddell, 'A New Clinical Model for the Treatment of Low Back Pain', in James Weinstein and Sam Wiesel (eds), *The Lumbar Spine* (Philadelphia, PA: W. B. Saunders Co., 1990): 38–56.
22. See Henry La Rocca, 'Failed Lumbar Surgery: Principles of Management', in Weinstein and Wiesel, *Lumbar Spine*: 872–81.
23. *Spine*, 1980; 5: 87–94.
24. *Journal of the American Medical Association*, 1992; 268 (7): 907–11.
25. *The Mount Sinai Journal of Medicine*, 1991; 58 (2): 183–7.
26. Waddell, op cit.
27. La Rocca, op cit.
28. *Spine*, 1986; 11: 712–9.
29. *Archives of Physical Medicine and Rehabilitation*, 1998; 79: 1137–9.
30. *Australian Journal of Physiotherapy*, 1997; 43: 91–8.
31. *Journal of the Canadian Chiropractic Association*, 1992; 36: 75–83.
32. *British Medical Journal*, 1994; 309: 1267–8.
33. *British Journal of General Practice*, 1997; 47: 653–5; 'Royal College of General Practitioners Clinical guidelines for the management of acute low back pain', (London: RCGP, 1996).
34. *Journal of Pathology and Bacteriology*, 1934; 38: 117–27.
35. *The Breast Journal*, Oct. 2000; 6 (5): 331–34.
36. *American Journal of Nursing*, 2001; 101: 11.
37. *The Lancet*, 1995; 346: 1334–5.
38. M. Baum, correspondence, *The Lancet*, 1996; 347: 260.
39. *Acta Radiologica. Supplementum.* Dec. 2001; 42 (424): 1–22.
40. *American Journal of Roentgenology*, Nov. 1999; 173 (5): 1303–13.
41. *Journal of the American Medical Association*, 1991; 266: 1280–2.
42. *The Lancet*, 1994; 344: 1496–7.

43. *New England Journal of Medicine*, 1989; 320: 822–8.

44. *British Medical Journal*, 1994; 308: 809–10. *New England Journal of Medicine*, 1994; 330: 1460, and 330: 1448–50; *The Lancet*, 1994; 343: 1049–50, and 343: 1496–7.

45. *New England Journal of Medicine*, 1995; 332 (14): 907–11.

46. *New England Journal of Medicine*, 1981; 305: 6–11; *European Journal of Cancer and Clinical Oncology*, 1986; 22: 1085–9; *European Journal of Cancer*, 1990; 26: 668–70.

47. *British Medical Journal*, 1991; 303: 1431–5.

48. Ibid.

49. Interview with surgeon Andrew Kingsnorth, October 1994; see also *British Journal of Surgery*, 1992; 79: 1068–70.

50. *New England Journal of Medicine*, 1973; 289: 1224–9.

51. *New England Journal of Medicine*, 2004; 350: 1819–27.

52. *Hernia*, 10 March 2004.

53. *Hernia*, 2003; 7: 185–90.

54. Ibid.

55. *The Lancet*, 1994; 344: 375–9.

56. *The Lancet*, 1994; 343: 251–4.

57. Cherald Chodak, *New England Journal of Medicine*, 1994; 330: 242–8.

58. *Journal of Pathology and Bacteriology*, 1954; 68: 603–16, as reported in the *British Medical Journal*, 1993; 306: 407–8.

59. *The Lancet*, 1993; 341: 91.

60. *Journal of the American Medical Association*, 1992; 267: 2191–6; *New England Journal of Medicine*, 1994; 330: 242–8.

61. *Journal of the American Medical Association*, 1993; 270: 948–54.

62. *Archives of Family Medicine*, 1993; 2: 487–93, as reported in *Journal of the American Medical Association*, 1993; 269 (20): 2676–7.

63. *Journal of the American Medical Association*, 1993; 269: 2633–6.

64. *Journal of the National Cancer Institute*, 2000; 92: 1582–92.

65. US National Cancer Institute Statement, July 2001.

66. *Journal of the American Medical Association* 1995; 273 (2): 129–35.

67. Interview with Reginald Lloyd Davies, July 1995; see also *The Lancet*, 1994; 344: 700–1.

68. *New England Journal of Medicine*, 1994; 330: 242–8.

69. *Journal of the American Medical Association*, 1995; 274 (8): 626–31.

70. *The Lancet*, 1995; 346: 1528–30.

71. *The Journal of Urology*, 1953; 70: 937.

72. *Obstetrics and Gynecology*, Feb. 2000; 95 (2): 199–20.

73. 'Hospital Episodes Statistics 1993–4' (HMSO) as cited in *What Doctors Don't Tell You*, 1996; 7 (1): 1–3.

74. *Obstetrics and Gynaecology*, 1993; 82: 757–64. See also *The Hysterectomy Hoax* (New York, NY: Doubleday, 1994).

75. *Fertility and Sterility*, 1984; 42: 510–14.

76. *New England Journal of Medicine*, 1993; 328: 856–60; *Cancer*, 1985; 56: 403–12.

77. *American Journal of Obstetrics and Gynecology*, 1982; 144: 841–8.

78. *Obstetrics and Gynecology*, Feb. 1993; 81 (2): 206–10.

79. *The Pulse*, August 14, 1993.

80. *British Journal of Urology*, 1989; 64: 594–9.

81. *British Journal of Obstetrics and Gynaecology*, 1994; 101: 468–70.

82. *American Journal of Obstetrics and Gynecology*, 1981; 140: 725–9.

83. *American Journal of Obstetrics and Gynecology*, 1993; 168: 765–71.

84. *Fertility and Sterility*, 1987; 47: 94–100.

85. For specific alternatives to hysterectomy, see *What Doctors Don't Tell You*, 1996; 7 (1): 3.

86. *The Lancet*, 1991; 337: 1074–8.

87. Ruditer Pittrof et al., *The Lancet*, 1991; 338: 197–8.

88. *Journal of the American Medical Association*, 1993; 270 (10): 1230–2.

89. Angela Coulter, correspondence, *The Lancet*, 1994; 344: 1367.

90. *British Journal of Obstetrics and Gynaecology*, 1996; 103: 142–9.

91. *World Journal of Surgery*, 1987; 11: 82–3.

92. 'Blood Technologies, Services and Issues', US Office of Technology Assessment Task Force, US Congress, 1988; 22/23: 121–9.

93. *Vox Sanguinis: the International Journal of Transfusion Medicine*, 1987; 52: 60–2.

94. Ibid.

95. *Transfusion Medical Reviews*, 1989; 3 (1): 39–54.

96. Ibid.

97. *The Lancet*, 1996; 348: 229–32.

98. *British Medical Journal*, 1994; 308: 1205–6; also 308: 1180–1.

99. Ibid.

100. *Journal of the American Medical Association*, 1998; 279: 1596–7.

101. *Journal of the American Medical Association*, 1998; 279: 1596–7.

102. *British Medical Journal*, 1998; 317: 235–40.

103. *Journal of the American Medical Association*, 2002; 288: 1499–507.

104. See Luc Montagnier, *AIDS: The Safety of Blood and Blood Products* (John Wiley & Sons, Chichester, West Sussex, 1987).

105. *Gastroenterology*, 1988; 95: 530–1.

106. *Monitor Weekly*, 7 April 1988.

107. A newly discovered virus that causes hepatitis has been detected in blood transfusions. TTV (transfusion transmitted virus) viraemia, is frequently found in the blood donor population, new research has discovered. The virus was discovered in 19 of 1000 regular blood donors when researchers from Edinburgh University analysed blood samples from the local transfusion centre. The virus has also been picked up in Japanese research (*The Lancet*, 1998; 352: 191–5).

108. *The Lancet*, 1998; 352: 191–5.

109. *British Medical Journal*, 1994; 308: 695–6.

110. N. Hallam et al., correspondence, *British Medical Journal*, 1994; 308: 856.

111. *New England Journal of Medicine*, 1989; 320: 1172–5.

112. *Annals of Otology, Rhinology and Laryngology*, 1989; 98: 171–3.

113. *Annals of Thoracic Surgery*, 1989; 47: 346–9.

114. *British Medical Journal*, 1986; 293: 530–2.

115. *Transfusion*, 1989; 29: 456–8. *British Journal of Surgery*, 1988; 75: 789–91.

116. *Annals of Surgery*, 1986; 203: 275–9.

117. *Vox Sanguinis*, 1989; 57 (1): 63–5.

118. *Journal of the American Medical Association*, 1986; 256: 2242–3.

119. *Journal of Bloodless Medicine and Surgery*, Spring 1986: 15–17.

120. *Journal of the American Medical Association*, 1973; 226: 1230. See also *Journal of the American Medical Association*, 1977; 238: 1256–8.

CHAPTER 11

1. *The Times*, 11 February 1990.
2. Ajay K. Singh et al., correspondence, *New England Journal of Medicine*, 1994; 331 (26): 1777–8; *New England Journal of Medicine*, 1994; 331 (17): 1110–15.
3. Dr David Lomax, correspondence, *The Lancet*, 1993; 342: 1247.
4. *The Times*, 21 September 1993.
5. *The Lancet*, 1996; 347: 527.
6. *Medical Journal of Australia*, 1997; 166: 172–3.
7. *Annals of Surgery*, 1997; 225: 31–8; *Journal of Laparoendoscopic Surgery*, 1996; 6: 311–17.
8. *New England Journal of Medicine*, 2004; 350: 1819–27.
9. *Journal of Hand Surgery*, 1997; 22: 317–21.
10. *American Journal of Surgery*, 1993; 165: 9–14.
11. *Surgery*, 1998; 123: 311–14.
12. *Journal of Gynecological Surgery*, 1989; 5: 131–2.
13. *The Lancet*, 1994; 344: 596–7.
14. *The Lancet*, 1993; 342: 674.
15. *Australian and New Zealand Journal of Obstetrics and Gynecology*, 1993; 31: 171–3.
16. *The Lancet*, 1993; 342: 633–7.
17. *The Lancet*, 1995; 345: 36–40.
18. *The Lancet*, 1994; 344: 596–7.
19. Ibid.
20. *The Lancet*, 1999; 354: 185–90.
21. David Lomax, correspondence, *The Lancet*, 1993; 342: 1247.
22. *Journal of the American Medical Association*, 1995; 273 (20): 1581–5.
23. *The Lancet*, 1993; 341: 1057–8.
24. *Journal of the American Medical Association*, 1994; 271 (17): 1349–57.
25. R. Treacy et al., correspondence, *British Medical Journal*, 1992; 304: 317.
26. The Guardian, 23 February 1993.
27. *Journal of Bone and Joint Surgery*, July 1991.
28. *Acta Orthopaedica Scandinavica* (Supplement), 1990; 61: 1–26.
29. *Journal of Bone and Joint Surgery*, 1994; 76A: 959–64, as reported in Minerva, *British Medical Journal*, 1994; 309: 888.

30. The Guardian, op cit.

31. *British Medical Journal*, 1992; 303; 1431–5.

32. *British Medical Journal*, 1992; 303: 1431–5.

33. *Journal of the American Medical Association*, 1994; 271 (17): 1349–57.

34. *The Lancet*, 1993; 341: 1057–8.

35. *Archives of Internal Medicine*, 2002; 162: 1465–71.

36. *British Medical Journal*, 1994; 309: 880.

37. The Guardian, op cit.

38. *The Journal of Bone and Joint Surgery*, 1994; 76B (5): 701–12.

39. *Clinical Orthopaedics and Related Research*, 1999; 369: 92–102.

40. *Current Opinion in Rheumatology*, Mar. 1994, 6: 172–6.

41. *Current Opinion in Rheumatology*, Mar. 1994; 6 (2): 161–71.

42. Journal of bound and Joint Surgery, 1994; 76B (5): 701–12.

43. *Journal of Bone and Joint Surgery*, 1992; 76B: 539–42; *Journal of Biomedical Materials Research*, 1977; 11: 157–64, as reported in *Journal of Bone and Joint Surgery*, 1994; 76B (5): 701–12.

44. *Fundamental and Applied Toxicology*, 1989; 13: 205–16.

45. *Science*, 1994; 266: 726–7, as reported in Minerva, *British Medical Journal*, 1994; 309: 1382.

46. *Journal of Bone and Joint Surgery*, American volume, 1997; 79: 1599–617.

47. *Clinical Orthopaedics and Related Research*, Aug. 1996; 329 (Supplement): S78–88; *Clinical Orthopaedics and Related Research*, Oct. 2000; 379: 123–33.

48. *New England Journal of Medicine*, 1992; 326 (1): 57–8.

49. *Journal of the American Medical Association*, 1992; 268 (21): 3092–7.

50. *The Lancet*, 1992; 340: 1202–5.

51. *New England Journal of Medicine*, 1992; 327: 1329–35.

52. *Journal of the American College of Cardiologists*, 1992; 19: 946–7; *New England Journal of Medicine*, 1991; 326: 1053–7.

53. *New England Journal of Medicine*, 1992; 326 (1): 10–16.

54. *Chest*, 1992; 102: 375–9.

55. *New England Journal of Medicine*, 1991; 325: 556–62.

56. *Journal of the American Medical Association*, 1992; 268: 2537–40.

57. *The Lancet*, 1993; 341: 573–80 and 341: 599–600.

58. *New England Journal of Medicine*, 1994; 331 (16): 1044–9.

59. *New England Journal of Medicine*, 1994; 331 (16): 1037–43; *The Lancet*, 1995; 346: 1179–84.
60. *Physicians' Desk Reference* (Montvale, NJ: Medical Economics Data Production Company, 1995): 2340.
61. *Medicines Compendium*, ABPI 2003.
62. *New England Journal of Medicine*, 1994; 331: 771–6.
63. *The Lancet*, 1993; 341: 234.
64. *The Lancet*, 1995; 346; 995–1000.
65. Report of the Interim Licencing Authority, sponsored by the Medical Research Council and the Royal College of Obstetricians and Gynaecologists, 1990.
66. *The Lancet* 1999; 354: 1, 1579–85.
67. *The Lancet*, 13 August 1994; Teratology, 1990; 42: 467; Les White et al., correspondence, *The Lancet*, 1990; 386: 1577; Lyn Chitty et al., correspondence, *British Medical Journal*, 1990; 300: 1726.
68. *British Medical Journal*, 1993; 307: 1239–43.
69. *Human Reproduction*, 2000; 15 (3): 604–7.
70. *The Lancet*, March 30, 1991.
71. *The Journal of Urology*, 2003; 169 (4): 1512–15.
72. *American Journal of Human Genetics*, 2003; 72: 156–60.
73. *American Journal of Human Genetics*, 2002; 71 (1): 162–4.
74. *The Lancet*, 1998; 351: 1524–5.
75. *Nature Cell Biology*, 2002; 4: (S1), S14–S18; *Nature Medicine*, 2002; 8: (S1), S14–S18.
76. *European Journal of Human Genetics*, 2003; 1 (4): 325–36.
77. P. Boulot, correspondence, *The Lancet*, 1990; 335: 1155–6.
78. *What Doctors Don't Tell You*, 1994; 5 (6): 7.
79. Robert H. Heptinstall, *Pathology of the Kidney* (Boston, MA: Little, Brown and Company, 1992): 1592.
80. *Nephron*, 1993; 63 (2): 242–3.
81. *Journal of Endourology*, 1994; 8 (1): 15–19.
82. *Journal of Urology*, 1993; 150 (6): 1765–7.
83. *Polskie Archiwum Medycyny Wewnetrznej*, 1993; 89 (5): 394–9.
84. *British Journal of Urology*, 1991; 68 (6): 657–8.
85. *Japanese Journal of Clinical Radiology*, 1990; 35 (9): 1015–20.
86. *Nephrologie*, 1993; 14 (6): 305–7.

87. *RoFo. Fortschritte auf dem Gebiete der Rontgenstrahlen und der neuen bildgebenden Verfahren*, 1993; 158 (2): 121–6.

88. *Acta Urologica Japonica*, 1993; 39 (12): 1119–24.

89. *Acta Urologica Japonica*, 1992; 38 (9): 999–1003.

90. *Urologica Internationalist*, 1993; 51 (3): 152–7.

91. *Journal of Urology*, 1993; 150: 481–2.

92. *Journal of Urology*, 1991; 145 (5): 942–8.

93. *Journal of Pediatrics*, 1994; 125 (1): 149–51.

94. *Journal of the Association of Physicians of India*, 1993; 41 (11): 748–9.

95. *Journal of Urology*, 1990; 144 (6): 1339–40.

96. *Scandinavian Journal of Urology and Nephrology*, 1993; 27 (2): 267–9.

97. *Nephrology, Dialysis, Transplantation*, 1990; 5 (11): 974–6.

98. *Acta Urologica Belgica*, 1994; 62 (2): 25–9.

99. *Journal of Urology*, 1994; 151 (6): 1605–6.

100. *Opthalmology*, 2003; 110; 748–54.

101. *The Lancet*, 2003; 361: 1225–6.

102. ASCRS Symposium, June 1996.

103. *The Lancet*, 2003; 361: 1225–6.

104. *New England Journal of Medicine*, 1999; 340: 1471–5; *Annals of Plastic Surgery*, 1988; 20: 562–5.

CHAPTER 12

1. The Netherlands 1986 Monthly Bulletin of Population of Health Statistics.

2. Norman Cousins, Deepak Chopra and Andrew Weil, are just a few of the authors who have popularized the mind–body connection. See also *The Lancet*, 1995; 345: 99–103 and *The Lancet*, 1994; 344: 995–8.

3. *The Lancet*, 1994; 344: 1319–22.

4. *The Lancet*, 1994; 344: 973–5.

5. *British Medical Journal*, 1992; 305: 341–6.

6. *What Doctors Don't Tell You*, 1995; 6 (4): 8–10.

7. *British Medical Journal*, 1991; 303: 1105–9; also 303: 1109–10.

8. Ibid. See also *British Medical Journal*, 1991; 303: 1105–9.

9. *British Medical Journal*, 1995; 310: 489–91.

10. *American Journal of Public Health*, 1993; 83: 1321–5, as reported in *Journal of the American Medical Association*, 1993; 270 (18): 2170.

11. Leon Eisenberg, MD, special communication, *Journal of the American Medical Association*, 1995; 274 (4): 331–4.

12. *Journal of the National Cancer Institute*, 1993; 85 (15): 1483–92.

13. *Journal of the American Medical Association*, 1994; 272 (18): 1413–20; L. McTaggart (ed) *The WDDTY Good Supplement Guide* (What Doctors Don't Tell You plc, 2003).

14. *New England Journal of Medicine*, 1994; 331: 141–7.

15. *Annals of Internal Medicine*, 1999; 130: 554–62; *Journal of Nutrition*, 1997; 127: 383–93.

16. *Prostaglandins, Leukotrienes and Essential Fatty Acids*, 2000; 63: 1–9.

17. *Archives of Opthalmology*, 2000; 118: 401–4.

18. *The Lancet*, 1994; 343: 1454–9.

19. *Journal of the American Medical Association*, 1995; 273 (20): 1563.

20. Interview with Dr Jonathan Wright, May 1996.

21. See Melvyn Werbach, *Nutritional Influences on Illness* (Tarzana, CA: Third Line Press, 1993) and *Nutritional Influences on Mental Illness* (Tarzana, CA: Third Line Press, 1991), for an extensive review of the medical literature and scientific studies which exist on the role of nutrition in causing or treating illness. Also see the *Journal of Nutritional and Environmental Medicine*, a monthly scientific review in the US, and the *American Journal of Clinical Nutrition*, two excellent sources of scientific papers on the subject.

22. *The Lancet*, 1992; 340: 439–43.

23. Natural Resources Defence Council, 'Intolerance Risk: Pesticides in our Children's Food' (Washington, DC: NRDC, 1989). See also *What Doctors Don't Tell You*, 1995; 6 (3): 1–3.

24. Dr John Mansfield, 'Chemical Crippling', *What Doctors Don't Tell You*, 1995; 6 (7): 12. See also the work of Professor William Rea, head of the Environmental Health Center in Dallas, Texas.

25. *Journal of the American Medical Association*, 1995; 273: 1179–84.

26. *The Times*, 28 March 1995.

27. *British Medical Journal*, 1995; 310: 1122–5.

28. *The Times*, 1 November 1994.

29. See Melvyn Werbach and Michael T. Murray, *Botanical Influences on*

Illness (Tarzana, CA: Third Line Press, 1994), and the 'Alternatives' column in *What Doctors Don't Tell You* and *Proof!* (both from The Wallace Press), which contain copious scientific evidence that alternative medicine works.

30. *Medical Biology*, 1977; 55: 88–94, as quoted in *New England Journal of Medicine*, 1995; 333 (4): 263.

31. See B. Pomeranz and G. Stu, *Scientific Bases of Acupuncture* (New York, NY: Springer-Verlag, 1989), as quoted in *New England Journal of Medicine*, 1995; 333 (4): 263.

32. *New England Journal of Medicine*, 1995; 333 (4): 263.

33. *New England Journal of Medicine*, 1994; 330 (3): 223.

34. C. Hewlett, correspondence, *The Lancet*, 1994; 344: 695. See also *What Doctors Don't Tell You*, 1996; 7 (3): 5.

VISIT OUR WEBSITE ...

If you enjoyed *What Doctors Don't Tell You*, and would like to find out more about medicine, or safer ways to treat your own specific ailments, visit our website at:

www.wddty.co.uk

For more about *The Field* and latest discoveries about how to live 'in the Field', visit Lynne's other website:

www.livingthefield.com

Index